In the Midst of Winter

Counseling Families, Couples, and
Individuals With AIDS Infection

REVISED EDITION

A NORTON PROFESSIONAL BOOK

In the Midst of Winter

Counseling Families, Couples, and
Individuals With AIDS Infection

REVISED EDITION

Gillian Walker

in collaboration with

The Ackerman Institute AIDS and Families Project

New York

W. W. Norton & Company · NEW YORK · LONDON

First edition

Library of Congress Cataloging-in-Publication Data

Walker, Gillian, 1940–
    In the midst of winter : counseling families, couples,
  and individuals with AIDS infection / Gillian Walker, in
  collaboration with the Ackerman Institute AIDS and Families Project,
  New York. — Rev. ed.
      p.   cm.
    "A Norton professional book."
    Previously published with subtitle: Systemic therapy with families, couples,
  and individuals with AIDS infection.
    Includes bibliographical references and index.
    ISBN 0-393-70204-9 (pbk.)
    1. AIDS (Disease)—Patients—Counseling of.   2. AIDS (Disease)—
Patients—Family relationships.   3. Family psychotherapy.   4. AIDS
(Disease)—Patients—Mental health.   I. Ackerman Institute AIDS and
Families Project.   II. Title.
RC607.A26W34   1995
362.1'969792—dc20   95-18597
                                                              CIP

W. W. Norton & Company, Inc., 500 Fifth Avenue, New York, N.Y. 10110
W. W. Norton & Company, Ltd., 10 Coptic Street, London WC1A 1PU

1 2 3 4 5 6 7 8 9 0

For Anita Morawetz
and Cal Berkowitz,
with love

In the midst of winter, I finally learned that there was in me an invincible summer.

Albert Camus, *L'Eté*

Contents

Acknowledgments

THE ACKERMAN AIDS AND FAMILIES PROJECT TEAM

THIS BOOK REPRESENTS THE collaborative work of a group of clinicians who have spent the last five years working with families of people with AIDS. The case material in the book has been gathered from presentations members of the project have made across the country. In that sense the therapists are the authors of these case examples.

There is no way that I can adequately thank my colleagues on the AIDS project for their endurance, compassion, and political passion, which have sustained all of us through the pain of the epidemic and the difficulties of incorporating an AIDS project into an outpatient mental health clinic.

John Patten and I were the co-directors of the Project. Together we worried about its finances, fought its battles at home and outside. John had worked with chronically ill patients for years. A physician, associate director of the family therapy program at Payne Whitney (New York Hospital), a founding member of AAMFT's Caucus for Gay, Lesbian and Bisexual Issues, and a Gay Men's Health Crisis (GMHC) volunteer, John cared deeply about people with HIV infection. He worked tirelessly to interview all families seen in the project, interpreting for them the arcane medical issues of the illness, negotiating with other physicians to provide clients with the most up-to-date protocols, visiting clients in hospitals and at home. He knows more about the interface of medical systems and families than anyone I have ever encountered. As a result of his ability to give clients information in clear, simple language and to help them build a more effective relationship with the physicians who treat them, many clients have moved from a sense of powerlessness and despair to feeling empowered to both fight the disease and to seek a better quality of life with illness. A skilled student of Milton H. Erickson's hypnotic techniques, John has taught patients techniques for dealing with pain and anxiety. This has been so successful that one patient reported utilizing John's teachings on the jolting RR train, one of the worst in the notorious New York City subway system. Finally, John has worked with the labyrinthine city bureaucracy to make a family systems approach available to many agencies working with people with AIDS. As the AIDS Project comes of age, John will head up a special project looking more deeply at issues for gay people, in their families of origin and of choice.

Unlike therapists who rely primarily on the gathering of verbal information, **Joan Gilbert** uses her sensitive attunement to the feelings the client elicits to guide her in shaping the session. Because she has the courage to face her own process, she is able to make us aware of the layers of meaning and emotion often concealed by denial in ourselves and in our patients. Joan's clinical work is as delicate and nuanced as her recognitions of the subtle countertransference that we unknowingly bring to many of the issues people with AIDS raise in us. Joan is currently writing about the emotional space that AIDS generates between the therapist and the client and how to enter it.

Laurie Kaplan, who serves both as the Project's administrator and as a clinician, had the courage to push us to begin to work with people with AIDS. Laurie's experience in hospitals and community agencies has made her a superb administrator as well as a teacher who can translate complex systems ideas to front-line workers. With Carol O'Connor she has begun to develop programs for training the staff of drug treatment agencies in family interventions. Her case in Chapter 15 is a representative example of her work, deceptively simple but profoundly true to the complex tasks that have to be accomplished.

Ruth Mohr joined the project as senior clinical supervisor—an act of courage, since she had recently lost her husband to cancer. Ruth has the sensitivity to become engaged with families and to find a way to share the humanness of her own experience as a mother, widow, and skilled therapist. Ruth gives us the perspective of generation and always senses when a team member needs comfort or courage. Her cases are both witty and touching as she moves from the planfulness of a strategic model to just being with the client. Ruth's current work is on the impact of AIDS on the elderly, as caretakers of orphaned grandchildren and as parents who have lost their own children.

Carol O'Connor, a therapist with many years of experience treating adolescents, groups, and alcoholics, brings her perceptions in a simple and direct way to her work with patients. Carol's strength is in helping families understand that they have far greater power to comfort and heal their own family members than any professional. Her belief in "minimal professional intervention"—that is, therapy that empowers families to find their own strength—has become a guiding principle of our work. Carol and Laurie's teaching of professionals and paraprofessionals working in the inner city and their advocacy for the needs of HIV-infected women form the basis of the next phase of the Ackerman AIDS and Families Project, which is sketched in the last three chapters.

Joe Rosenthal has forced us to become aware of the therapist's own emotions as they play out in work with patients who are ill. Because of his interest in Buddhist practice and long experience in working with stress and illness, he has constantly pushed us to define our own values around death and suffering. In this way he has helped us open ourselves to the patient's experience at the mysterious level of the spiritual.

Nellie Villegas joined us as the epidemic began to ravage the Hispanic population of the city. Nellie was raised in a Latino family, speaks fluent Spanish, and is dedicated to finding ways to facilitate outreach to Latino families. She has taught us that, while learning about the traditions and beliefs that various groups of Latino families have brought with them to this country is important, we might overcompensate and impose cultural stereotypes, which would lead us to underestimate a family's potential to grow and change. Knowledge about culture is merely the basis for inquiry into the unique and particular way each family interprets its own cultural inheritance. Once, when an "expert" on Hispanic families was warning us about the cultural inhibitions we would encounter in asking families for sexual information, Nellie said quietly, "I don't seem to have trouble with that." Her exquisite sense of timing enables families to deal with so-called taboo areas because they feel her support, respect, and belief that it is safe for them to do so.

Sippio Small, an African-American therapist with extensive experience with drug users and their families, was the last person to join our team. He was immediately overwhelmed by requests of African-American families that he work with them and their children. Until he joined the team, we were blind to the pain for many families of meeting only therapists not of their own race and culture. For single-parent mothers, many infected with AIDS from a drug-using spouse, Sippio became someone who understood from his own experience their struggles with racism, poverty, and social neglect. He had a way of helping them to see a way out of the desperate places they were in and to believe in a different future for their sons and daughters.

My discussions with Sippio about the politics of racism and political neglect as they affect inner-city communities and the delivery of social services have informed the book's last chapter. Sippio has become a key figure in Ackerman's collaborative provision of family services to Montefiore Hospital's Women's Center. His deep feeling for the people of his community has had an extraordinary impact in creating support networks for HIV-infected men as well as women and families.

SUPPORTERS OF THE TEAM

I am grateful to Bob Davis and Richard Gelb, who joined the team to give help in specific areas. Bob Davis is a psychologist with much experience in community organization, Richard Gelb a family therapist who over his long career in drug treatment has always tried to build family systems approaches into various hospital-based methadone maintenance programs. Bob worked tirelessly in the beginning of the project to foster our relationships with community agencies. Richard helped us understand the maze of city bureaucracy as we began to work with drug users and their families.

Marcia Scanlon, our assistant administrator, not only handled our mail but also brought an artist's sensibility to the work of keeping a group of very different and sometimes very stressed people organized for the tasks of fundraising. More importantly, she began to build connections with many city programs by representing us at critical meetings.

Carol Maslow helped us raise money when it counted most. But more than that, Carol, a clinician in her own right and a volunteer at GMHC, saw the need for our agency to reach out to the community.

Clymene Wykoff, Emily Davidson, and Nan Jones spent years filming our families and editing our training tapes.

Ackerman staff who always made us feel their support include Erlynne Evans, who fielded telephone emergencies with compassion and tact and made each client feel respected and welcome. Carol Tofel always figured out ways to comfort us when things were hard. My colleagues, Virginia Goldner, Marcia Sheinberg, and Peggy Penn, lovingly (albeit sometimes crossly) put up with my distractions. My thanks to Peter Steinglass, who has been generous with his support and ideas during some dark days, and to Donald Bloch, who supported the writing of this book and gave us our home.

Among those outside Ackerman, my thanks to Daniel Corte, who made us welcome at GMHC, and especially to Ernest Drucker, Cathy Eric, and Anitra Pivnick of Montefiore Hospital's department of epidemiology and social medicine, whose comments have shaped my ideas about service provision. Roger MacFarlane, a tireless warrior for human rights from the earliest days of the AIDS epidemic, was an early supporter, a challenging but just and witty critic, and always an inspiration to those of us who worked with people with AIDS.

Thanks to Susan Barrows Munro, whose faith that authors will finally do what they promise is inspiring and who read and reread many drafts of this book, and to Margaret O. Ryan, who shaped it.

My loving thanks to my family, my husband Albert Maysles and children, Rebekah, Philip, and Sara, and Milly Addolarato. They have put up with what Sara, my youngest daughter, sees as the decimation of forests as the printer churns out drafts, and have brought me endless cups of tea and love.

This book is dedicated to the memory of Anita Morawetz and Cal Berkowitz. Cal's courage, humor, and lovingness was an inspiration to all of us as he fought to live fully and joyfully each moment of his foreshortened life. Each Christmas, John Patton and Cal sent us hilarious Christmas cards which both celebrated their love and reminded us of the tension of being gay and in love in a world cruelly shadowed by AIDS.

My friend and colleague Anita Morawetz shared the writing of my first book. Her fine essay "Personally Speaking," written when she was ill with cancer, is a beautiful and subtle description of the process by which the ill person creates a meaning for a life with illness. It became a touchstone for helping me understand what people with AIDS experience as they enter the medical system. As I reread it, I hear again Anita's strong, spirited, and wise voice. In the last years of her life, Anita chose to work with people with AIDS. I only wish that we had been able to write this book together.

Finally, there is no way that any of us can really pay tribute to our clients and their families who have shared their experiences with us. We have tried to go with them on *their* journeys, only to find that they have redefined in a thousand ways the meaning of our own life journeys by their spirit, humor, courage, and honesty.

CORPORATE SUPPORT

The AIDS and Families Project has received support from the following:

United Way
United Hospital
Warner Communications
Tisch Foundation
Samuel and May Rudin Foundation
Dancing for Life
James Taylor
U.S. Trust Company of New York
Gladstein Foundation
Gay Men's Health Crisis
Broadway Cares
Diffa
Charles E. Culpepper Foundation
New York Community Trust Foundation
Liz Claiborne Foundation
Normaltown Music International, Inc. (B52 concert)
Cissy Patterson Trust
MONY Financial Services Foundation

Introduction

WRITING THIS BOOK, I cannot seem to find a form to capture the experience of working with families of people with AIDS. Often I feel I know nothing and have nothing to say that will be of use to other professionals. AIDS seems closer to a novelist's experience than to a professional's. Then I realize that that is the point: AIDS strips you of all preconceptions; it takes you to the edge of experience where there are no guideposts. It is this stripping away of one's professional persona, this confrontation with one's deepest beliefs, fears, and values, this opening of unanswerable questions that is the essence of my experience of the past five years.

Family therapy with HIV-infected people is like night sailing in stormy, uncharted waters. The comforting guidelines of structural, systemic, and strategic therapy do not apply. Each situation seems unique, puzzling, fraught with paradox and desperately urgent. The emotions raised in sessions are more powerful than in any other family work we have done. I find myself grateful for the relief of my other clinical work, even when I am supervising difficult cases in which patients are anorexic or schizophrenic. At least there I have some idea of what to do and the pain is not unmanageable.

If one is willing to endure a sense of confusion and helplessness, working with HIV-infected patients presents the most profound issues of living and dying. The comfort of assuming a neutral stand is impossible. The themes in these families and couples include a dizzying range of emotions and behavior—murder and heroic sacrifice, fury and despair, helplessness together with transforming love, and hope in the face of the unbearable physical and emotional pain.

We are in the throes of an epidemic that touches us all, that brings seemingly unbearable pain. And yet working in the trenches of this epidemic is often joyful. As Camus wrote, "In the midst of winter, I finally learned that there was in me an invincible summer."

I cannot remember where I stood when the journey began—only that it began casually in 1985 with a group of Ackerman Institute graduates who wanted to work together. One of them, Laurie Kaplan, asked the question, "Who is working with the families of people with AIDS? I would like to do that."

At that time I knew very little about the people who got AIDS. I didn't know that it had spread to intravenous drug users. I certainly did not think it could touch my family. I had followed the course of the epidemic with more than passing interest, however. Two close friends were AIDS researchers and I had many gay friends, some colleagues; but we did not talk about the disease, just as we avoided talking about the experience of being gay. I worried about my friends at times, but then denial crept in (on both sides)—denial both merciful and dangerous. *He looks fine . . . he has had a lover for years . . . he isn't interested in sex.*

Laurie's question began the project. Bob Davis, Carol O'Connor, Joan Gilbert, and Ruth Mohr joined her as team members, and John Patten joined me as the project's co-director. Later, Joe Rosenthal, Sippio Small, Nellie Villegas, and Richard Gelb would work with us. From the beginning we expected to confront many issues for which we had no answers. We were working with people with a catastrophic illness that might infect several members of the same family, a disease that could be spread to the person one loved most in the act of love. We sensed that we would have to be open to learning about our clients' often unfamiliar worlds.

We were grateful for the accidental diversity of background and experience among those who comprised our team. We came to believe that giving each therapist permission to find his or her own voice and to draw on personal life experience in creating deep bonds with clients was more important than any strategy and technique.

There were to be no rules about who should be seen or how an interview should be conducted, no emphasis on hypothesis-gathering, and no preordained structure for the therapy itself. Initially, I became impatient with the meandering feeling of this lack of structure and pushed for focus. The team often reminded me that my need for structure was often a wish to do something in order to alleviate my own helplessness. Over time, we learned that so much of our work involved simply being with the client on the difficult journey. Even then, we were not always successful in respecting each other's way, in finding the time to listen to each person's concerns, or even in coming together to mourn our losses.

What is miraculous is how this most demanding of illnesses brought into focus the gifts that give each of us a unique therapeutic style. Without the dedication of my team members, working long hours most often without pay, this project and this book could not have existed. Their ideas and the philosophy of treatment that we created together are at the heart of my writing.

This book is about the work we have shared—the ideas developed in the heat of writing grants, listening to each other teach, creating training tapes, wrestling with the seemingly intractable problems of AIDS patients in the consulting room, behind the mirror, even in hospital rooms and clients' homes.

The first section, "Systemic Therapy With HIV-Infected Persons," deals with the application of a systems approach to working with people who have AIDS infection. The first chapter of this section describes our thinking about the impact of multiple systems on the infected person, including the beliefs of the larger culture about AIDS. It argues for systemic approach as the counseling treatment of choice. In the next two chapters we look at ways in which family therapy has been adapted to work with people with HIV infection. The second chapter deals with the resistance to conjoint sessions that has to be overcome before family therapy can take place. The third presents a model of therapy that has been developed over five years of practice by the Ackerman team.

The second section, "The Illness Journey," examines the psychosocial issues raised by each stage of HIV infection, from the decision to be tested through the chronic phase of AIDS illness. Chapter 8 explores the ethical and legal issues for the clinician as she or he makes decisions that must balance conflicting rights: the client's right to confidentiality and the right of a person who may unknowingly be placed at risk by a client's behavior to protection by the clinician who is aware of his/her situation. The second half of this chapter explores the effect of AIDS secrecy on families. It suggests that the ramifications of enforced secrecy for family functioning may not be fully understood for another generation. Chapter 9 explores issues of sexuality in the context of AIDS as they affect couples, families, and individuals and spells out safer-sex guidelines.

The third section, "Journey's End: Beginnings" describes the terminal phase of AIDS illness and the reorganization that begins with the work of grieving.

The fourth section, "AIDS: The Inner-City Experience," explores AIDS as it affects poor families and people of color. Included is a discussion of the development of an in-service training program in a city hospital that deals with pediatric AIDS. The chapter on "Dislocations" describes a major task for inner-city families, particularly for grandparents, healing the wounds of a generation of orphaned children.

The final section, "AIDS and Larger Systems," looks at the way service delivery is organized and proposes that family systems thinkers become involved in designing ecosystemic, community-based and community-directed programs, drawing on models such as GMHC and Auerswald's crisis intervention unit at Gouverneur Hospital.

In the Midst of Winter

Counseling Families, Couples, and
Individuals With AIDS Infection

REVISED EDITION

PART I

Systemic Therapy With HIV-Infected Persons

CHAPTER 1
The Family and Cultural Context of AIDS

IN 1985, AS WE BEGAN the Ackerman AIDS and Families Project in New York, we observed that there were almost no counseling services for gay couples in which a partner had HIV disease.* There were no counseling services that addressed the needs of the parents and siblings of the gay person with HIV disease as they processed both difficult and often painful information and tried to negotiate medical care for an ill family member. We also observed that an increasing number of poor people, mostly people of color, were being diagnosed with AIDS. Although in most of these cases more than one family member was ill, infected, or at risk, most health-care settings conducted "business as usual": Counseling was delivered to individual patients, and family members were seen only if they came in with the patient or were involved with practical issues of care. Even now, five years later, while most people recognize that AIDS affects whole families,[†] in the majority of cases a family systems approach is not the treatment of choice, nor does treat-

---

*The term "HIV disease" will be used throughout the book to describe people who are infected with HIV virus. The disease commonly called AIDS should be conceptualized as a spectrum disease following from infection with the HIV virus; however, here the term "AIDS" will be reserved for the phase of the illness marked by the appearance of opportunistic infection.

[†]Throughout the book, "family" is conceptualized in its broadest sense as any intimate network that constitutes the significant relationship context of the patient's life. "Family" thus includes gay or straight couples, nuclear families, a gay man's friendship network, professionals who are providing care, and loosely defined extended families, possibly including non-blood kin members.

ment target the family unit as the location for effective intervention. Furthermore, family systems techniques for empowering families to marshall resources, such as meetings that systematically include extended family members or convene all the health-care and social service workers involved with a patient, are alien to most treating systems.

From previous experience with chronically ill families,* we knew that when a family member was ill, family needs had to be assessed and family counseling routinely provided. Optimally, counseling would involve a family case management approach, where one counselor trained in family systems work identified the complex psychological and concrete service needs of all family members and coordinated care. Individual counseling might be indicated in some cases or for periods of time during a person's course of illness.

HIV-infected people and their families need help with a wide range of issues. These issues include adjusting to a life-threatening diagnosis, obtaining concrete services, organizing to meet needs for care, managing the reactions of children to a parent's or sibling's illness or death, future planning for loss and bereavement, and reorganizing family functioning following loss (Tiblier, Walker, & Rolland, 1989). The emotions generated by HIV infection run high, and family conflicts often escalate as family members experience feelings of depression and hopelessness. Isolation, secrecy, stigma, and discrimination further compound and intensify family difficulties. The family must learn to attend to the needs of the ill individual while also putting illness in its place, so that the family as a whole and its members can continue to master normal developmental tasks. In addition, family members must deal with feelings about homosexuality or drug use in order to care for the ill person and to prevent the spread of infection, and they must make difficult behavioral changes in sexual and drug-use practices.

Often HIV infection results in a roller-coaster disease course that makes constantly changing demands on both patient and caregiver. In the face of uncertainty, long-range planning becomes difficult. Some seemingly healthy patients succumb rapidly to an opportunistic infection, while others, though weakened by illness, overcome one infection

---

*For several years, the author had been involved with the Ackerman Institute's chronic illness project in which the impact of illness on families and intervention strategies were explored. The co-director of the AIDS and Families Project, John Patten, had been a consultant to Memorial Sloan-Kettering Hospital on family aspects of cancer and had extensive experience with hypnotherapeutic management of pain associated with illness.

after another. A severe initial illness may be followed by years of good health and then a sudden rapid decline, as the patient is bombarded by opportunistic infections. Some opportunistic infections leave permanent damage to vision, mobility, or brain functioning but are not in themselves life-threatening, so that the patient must adjust to physical limitations. But by 1991, for most people, increased knowledge of the clinical course of HIV infection, better early diagnostic procedures, and the advent of both more effective antiviral medications and medications targeted to opportunistic infection have made HIV infection a chronic illness that requires only brief periods of hospitalization and includes long periods of time when the person can resume normal activities.

Despite improved diagnosis and treatment, the opportunistic infections that mark AIDS are an ever present Damoclean sword over families. Because opportunistic infections not only are terrifying but also may require intensive hospital care, family members may need repeatedly to prepare emotionally for what seems to be a fatal episode. Continual reorganization of family roles is required to meet the shifting demands of hospital or home care and to help the recovering patient resume normal activity. For example, during some home-care periods the person-with-AIDS (PWA) who has suffered an opportunistic infection might be severely incapacitated, so that the family needs to organize to provide intensive nursing care. Following another brush with death, he may recover rapidly and be ready to resume normal functioning, while the family members, remembering the last episode, anticipate providing round-the-clock care.

ILLNESS DEMANDS: FAMILY FIT

How a family manages an illness depends both on the nature of family organization and on the belief systems that govern the family's response to illness. HIV disease not only makes extraordinary demands on family organization but also carries an extraordinary burden of social stigma.

As we have attempted to understand a family's capacity for providing care and adapting to the demands of AIDS illness, we have been guided by David Reiss's (1986) work on chronic renal disease families and his earlier work on the ways families construct meaning systems around illness (Reiss, 1981). In his work on chronic renal disease Reiss noted that the demands of normal middle-class life require families to become complex goal-oriented structures, structures that may be ill adapted to meeting the needs of a chronically ill person over long periods of time.

The middle-class families in his study did well in the initial diagnostic and treatment development stages of the illness. However, during the chronic phase, illness caused increasing disruption in family life. This was followed by a final coping effort and a major realignment in the family. Eventually, the well family members in this study pulled together, becoming more invested in each other, while the ill person was extruded from the family to the world of the medical system.

Reiss hypothesized that this process of extrusion from a system that represents life and attachment to a system associated with fatal illness hastens death. One way of viewing this dynamic, which has become crucial in our thinking about AIDS, is the systems-oriented concept of "fit": For the middle-class family the illness did not "fit" the family's life trajectory; however, it did fit the medical system organized to serve it (Reiss, 1986).

Interestingly, Reiss found that, while seemingly "disorganized" poor families were not as effective as middle-class families in the early stage of the illness, they were able to adapt over time to the chronic demands of the illness. These families were less goal-oriented and had access to a loosely organized extended kin system that could absorb care needs. Because the family's survival routinely depended on its ability to absorb tragedies and life crises, it could create a niche for the ill person, allowing nourishing attachment to the life force of the family.

Family organization is a critical factor in a family's ability to "fit" with illness demands. But family organization can be affected by issues particular to this disease's location within the larger culture. For instance, in a large city with an active gay community, a gay man's family of choice may be organized to comfortably embrace the person with AIDS. This family welcomes AIDS organization volunteers who lighten the caregiving tasks and utilizes the resources of the gay community for recreation, health preservation classes, support groups for patients and caregivers. However, if the gay man's family of origin enters the picture, the fit may become stressed, as conflicts arise between care systems with different organizations and beliefs.

Similarly, a "disorganized" African-American family, such as those in Reiss's chronic renal disease study, may have the internal organizational flexibility to "fit" with the many illness demands of AIDS. However, when the illness carries a stigma in the community, the family may find itself cut off by enforced secrecy from community supports and rituals, church groups, kin and friendship networks that are necessary for its continued functioning and would mitigate its pain. If the secret is out, the stigma of AIDS may result in ostracism from the community and may jeopardize employment, financial stability, or even housing, thus threatening the family's very survival.

Reiss's findings provide a template for clinicians analyzing a family's capacity for organizing to "fit" with illness demands. Since AIDS fears may sever family ties to vital natural community resources, the clinician may have to improvise and build links to other supports, such as networks of families dealing with HIV infection, peer support groups, AIDS organizations, and AIDS-sensitive church groups. Reiss's model also underscores the importance, in terms of the family's continued ability to deal with crisis, of balancing illness demands with the goals of normal life.

CONSTRUCTING MEANINGS FOR ILLNESS

Even families that have the flexibility to adapt to illness needs have to overcome powerful messages transmitted through the generations and from the larger culture if they are to fully embrace the sufferer in all aspects of his disease. In the pages that follow, we will look briefly at the ways in which cultural and family meanings given to AIDS and to the behaviors associated with it influence adaptation to HIV illness in three affected populations: gay men, drug users, and hemophiliacs. But first let us look more generally at illness meanings.

In *The Family's Construction of Reality*, Reiss looks at the ways in which family belief systems shape the illness experience and how the illness experience reconfigures or rigidifies family beliefs. He writes:

> Families develop shared explanations of a wide range of events in the perceptual world . . . the sharing process itself strengthens the system and sharing avoids the severe challenges that intense face to face encounters . . . would provide for the explanatory systems which were fashioned and believed in by individuals alone. (1981, p. 173)

Some families in Reiss's study were able to utilize the experience of illness to set in motion "processes of recognition and growth through experience" (Reiss, 1981, p. 192). For these families the illness crisis was a time of experiencing, questioning, and learning. During the course of illness they were open to utilizing information from the other systems that interacted with them to broaden their understanding of themselves, their capacities, and their deficiencies. Other families operated on what Reiss calls a "template for reorganization" that centered on "revelation and the discovery through meaning." These families did not emphasize the acquisition of new experience, knowledge, and skills; rather, they became "engaged in decoding the symbolic meaning of the crisis and subsequent disorganization" (1981, p.193). These decodings were often tied to a reiteration of past beliefs that were organized to give meaning to the crisis.

While Reiss seems to imply that families able to use the crisis as an opportunity for learning do better in the aftermath of illness, many of the families seen in the AIDS project were "revelation" families whose connections to their past were critical to maintaining a sense of family cohesion. Tying the illness event to these shared connections served to create meanings important both to the family's management of illness and to its recovery.

The Meanings of AIDS

In order to understand how the person-with-HIV-infection and the family evolve a fit or not, it is necessary to remember that the experience of HIV infection cannot be separated from the history of family beliefs, both about the illness and about the behaviors that caused it, and from the societal meanings given to AIDS. Both the ill person and the family have to construct two sets of meanings: one for the behaviors that led to contracting the illness and the other for the illness itself.

Many people who contract HIV disease have belonged to socially stigmatized subgroups: drug users, bisexuals, gays. Many have concealed their membership in these subgroups, until it is revealed by diagnosis. At the point of revelation (coming out), the person becomes defined by the stigma itself; "an individual who might have been received easily in ordinary social intercourse" is now seen as possessing a trait "that can obtrude itself upon attention and turn those of us who meet him away from him, breaking the claim his other attributes have on us" (Goffman, 1986, p. 7). Both family of origin and the infected person have to deal with this change in perception as the stigma subsumes other identities.

The stigmatized person's movement between two worlds – the world of his fellow stigmatized and the world of "normals" – creates two narratives about the self, a narrative of shame and a narrative of pride. As he strives for acceptance by "normals," he internalizes their beliefs about his condition, which makes his failings painfully evident, giving rise to a deep sense of shame and ultimately to a "spoiled identity" (Goffman, 1986). However, a second narrative may be constructed when the stigmatized person becomes involved in organizations of people sharing similar stigmas or sympathetic to their struggle, organizations with the political goal of changing the narrative of shame to one of pride. As we shall see, this positive alternative narrative must also be constructed about HIV infection to counterbalance society's stigmatizing account.

HIV disease, like TB and cancer before it, has deeply stigmatized cultural meanings. The disease is associated with those areas where society has the most complex ambivalence and dread: drug usage, sexual deviance, sexuality itself, physical disfigurement. Given the plague tradition, the specific location of HIV in social subgroups considered to be marginal or deviant, as well as with the modes of transmission and the terror engendered by its extraordinary fatality, it is not surprising that the most common initial meaning given to HIV infection is that it is a punishment for past sins violating the normative social order. Its first cultural meaning, then, is a disease that the sufferer has brought upon himself through deviant behaviors.

Sontag (1989) points out that identifying plague with either moral laxity or otherness has traditionally been a way of mastering the potential terror engendered by epidemics of fatal diseases for which science has not yet discovered a cure. One way of mastering terror is by imagining that the disease belongs to others and not to ourselves and that an imagined moral rectitude will operate as a shield between ourselves and the disease that terrorizes us. As a result, diseases thought to be fatal, such as cancer, tuberculosis, and more recently HIV disease, must be associated with sin or some moral failing of character. Because of confusion or myths about how the disease is transmitted, the infected person is seen as potentially polluting in both the literal and the moral sense and must be avoided. Fears feed on fears and replace compassion. Hysteria and demands for containment and identification of those who are polluted replace thoughtful epidemiology and the advocacy of reasonable precautions. Society alternates between a moral compunction to provide compassionate care for its ill and to protect its members by allocating monies to finding a cure, on the one hand, and, on the other, a Malthusian sense that deviant elements of the population will be eliminated if the disease is allowed to continue in those groups but prevented from entering the general population.

HIV infection not only challenges us to acknowledge our common identity with the infected as sufferers from a terrible illness, but also forces us to deal with our beliefs about what is normal and what is deviant. For example, in providing compassionate care for a gay child, parents must begin to challenge their own assumptions about gayness, as they construct with the ill person a shared, affirmative meaning for the illness. The meanings that family members are able to give to AIDS will define their participation with the patient and the healing of their own system throughout illness after the patient dies.

Families meeting this personal challenge may in turn develop increased political awareness. Gay rights leaders (ACT-UP, for example) and progressive drug treatment advocates (Drucker, 1990) challenge the ways in which the state, by maintaining strongly demarcated and scrutinized categories of normal and abnormal behaviors, maintains the hegemony of patriarchy dominated by white, heterosexual citizens. It is no accident that AIDS marches and gay rights marches are inextricably linked and that in the 1980s AIDS became a rallying cry for other kinds of political protest. When one thinks about "AIDS," there is no way that the meaning of personal experience can be separated from the belief systems of the larger political context.

Meaning, Politics, and Illness in the Gay Community

Families dealing with a gay son or sibling with AIDS must confront the interconnected stigmas of homosexuality* and of a disease whose contamination mythology increases its aura of pollution. As we have said, stigma implies deviation from a socially constructed norm, whether it be of beauty, of health, of sexuality, or of socially accepted habits. These norms are so deeply ingrained that they achieve a truth status; that is, they are not seen as having been socially constructed but as having an essentiality, for some resting in revealed truth, for others documented by science.

From the late nineteenth century until the late 1970s, homosexual behavior was categorized as a disease. The etiology, genetics, biology, and psychodynamics of homosexuality considered as a deviant sexuality

---

*The problem of usage of terms *gay* or *homosexual* has been addressed in the following way. "Gay" is used in its affirmative sense, when talking about client's experiences or pointing to a wider cultural and communal identity; "homosexual" is used when the subject is negative societal attitudes towards same-sex orientation or the historical subject of clinical inquiry.

have occupied many volumes of psychiatric inquiry, despite anthropo-
logical evidence that attraction to the same sex is widespread (Kinsey,
Pomeroy, & Martin, 1948), and has had different status and meaning in
different cultures and at different stages in history (Boswell, 1980; Foucault, 1980; Greenberg, 1988; Weeks, 1985). Because same-sex attraction,
if not activity, is familiar to most of us, and certainly a part of erotic
literature, heterosexual dominance is maintained by the fear that stigma
will follow the revelation of deviant sexual behavior. Within most
Western cultures, the construction of homosexuality as a psychiatric
disease or deviancy coexists with beliefs that same-sex sexual attachments violate secular and religious laws and thus should be subject to
punishment. It is critical in thinking about HIV disease as it affects gay
men to realize that the disease is located in a homophobic culture and
that most gay men's families of origin start with one or another of these
assumptions.

One way of looking at the prevailing negative attitudes towards
homosexuality is that they support the hegemony of heterosexuality and
traditional patriarchal structures. Foucault (1979) has noted that the
operations of power require the maintenance of strict categories of
difference. In other words, cultures considered to be deviant are ghet-
toized and information about their workings are limited to dominant,
stereotyped, often problem-saturated narratives, as, for example, gay
men are promiscuous, wish to seduce straights, are effeminate, and so on
(or drug users are criminals by nature, poor parents, have little else in
their lives but drugs, are dangerous and tough, etc).

While gays fear that homophobic views will be fueled by AIDS fears
and by the accompanying political rhetoric of rightwing conservatives, at
the same time gay writers, artists, and film-makers are challenging
deep-seated myths about gays. AIDS opens the closet of gay culture, as
the faces and lives of the afflicted and their caregivers become visible,
human, and ordinary (for example, Paul Monette's *On Borrowed Time*,
Michael Cunningham's *At Home at the End of the World*, Edmund White
and Adam Mars-Jones' *The Darker Proof*, Larry Kramer's *The Normal
Heart*, and the movie *Longtime Companions*). "AIDS has mobilized more
gay men into political and community organizations . . . than any other
event in the short history of the gay movement" writes Dennis Altman
(1988, p. 309).

Positive narratives about gayness emerge as the person-with-AIDS
insists on being seen not as a representative of a political category but as
a member of a more inclusive category of human suffering, which

includes sexual difference. When the "homosexual" is seen in all his humanness and the fundamental ordinariness of his emotional relationship is acknowledged, a paradigmatic change is threatened, which strikes at power relationships to which many families subscribe.

HIV disease in a gay family member forces the family to construct a meaning for his sexual orientation. The continuous discourse about sexuality that is central to twentieth-century culture (Foucault, 1980) has given a person's sexual orientation a defining importance. The array of ideas and myths that has accumulated around homosexuality— such as "gender inversion," parental failure to help a male child develop an adequate sense of masculine identity, overclose mothering, distant fathering, and overintense father-son rivalry—makes it difficult for the family to arrive at an affirmative meaning for the child's sexual orientation.

The family's confusion about constructing a meaning for homosexuality is made more complex by the essentialist-constructivist controversy over the origins of gayness. Sexual orientation is held by essentialists to be fixed at birth or in the first years of life and to have incompletely understood genetic, biological, temperamental, and psychological components. The constructivists hold that sexual orientation arises from a complex matrix of interactions and experiences, as well as the meanings given to them. From a constructivist perspective, sexuality is seen as contextual, fluid, evolving, subject to change, and involving elements of choice. Meanwhile, essentialists see sexual orientation as inevitable and predetermined, as the person comes to uncover his or her essential sexuality and claims membership in one or another category of the sexualities.

The constructivist position may feel more comfortable to family therapists, who generally renounce diagnostic categories, instead adopting a mode of thought that identifies the multiple narratives available to people, and whose interest is in deconstructing the multiple meanings of experience. Yet, many people who define themselves as gay prefer an essentialist position, which may also be more readily adopted by families living in a homophobic culture. Within a heterosexist culture, a constructivist explanation may lead to parents' feeling blamed for not having managed defining events differently, to a self-lacerating search for causes, or to assumptions that, if sexuality has some fluidity and involves some element of choice, the child, without too great cost, could have chosen heterosexual relationships. By contrast, an essentialist position lays these questions to rest. This opens the way to rebuilding the relationship by encouraging conversations around more fruitful, less controversial topics. However, a constructivist approach may be useful in decoding the meaning of erotic experience. We have found it to be particularly helpful in working with bisexual men to construct positive meanings for erotic experiences with both genders.

A major task for the gay person is to create an affirmative meaning system around sexual orientation. Because a gay person must maintain the legitimacy of his sexuality within a homophobic culture, he constantly has to fight his own self-loathing and shame about sexual difference, which mirrors the larger culture's attitudes. This wound of internalized homophobia will never completely heal. One strategy for building a positive sense of identity (a narrative of pride) is to enter gay culture, build gay friendship networks, and become active in gay professional, political, or community organizations. Gay culture itself has a cohesion promoted precisely by its adversarial relation to the larger "straight" culture, as well as by the enforced secrecy of the "closet" and its rituals. This adversarial relationship can give the gay person a powerful sense of belonging, which counterbalances his sense of not belonging to the dominant culture.

The advent of AIDS in the gay community threatened a carefully constructed, positive communal identity. After the Stonewall riots in 1968, the emerging gay liberation movement identified gay role models, organized to combat discrimination, and developed ways to foster gay pride. The celebration of gay culture included embracing its sexual hedonism, both as an expression of normal sexuality liberated from heterosexual puritanism and as a political expression of community. AIDS, a sexually transmitted disease the majority of whose victims seemed initially to be gay men, reinvoked a powerful set of negative meanings, those spoken by the homophobic voices promising punishment for violating the laws of God, nature, and state. As one client said, "How could I even be interested in sex with my lover when what was supposed to be an act of love has brought us this punishment?"

A major struggle for gay people was to find a meaning for illness that restored a positive sense of gay identity. One image that emerged was of the person with AIDS as emblematic of the wounding of gay men by straight society's homophobic discriminatory practices. In this construction the very hedonism that had spread the disease could be seen both as a reaction to years of persecution and repression of gay sexuality and as an assertion of masculine sexual potency in a culture where gay sexual orientation was often conflated with gender inversion. In the absence of the legitimacy of open gay marriages, anonymous sex that took place within the privacy of gay meeting places and away from the scrutiny of the straight world could be seen as a solution for the need both for sex and for community. By contrast, the visibility of committed relationships might compromise the gay person in the straight world where he had to make his way.

The person with AIDS, visibly disfigured by the ravages of illness, creates a meaning for illness as he becomes a powerful image of gay suffering and the ravages of discrimination. He leads gay rights marches and joins organizations like ACT-UP. His courage becomes celebrated and mourned in the new gay literature. The long-term survivor becomes a metaphor for the battle of a whole community to survive both literally and psychologically—not just AIDS but discrimination, including violence against gays. The ritual meanings given to care, to remembrance of the dead, and to celebrating ongoing life and gay pride in memorial services reinforce the gay culture's need to protect and embrace its own. The thousands of colored balloons rising from memorial services symbolize the fragility of gay life, its aspirations to a freedom of the spirit that always remains elusive.

Although gay men may have constructed a fit between illness and community that promotes care and gives meaning to illness, the PWA is still faced with the problem of fit between his gay sexual orientation, his disease, and his family of origin. Many gay adult children have moved to another city in order to make sure that their gay lifestyle is hidden from their family of origin. This move away from what is experienced as a homophobic context helps the gay person consolidate a meaningful adult identity. But the task of conveying that meaning to his family is often a terrifying one, so that frequently, when he returns home, it is as son or sibling, with the markers of his adult gay identity left behind. The following composite case illustrates the complex interaction between family organization and illness meaning often encountered as the family of origin and the gay man try to evolve a fit with illness needs that promotes care.

CASE EXAMPLE

Joseph, a young gay man, has successfully achieved an accommodation between sexual difference and social identity, concealing gayness in areas such as work and family, revealing it only to gay and trusted straight friends. At first, diagnosis with HIV infection floods him with the reality of difference. He fears that his friends will see him not as Joseph but as an ill person, ill and infectious. Like many gay men, Joseph has moved far from home to conceal homosexuality from his conventional, church-going parents.

He is diagnosed with pneumocystis pneumonia. Worries about declining health force him to consider a double "coming out" to his family. The fragile structure of accommodation may shatter. Profound feelings of guilt may overwhelm his carefully constructed social identity as a gay man. He knows that, in order to care for him, his family will enter not only the arena of his life with AIDS but also the arena in which his gay identity takes place. Although he takes an essentialist position and reassures his family that he has known of his attraction to men since early childhood, he realizes that his parents will still have to confront their deepest fears about his sexual orientation. Joseph's mother is understanding, as is his sister. His father, however, is angry and feels strained when he has to be alone with his son.

It is common for fathers to have great difficulty in overcoming ambivalence, hostility, or perhaps even fear of a son's homosexuality. Many mothers find themselves shouldering the burden of a child's illness almost as a single parent or engaging in painful confrontations with their husbands as they try to negotiate a more positive relationship between father and son. These confrontations may resonate with unresolved sexual issues for the parents. It is common to find that the most homophobic of fathers have had same-sex relationships. Frequently, as we work with young gay men to help them understand their fathers' hostility, they remember hearing stories or seeing photographs that indicate that their fathers may have had same-sex relationships or powerful erotic feelings towards other men. It should be remembered that many of the young men now dying of AIDS had fathers who were in World War II, a time when many men and women engaged in same-sex relationships and then returned to marry and live "normal" heterosexual lives (Scagliotti, 1985). Often, in order to discount the meaning of such a relationship, the father explains it to himself as the exigency of war. But its pleasure and tenderness may continue to haunt him, raising questions about his own sexuality, which he answers by rejecting his son's gayness. These possibilities should be kept in mind as the clinician helps the parents both create a meaning for their child's sexual orientation and negotiate a family structure that can provide care and support for the PWA.

Joseph's parents arrive at an uneasy peace, with his father agreeing to try to tolerate his son's homosexuality. They agree, however, that if they are to care for their son, he must return "home." Joseph's parents are actively involved in midlife careers, making it impossible for them to arrange for Joseph's care if it means visiting a distant city during the course of an unpredictable and possibly protracted illness. Furthermore, if they were to care for him where he lives, they would constantly have to face evidence of his gay life. When he returns home, he returns as an ill son and not as a young gay adult.

Joseph is thus faced with an intolerable choice. If he does not return home, he may die without healing the wounds caused by his original separation from his family. He is afraid to be subject to the vagaries of care by a patched-together network of friends and AIDS volunteers. If, on the other hand, he returns "home," he must leave the familiar world that defines his adult identity as a gay man. Furthermore, he senses that, while his parents can organize their life to "fit" with the course of his illness and dying, they cannot fit with his living as a gay person. In that sense, returning "home" may mean an emotional death, which may hasten physical death. Joseph knows that his family will be fearful that the community will learn the nature of his illness and that living in a community where his disease and his orientation must be concealed can affect his will to live. In Reiss's words, he and the family may rapidly reach a "set-point" where they begin to detach emotionally from each other in preparation for his death, Joseph becoming more dependent on the medical system and the other family members attempting to resume the trajectory of normal life.

Joseph returned home because, like many gay men, he did not have a relationship he could define as his primary commitment. But other gay men insist that if family members become involved, they must provide care where the men live. This decision may create another set of problems, disrupting the organization of both the family system and the gay man's caregiving system, which often includes gay friends and a partner. The PWA's care partner, who has led a fairly exclusive life with his lover, may have to adapt to what feels like the intrusion of often hostile parents, who in many cases do not regard the couple's relationship with the same respect that they would accord a heterosexual marriage.

The parents, in turn, must face the thorny issue of accepting a son's "coming out" while dealing with a terrifying illness. Without having had the ritual of a marriage to mark the transfer of power from the parents as principal caregivers and decision-makers to a spouse, they must nevertheless accept that their son has designated decision-making power to his gay partner. In addition, the parents' belief that they are there to give compassionate care to a dying child may contrast sharply with the gay community's commitment to "surviving and thriving with AIDS"—a belief about illness with strong associations to celebrating gay sexual orientation.

If, however, family members have the flexibility to use the occasion of illness as a template for "recognition and growth" (Reiss, 1981), the experience of entering into the gay world—of learning about their child's life, his friendship network, the meaning that being gay has had for him, and of caring for him within this context—can be transformative, deeply enriching their lives, their sense of themselves as individuals and as a family. It may even transform their politics.

Meaning and Illness in Communities of Poverty and Drug Use

The joint stigmas of drugs and AIDS shape inner-city attitudes and create problems of fit between the needs of the ill drug user and the family's ability to organize to provide care. At the same time, long-standing conflicts between the drug user and his or her family also affect family members' willingness and ability to provide care.

Drug use is the scourge of inner-city communities. Few families have not been victimized by a drug user; few families do not have close relatives who use; few families do not fear that their children may become ensnared in the drug culture. Embracing the drug user with AIDS means overcoming strong negative feelings toward drug use. To quote African-American writer Harlon Dalton,

> For us, drug abuse is a curse far worse than you can imagine. Addicts prey on our neighborhoods, sell drugs to our children, steal our possessions, and rob us of hope. We despise them. We despise them because they hurt us and because they *are* us. They are a constant reminder of how close we all are to the edge. And "they" are "us" literally as well as figuratively; they are our sons and daughters, our sisters and brothers. (1989, p. 217)

The families of drug users, the communities in which they live, as well as the helping systems they turn to, dehumanize them. They are "junkies," with their social identity defined by their stigmatized habit. Punitive attitudes create a recursive cycle whereby the drug user becomes increasingly disenfranchised and alienated from mainstream society and is driven deeper into the subculture of crime, drugs, and AIDS. The deeper he goes, the more punitive family and community become (Goldstein, 1989). This subculture is not without its own rituals of community: shared needle use, after-hours clubs, particular language, family-like relationships such as the "running partner" (Williams, 1989). But because social stigma cuts a wedge between the drug user and straight society, the drug user may experience his hold on relationships with non-using family members as tenuous. As a result he or she may be afraid to risk revealing HIV infection to loved ones, even to a sexual partner, for fear he will lose them. AIDS counseling programs that hope to be effective in reaching drug users must reach out to the drug user even if he or she wishes to continue using drugs. Drug treatment and AIDS prevention are not synonymous, just as ongoing drug use does not preclude "good enough mothering." Providing information about measures the drug user can take to protect himself against HIV infection—for example, rinsing needles with bleach and using condoms—has been shown to be effective in reducing infection rates in drug users who are not interested in stopping drug use (Zinberg, 1989).

The ubiquitousness of drug use, the absence of on-demand treatment programs that can respond when the drug user is ready to stop, and more importantly, the lack of alternative economic opportunities to drugs leave families of the inner city with a sense of despair. The addition of HIV disease to drug use, especially as it spreads to women through needle-sharing, sexual contact with drug users, and more dangerously now through crack use and the exchange of sex for drugs, is leaving the community with the unbearable burden of caring for a generation of traumatized and orphaned children.

AIDS piles stigma onto a community already stigmatized by racism and prejudice against poor people. Unlike the gay community, the inner-city community has not been stimulated by AIDS to collective political action against government neglect and discrimination, as represented by the absence of social programs to check the spread of the disease. The reaction of the community has been largely silence and shame, as anger turns into fatalism and depression. An invisible virus is low on the list of priorities for a community ravaged by drugs and violence, a community denied adequate housing, nutrition, health care, education, and jobs. Furthermore, AIDS is associated not only with drug use but with homosexuality. There are strong currents of homophobia among people of color, strengthened perhaps by African-American sensitivity to Jim Crow stereotypes of the weak black male and the strong black woman, stereotypes reinforced by a social context that denies black men economic opportunities (Dalton, 1989).

Family stigma about an AIDS-infected member mirrors community stigma. A mixture of fear, shame, and anger pushes the family towards concealment and secrecy. The reality is that revelation may bring social ostracism, discrimination in schools against healthy children of an AIDS-infected parent, and even loss of housing. What is remarkable is that, given the risk to the family of embracing the person with AIDS, most families of drug users do continue to care for the ill person throughout the course of the illness.

The families of drug users often have some of the organizational flexibility that Reiss saw as enabling a family to absorb chronic illness. Most families have large, loosely organized kin systems, including non-family members who have kin status (Boyd-Franklin, 1989). They have experience dealing with illness and loss and show a high degree of loyalty to their members. But drug use has often created deep intrafamilial conflicts that become exacerbated at diagnosis. While all studies show that drug users have more contact with their families than non-users (Stanton & Todd, 1982), they usually have had stormy relationships with parents and siblings. Generational boundaries are seldom clear in drug-using families, and conflicts that are ostensibly about drug use often pit the family of origin, from which the drug user seldom separates, against the partner or nuclear family. Family members frequently reject the drug user's partner, who may be blamed for the family member's continuing drug use and HIV infection; in turn, the partner may blame the family of origin. As a drug-using couple agreed, "We have to keep away from both our families. Going back home is the surest way back to drugs. It is like a magnet." (Perhaps not surprisingly, conflicts in their relationship propelled both of them back to their respective families within a few weeks of this statement.)

If both partners are infected, one family of origin may agree to allow the adult child and the grandchildren to return home, often on condition that he or she separate from the partner. In one such family, a daughter and her children returned "home"; however, she carried on secret trysts with her drug-using husband, even while publicly condemning him to her mother. The children, who often went with their mother to see their father, were sworn to secrecy. Grandmother, who saw the husband as having destroyed her daughter's life, was implacable in her hatred of him, which caused great difficulties for the children when their mother died and their father was still living. Ongoing therapy with the grandmother and the children after their mother's death made some degree of reconciliation with their father possible before he died.

Conflicts such as these may interfere with the family's ability and willingness to provide adequate care for the ill person and with the drug user's willingness to receive it. These conflicts may also generate stresses that are medicated by increased drug use, which in turn compromises immune functioning. And they may make the healing process for orphaned children more difficult to manage.

A family's relationship to a drug-using member may have been organized around attempts of one or both parents to rescue him/her from drug use. The fatality of AIDS forces family members to face the futility of their efforts to save the drug user, to accept that there will be no more chances. As hopelessness and anger mount, blame is tossed about like a hot potato: Father was too harsh; mother was too close and protective; a lover caused the user's downfall. A parent's anger is often exacerbated by his or her history as a rescuer for the addict and frequently for a family member in the previous generation.

Scapegoating a spouse or care partner as the cause or supporter of the ill person's addiction may temporarily stabilize family stress by alleviating frustration and powerlessness. If the partner of the ill drug user is not also addicted, he or she has often spent many years trying to rescue a partner from addiction. In the heat of the terror generated by what is seen as the diagnosis of a fatal illness, the non-addicted partner may blame the drug user's family of origin for having caused the addiction, thus exacerbating tensions between the two systems to which the ill person belongs.

CASE EXAMPLE

Mary shipped her husband Jeff, a drug user, home to his mother when he began to develop open sores from Kaposi's sarcoma.* Their two children were bewildered about why, since their father was ill, their mother was always so angry and no longer wished to care for him. After he left, they began to show symptoms. They had never been told directly of their father's drug use or of the fact that he had AIDS and had infected their mother and a sibling who had died. Nor could they know that as their mother became more angry at him for what had occurred, he became more coercive about having unprotected sex with her. Jeff's mother was

---

*The therapist in this case was Ruth Mohr.

bitter that Mary blamed her for her son's addiction and that her daughter-in-law hurt her son by refusing to care for him. Mother reasoned that, since Mary had met Jeff while he was in a drug program, she should have known what his problems were.

Old angers between the two women resurfaced. Jeff, caught in the cross-fire, no longer had the will to live and resumed heavy drug use, both as a way to medicate his terror and guilt and as a suicide tactic. He died shortly after he returned to his mother's house. In this case the family and the drug user were unable to construct any positive meaning for illness. Mary saw illness as a punishment for Jeff's behavior and her in-laws' poor parenting. She felt that she was unfairly punished for her attempts to help Jeff and build a family with him. Betrayal became the dominant narrative.

With ongoing therapy, however, Mary began at least to find meaning in her own life, as she dedicated herself to raising her children in the shadow of HIV infection. Her loss in some ways made her closer to members of her own family, although she could never talk with them directly about what had happened.

Despite intense family conflicts that have accompanied drug use and are exacerbated by an HIV diagnosis, many families are able to care for their ill family member and to find in such caretaking an enriching spiritual experience. Positive meaning is often found in religion. For many minority families with a tradition of enduring suffering by finding in it religious meaning and evidence of God's plan, the revelatory template that Reiss described is used to give spiritual meaning to the illness. Members of one family were able to reorganize when the therapist suggested that they turn in silent prayer to the memory of a beloved deceased grandmother; in this remembrance they found the spiritual strength and consolation they needed to endure the death of a baby. In another family the mother was able to recover from the death of a daughter and a granddaughter when she was able to talk with her dead daughter in church about her worries for her other daughter and her son. In families where religion has always been a potential joining force, the restoration of prayer as a means of family connection and the redefinition of AIDS as a trial sent from God rather than as a punishment may help the family transcend bickering and bitterness.

For many families from African-American and African-Caribbean backgrounds, tapping into spiritual beliefs is a traditional way of mastering suffering (Boyd-Franklin, 1989). The stigma of HIV infection and the forbidden behaviors that have caused it frequently cut the family off from sources of spiritual strength and healing. The following case demonstrates the way in which a family assigns a meaning to AIDS that fits with its deepest spiritual beliefs. This meaning allows family members to become committed to caring for each other with a sense of God's forgiveness, direction, and blessing.

CASE EXAMPLE

Joan and Thomas are a dignified West Indian couple, church going, with many grown children from previous marriages.* Both have AIDS. Since Joan has been been monogamous, Thomas most probably infected her, but it is not clear how he became infected. He told Joan that he had had an affair, but it seems likely that he may be bisexual. Joan is a forceful, emotional woman, voluble in her expressions of feeling. In early sessions she is enraged at her husband for giving her the disease. Thomas is quiet, sensitive, and ashamed of the suffering he has caused her. He speaks about moving away to a place where no one will know anything about them, starting over. His family knows that he has AIDS; hers does not. She has spoken of the great shame of AIDS, her fear that the secret would come out if she or he were to have a traditional family funeral. She wants just to be buried quietly, with no one knowing.

As this evening's discussion turns to the most dangerous subject of all—how Thomas had contracted the disease—Joan seems upset, alternatively edgy with her husband, who is quiet and sad, and protective of him. Her anger comes in passionate, rapid outbursts. Is she angry because of the disease itself or because the secrets still hang between them? He tells us that they spend almost every evening alone together, because she is afraid to go out with her friends, lest someone find out. He wonders what she is thinking during those long silences, whether she blames him, but he is afraid to ask her and she does not bring up the subject.

The therapist pushes the couple for a more open conversation about how he became infected. They resist. Thomas shifts the subject to the possibility that a cure will be found, "I've not heard of anyone being cured before. But a cure will come soon, like syphilis." Quite suddenly, Joan leans forward towards the therapist and says with intensity, "Doctor, do you believe in God?" Somewhat startled and harboring some doubts on the matter, he hesitates. "I have many beliefs," he says, "What

---

*This case was treated by John Patten. The consultant was Sippio Small.

is important here are *your* beliefs." "Do you read the Bible?" she pursues. He passes the question back, as therapists are taught to do. "I know religion is of great importance to you and to your husband." She pursues, "But not to you. So if you do not read the Bible, you will not know who I am. You have different beliefs, you say." Her determined, almost aggressive stance is in contrast to her usual deferential demeanor towards a doctor who has helped her greatly by patiently hearing her unhappiness and making sure that she and her husband get proper medical care. Thomas, who is attached to the doctor, murmurs reassuringly to his wife, "Of course he reads the Bible. Of course he does." And then, realizing that perhaps the doctor doesn't, he attempts to improve the situation by persuading the doctor that he should read the Bible because a doctor's profession and a minister's go hand in hand, since they both deal with death.

Seeing that Joan has had her say and is buttoning up her coat, the African-American consultant behind the one-way mirror telephones the doctor, "I think if you want them to come back, you will have to join their religious beliefs." While the doctor can't quite overcome his religious skepticism to announce his fervent belief, he is able to describe his upbringing in the great Anglican tradition, with much Bible study. Joan seems satisfied. "Then," she says, "I didn't ask a sharp question but an important question. As you know, if you read the Bible, the Bible says we are living in the last days. This is the last days. I'm a poor learner, just strong in the Bible. And Revelation tells you, in the last days, there will be pestilence and incurable disease, sickness that no man will be able to cure. This is it, I believe, this is it. If this disease did not come, God's word would not be fulfilled. Somebody got to have it. Somebody got to die. For the word of God to be fulfilled, people have to have it." As her husband repeats his hope that she will be cured, and the therapist adds that he hopes they will discuss all these issues at the next session, she firmly closes the subject, "There's no need for discussion. The subject's closed."

The wife's designation of a religious meaning to their illness, within the belief system that the innocent and good often suffer in the service of the greater scheme of God's wisdom, closes the book on how her husband contracted the disease, on the subject of his betrayal of her, and on the more deeply troubling question of his bisexuality. And true to the structure of their relationship, Joan both protects her husband and wins the argument. After all, how can there be a cure if, in fact, they are living out the prophecies of Revelation? In the tradition of oppressed people, she finds consolation and meaning for her suffering in her religion. But more important, the meaning she finds exonerates her husband from blame. After all, whatever he may have done in the past, he was only acting as God's agent.

Meaning and Illness for Hemophiliacs and Blood-Product Users

The experience of stigmatization may be more devastating if the person has not had past experience of being, in Goffman's term, "a discredited person" or if he has hitherto been able to successfully conceal his difference from the normal world. For another affected population, hemophiliacs and other blood-product users, AIDS is an illness at odds with the family's previous experience of living with a chronic illness.

The shaping of the family organization to create a functional fit with the demands of hemophilia has constructed a set of beliefs about illness, personal control, and the medical system. These are all challenged by AIDS. Hemophiliacs have learned to put their faith in medicine and have been rewarded by technological advances that have made normal life possible. Modern treatment of hemophilia represents the triumph of medical technology over a condition that had been excruciatingly painful and frightening and had led to shortened lives. The fact that many hemophiliacs had grown up in families where hemophilia played a tragic part added meaning to this triumph (Rolland, 1987b; Tiblier, Walker, & Rolland, 1989).

In contrast to hemophilia, the HIV virus is an incurable infection that leads to death. For the past 20 years, injured hemophiliacs could be infused with the vital blood-clotting factor at home, thus allowing patients to avoid time-consuming and often frightening emergency room visits. Mothers, who carried a burden of guilt because they had genetically transmitted hemophilia to their male child, felt empowered as they actively intervened to alleviate pain. But with HIV infection the mothers learned that the life-saving infusions they had administered carried a deadly retrovirus, a discovery that brought unimaginable pain. Furthermore, this knowledge challenged the mothers' relationships with primary-care physicians, who over years of managing a child's illness had come to play an important role in family life.

That HIV infection of hemophiliacs could be attributed to the failure of the medical system to adequately predict the risks to this population was devastating knowledge for physicians, patients, and their families.

For patients, this knowledge aroused intense feelings of rage, helplessness, despair—emotions they had learned to control during years of practice in living with an illness in which bleeds were believed to be triggered by stress. For physicians, the knowledge poisoned deep personal relationships they had formed over the life span of chronically ill patients and challenged their beliefs in the power of technology to heal. Initially, these beliefs prevented them from even conceiving of such an enormous calamity, despite the evidence of African epidemiology, which was denied by the Centers for Disease Control. Research studies showing that hemophiliacs would become ill with AIDS at a slower rate than those infected by sex or drugs may have given affected persons and their physicians some hope; at the same time, they encouraged continued denial.

HIV shattered families' beliefs that illness—that is, hemophilia—could be mastered. For hemophiliacs mastery meant passing as "normal" in the outside world. HIV brought stigma to the public perception of hemophiliacs. To grapple with these assaults on fundamental belief systems, many hemophiliacs and family members denied the full meaning of infection. In one middle-class family seen at the Ackerman Institute, the husband, who had hemophilia, was infected with HIV through an infusion. He then infected his wife, who in turn transmitted HIV perinatally to her baby. They have two other children who are not infected. When they entered therapy because of behavior problems in one of the other children, the wife was once more pregnant. Despite the potential fatality of their HIV infection, it could not be discussed. To acknowledge HIV was to destroy their relationship with the medical system, which had been their lifeline to normalcy, and their perception of themselves as able to live a "normal" life unnoticed in a middle-class community. In this case the couple's desire to define themselves as "normal" led to denial, which in turn led to continued practice of unsafe sex. The "conspiracy of silence" about HIV, which is characterisitic of many hemophiliac families (Tsiantis, Anastasopolos, Meyer, Pantiz, Lanes, Platakouk, Aroni, & Kattamis, 1990), also led to the emotional isolation of family members. It also prevented this family from processing its underlying anxieties. As a result, family members were not able to comfort each other and make realistic plans for dealing with a possibly fatal illness. Indeed, in the AIDS-infected hemophiliac families we have seen, denial has been reinforced at all levels of the system, with tragic results.

Other blood-product users have to deal with a catastrophic and unexpected "bolt from the blue," which dramatically changes their life experience from normal to stigmatized. As with hemophiliacs, much energy goes towards concealment of the stigmatized infection for as long as possible.

BREAKING THE RECURSIVE LOOP
BETWEEN CONTEXT AND ILLNESS

A systems approach defines the family as the unit of intervention and the entire course of illness as the time-frame for intervention. Using a systems approach to HIV infection, one can identify the intricate recursive loops between context and illness that AIDS dramatizes. Our brief survey of three populations with high incidence of HIV infection shows how belief systems, history, culture, position in society, and family structure affect illness course, and in turn how the diagnosis of HIV infection and the subsequent illness shape family life. Such a systemic approach to chronic illness, which emphasizes the co-evolution of context and illness, has been proposed in recent years (Bloch, 1985, 1989; Penn, 1983; Ransom, 1985; Rolland, 1984, 1987a, 1987b, 1987c; Sheinberg, 1983a; Walker, 1983).

HIV infection forces the family to interface constantly with larger systems. A systems approach not only examines the levels of patient and family experience, but also attempts to create an ecosystemic or holistic approach to intervention. Families may need help in making their needs and beliefs about the illness clear to the medical team, in negotiating services, and in obtaining necessary medical information to ensure that they have the correct protocols or are able to make informed choices about treatment. One of the advantages of an ecosystemic approach is that it provides a model of coordinated care. By contrast, in most medical systems the delivery of counseling follows the organization of the medical-care delivery system. Counselors serve discrete categories of disease entities, with little coordination among services and with little or no provision for following the patient and his family through the course of a disease. As a result, although health-care workers who provide psycho-social services to AIDS patients are gravely overburdened, redundancy of worker involvement also exists. This inefficiency increases overburdening and burnout and results in a fragmentation of care, which is frustrating to both patient and staff. For example, in one case described in Chapters 16 and 18, fourteen caseworkers or counselors attached to different medical programs were involved with a family of three AIDS patients. These workers included methadone maintenance counselors, social workers from pediatric AIDS units in two different hospitals, inpatient social workers, a liaison psychiatrist, and a child welfare worker, among others. Yet, when the mother died, no provision had been made for the child's care because information exchange among these professionals did not exist.

Our work with AIDS patients over the past five years has trained us to be ecosystemic therapists, conceptualizing AIDS in ever broadening circles of social interaction. We have learned to be sensitive to the evolving fit between illness and the family system and to recognize how disease meanings particular to the family and patient have shaped that fit. We have come to pay attention to social constructs such as culture, sexuality, and ethnicity, which define how our clients perceive themselves and their suffering. We have moved into the communities in which our clients live, as it has become clear to us that intervention can no longer be wedded to the consulting room. Although mental health clinics have a role to play, particularly if professionals are willing to advocate for concrete services as a part of treatment, community-based primary-care facilities, hospitals, health clinics, and even schools remain the most efficient locations for family systems care delivery.

Although this book contains many accounts of families seen at Ackerman, we have come to focus our energy on designing community-based programs where a holistic approach to families assures the provision of needed services. Without such services, counseling will have little effect.

CHAPTER 2
Introducing a
Family Systems Approach

A T PRESENT THE MAJOR populations afflicted with HIV infection are gay men, IV drug users and their sexual partners, and hemophiliacs and other blood-product users. Each of these populations has its own difficulties in seeing family therapy as the treatment of choice. While family, partner, and the ill person may all have reservations about family therapy, we must also look at the hesitation of the professional to enter the stormy waters of the PWA's family context. The intensity of the illness can push us to feel overresponsible and overprotective of our patient against the prejudiced world in which he must suffer his illness. We may decide that it is better that we ourselves do the comforting, protecting, and working-through. This may even involve taking on the pain and burden of our patient's emotional life, thus shielding him from family members who may not be able to understand his life choices or the illness itself.

Conjoint therapy may be easier to introduce if whoever seeks treatment is accepted as the family therapy client and the client's rhythm about the introduction of other "family" members is followed. We have learned never to insist on family members' presence in therapy and have done complex systems work with the single client, even if he is living in a relationship in which the partner refuses to enter the therapy. However, we do talk about the desirability of seeing as many people as possible. In the intake telephone call, we discuss with the client who has been told, what they know about the disease, and who he or she still wishes to tell. This information permits us to have a session with the whole family, including children who have not been told, while still observing the parents' wish for secrecy. One man, for example, brought in five relatives over time, one by one. These sessions served as practice rounds for revealing his secret to his only daughter, a teenager who did not know the nature of his sickness. As he and his relatives discussed their feelings about his diagnosis, which they had learned shortly before the sessions, he saw that the therapist was able to engage his relatives and handle their emotions. Several months into the therapy he was able to tell his daughter and bring her to sessions.

GAY MEN

Despite the fact that large numbers of PWAs are in relationships or have relatives who could become involved, the majority of counseling services have focused only on the patient. Prior to the Ackerman AIDS project, only individual counseling or support groups were available in New York. If a lover and/or family members asked to be involved in psychotherapy, they were frequently referred to care partner support groups, rather than being seen with the PWA.

In organizations like Gay Men's Health Crisis (GMHC), volunteers have taken over many functions that otherwise would have fallen on family members. Indeed, volunteers often take the role of family members. Although crisis intervention teams and buddies are effective caregivers, they are not trained to be attentive to the fragile balances of the PWA's larger network of relationships. As a result, the powerful emerging relationship with the volunteer may inadvertently disrupt the balance of a marriage, or the volunteer may form an unwitting coalition with the PWA against the family of origin, thereby impeding the resolution of family issues. Such coalitions are not unexpected, since volunteers are often HIV-infected and dealing with the same issues of shame and hostility as the client PWA. Yet, the presence of volunteers may have alleviated the need for the PWA to confront issues with families perceived to be hostile and homophobic and to effect reconnections with family members.

Fear of Self-Expression and Confrontation

As we have struggled with advocating a systems approach in counseling HIV-infected gay men in the agencies and hospitals with which we consult, we have come to realize that the initial resistance to conjoint therapy with a partner or with the family of origin represents more important underlying concerns than can be explained by the predominance of individual therapy in the medical and mental health fields. The PWA and the professionals treating him often believe that conjoint therapy will encourage the expression of negative feelings—feelings that might rupture fragile relationships with family of origin or care partner or subject the person with AIDS to painful encounters at a time when emotional stress could exacerbate health problems. Diagnosis with AIDS often triggers an eruption of self-doubt, reviving repressive, homophobic voices that the gay man has tried to subdue. Some men view their illness as punishment for their lifestyle, sink into depression, stop fighting back, fail to take medication. Others project their self-hatred and anger onto the outside world; still others deny their illness and act in ways that put others at risk. The patient who blames himself does not want to face his family or even the feared reproaches or disgust of a lover; the patient who projects his self-hatred outward does not want to sit down with his enemy; the patient who denies the social consequences of his illness does not want to be confronted by others about his behavior.

Because a diagnosis with HIV infection affects both partners, it would seem natural for a couple to seek help in conjoint therapy rather than individual therapy, where couples issues can not be as easily resolved. For gay men, however, the prospect of coming to therapy as a couple may add a definition of commitment to the relationship with which neither partner is comfortable. In addition, there is a fear that the exploration of feelings never before plumbed may threaten dissolution of a bond experienced as all the more fragile for having no legal standing. Diagnosis raises issues of contamination, sexual betrayal, anger, and helplessness. The lover or spouse is often afraid of his own feelings about the illness, while the person with AIDS may feel unworthy of love. George, speaking about the difficulty in engaging in sex with his lover, sums up the feelings of many PWAs when he says, "I don't feel good about myself. I feel contaminated. I feel dangerous. I just cannot get close to my lover because I am so fearful for him. It's not sex that is the problem; it's the thing festering in me."

The care partner may feel cornered by feelings of love mixed with questions about whether he would have chosen this relationship had he known its future. He may be afraid to share these feelings with his lover for fear of distressing him at a time when he seems so vulnerable to illness brought on by stress. In some situations couples therapy is avoided because the lover or dying patient cannot tolerate expressions of feeling about the illness or impending loss.

The PWA may have maintained a longstanding pact of silence with his family of origin, guarded by the taboo against discussing or disclosing homosexuality. The pressure of illness exacerbates the conflict between the longing for disclosure and reconciliation with parents, on the one hand, and the fear that disclosure will stir up irresolvable issues about values and beliefs, on the other. The pact may be based on beliefs about what the other person wishes or could tolerate, whispered to a sibling, often a sister, or a sympathetic relative, but never confronted in a face-to-face encounter with the parents.

For instance, a mother may protect the silence she believes her son wishes by confiding to the therapist that which she and her son cannot confide to each other: that she knows that he is gay and that he is ill with Pneumocystis carinii pneumonia, not with ordinary pneumonia. She may have internalized cultural myths about homosexuality and as a result feel guilty that her parental "failings" caused her son to become gay. She may blame herself for being too close to him as he grew up. Her husband may have accused her of making their son into a "mamma's boy." Or she may worry that her son will not be able to deal both with his own upset and with her anticipatory mourning, so she may conceal her feelings from him.

Her son with AIDS may in turn fear that talking with his mother openly will upset her, that his illness and probable death from AIDS will be experienced by her as the final disappointment he inflicts on her. He may feel as guilty about dying of AIDS as about his sexual orientation, which he has never discussed with her. Or he may believe that, while she might be capable of understanding him, to disclose his illness would leave her with an unbearable secret in a straight world, where such disclosure would bring hostility and shame upon her. Both mother and son may secretly long to heal the rift but be afraid to move, each looking to the other for a sign.

Loyalty Conflict

Another issue that is sometimes involved in resistance to family therapy is the loyalty conflict between two very different families, which may play key roles in a gay person's life. The separation from his biological family may have resulted in his forming alternative "families" composed of intimate friends who are deeply connected and have long histories of shared events. In many cases, if a gay person is to belong to one family, he feels he must renounce the other. Reconciliation with the family of origin then represents a betrayal of the adoptive family of adult life.

CASE EXAMPLE

Chuck, a gay man in his thirties, arrived for the intake interview with four of his closest gay friends. The friends surrounded him, initially spoke for him, and seemed anxious and protective when I asked him about his relationship with his family. When he described the time he had spent recuperating at his mother's home after a serious bout of pneumocystis, he stated that he had disclosed neither his sexual orientation nor the nature of his illness. When he expressed a wish to open the issue with his mother and his brother, his friends became anxiously and lovingly protective and warned him strongly against doing so.

It became clear that Chuck was caught in a web of conflicting loyalties to these good friends, who had become a loving family to him, and to his family of origin, from whom he had long been separated by lifestyle and sexual orientation. His friends, who had experienced similar conflicts, were afraid for him, as they were afraid for themselves. Were he to seek help in healing the rift with his family before he died, his attempt, whether failed or successful, would reverberate through this network of friends, throwing into conflict their own beliefs. By keeping the secret of his gayness from his mother, the PWA maintained his coalition with his gay friends, who experienced revelation as endangering this valued, protective coalition. Family therapy would have forced a definition of the relationship between these two families, which were experienced by the ill person as mutually exclusive. Chuck needed a referral to a systemic individual therapy, which protected him from having to make a decision between the two systems as it worked to give him strategies for negotiating his relationships with both. Often, working with the individual in a systems model is the best way to eventually engage the family.

Peer Groups

Other social phenomena that have contributed to resistance to family therapy are the informal and formal peer groups that have traditionally provided support and affirmation for gay men. Organizations such as GMHC, ACT-UP, and the PWA Coalition help gay men develop a positive self-image and an optimistic view of the possibilities for a rich and fulfilling life with AIDS. These peer proups are protective of their members. Many participants have experienced painful rejections by the family of origin when they have revealed that they are gay, and still more negative responses when they have revealed that they have AIDS. Such stressful negative responses are seen as further endangering an already compromised immune system. As a result, peer support groups are regarded as safe havens from insidious homophobia and as family-like groups where a person can build a positive gay self-concept and an optimistic attitude towards living with AIDS.

Individual Therapy

Another option often experienced as safer than family therapy has been finding solace with a caring individual therapist. Individual therapy offers confessional privacy where even the most disturbing thoughts and feelings can be disclosed. Work with AIDS sufferers often contains many of the rituals of the traditional, religious, confessor-penitent relationship: from the confession of guilt, to the statement of resolution to lead a better life as a barter with God for time, and finally to the therapist's preparing the patient for death. The patient may use the individual session to explore feelings of desolation and despair that he wishes to conceal from his loved ones or to ventilate negative feelings about those taking care of him—feelings he may be reluctant to share with them because of his dependency on or gratitude for their care. A systems-oriented individual therapy may be the first step in helping the gay person feel enough support to ask family members to join him in treatment.

DRUG USERS

Drug users have typically felt more comfortable with others who share their compulsion and life experience, both in the street and in drug treatment programs. Ex-drug users are often the only people whom drug users trust to help them change their drug-taking behavior. When we began our project, there were few services for HIV-infected persons who used drugs or for people struggling both with drugs and with the limitations created in their lives by HIV infection. Denial was a major factor in the failure of drug programs to become leaders in organizing HIV-infected drug users to obtain services and special counseling tailored to their needs: Drug counselors were often ex-drug users who themselves were at high risk for carrying the virus. Recently, however, some drug programs have set up special sections for HIV-infected patients.

The infected drug user who seeks counseling is likely to choose peer-oriented drug-free treatment programs or to enroll in a methadone or detox program where he will receive minimal individual counseling. The drug counselor will see the individual but rarely the collaterals. In this sense there is a perfect fit between the structure of methadone and detox programs and the reluctance of the drug user to involve family in situations where his drug use could be challenged. For example, in the interests of preserving confidentiality, methadone workers are not permitted to speak to other family members or to engage them in treatment unless the client expressly asks for their involvement. For the most part, clients fear family anger and the repercussions that could result if ongoing drug use is revealed during the course of counseling. Drug-free programs seldom engage families in conjoint therapy with the drug user on a regular basis. In fact, they may attempt to sever the drug user's contact with the family, which is seen as infantilizing the client and enabling his drug-using behavior.

From the perspective of African-American and Latino families, the drug user may be seen as a criminal and not as a patient. Theft from the family, introduction of other family members to drugs, violence, and neglect of children are common by-products of drug use. HIV infection constitutes an even more dangerous stigma for the family. Even though family members may feel strong ties of loyalty to the drug user, they may not see the usefulness of therapy because they see him as "bad," not "sick." Furthermore, the style of many families where there is drug use is to avoid the very emotions, particularly those concerning loss and mourning, that therapy is designed to elicit. Since drug-using families seem to have experienced greater degrees of tragic, untimely loss than other families (Stanton & Todd, 1982), unresolved mourning for past losses is triggered anew by their fears that they may lose the drug user to AIDS. Family therapy is then experienced as an emotional context that is simply too painful to risk.

Careful outreach to family members is needed to persuade them, first, that therapy can be a path to obtaining needed concrete services and, second, that they can be helped to manage the recurrent problems caused by a family member's addiction. The worker must be sensitive to the fact that family members will need a forum to speak about their anger and disgust at the infected drug user and that initially they may be more comfortable in doing so if the drug user is not present. In a program with which Ackerman's AIDS project has been associated, the Women's Center of Montefiore Hospital's Department of Social Medicine and Epidemiology, community people have organized peer support groups of infected drug users. These groups have served as a clearinghouse for information about necessary resources and have been able to demonstrate to families that the drug user is serious about getting help. These groups have monthly informal dinner meetings with family members who wish to attend; these family nights have served as an effective entry point for conjoint therapy (Eric, Drucker, Worth, Chabon, Pivnick, & Cochrane, 1988). Issues of transmission of HIV infection present problems that argue strongly for counseling the drug user with family of origin and/or sexual partner. Often drug counselors have information that a client may be infecting his sexual partner, but are not permitted to break confidentiality to disclose a client's HIV status to the person(s) at risk. Since drug users are often notoriously irresponsible (particularly when using a drug like crack, a drug which stimulates sexuality and is popular with methadone users), the counselor is faced with the likelihood that the client will neither disclose his HIV status nor refrain from unsafe sex. In response to this problem, some states are developing statutes mandating contact tracing of sexual partners, but epidemiologists warn that the punitive aspects of contact tracing will drive people from seeking testing and treatment. An emphasis on conjoint counseling as the treatment of choice for drug users would make such policing unnecessary.

Families where there is drug use often contain many people who are at risk for HIV, through active use or as sexual partners of people at risk. Were drug users to include their families in treatment, the family session would provide a location for disseminating safer sex information and helping people work through the beliefs, emotions and relationship issues which impede taking protective measures. Multiple couples groups are an effective way of providing safer sex information and of utilizing both peer pressure and support to motivate infected or at-risk men and women to change sexual practices.

HEMOPHILIACS

Psychotherapy is often refused by hemophiliacs because the patient and his family wish to be perceived as normal. Seeking psychotherapy implies stigma and the admission of abnormality. In general, people who are dealing with a chronic physical illness do not want to be labeled as emotionally ill as well, and so they frequently avoid proffered psychotherapy unless it is task-oriented or disguised as a concrete service. Thus, in a successful program for hemophiliacs at the Philadelphia Child Guidance Clinic, rather sophisticated family group intervention could take place in the context of parents learning hypnotic relaxation techniques to apply when children were undergoing home infusion (Rosman, 1988).

SHIELDING THE CHILDREN

Another major source of resistance to conjoint family therapy comes from parental needs to shield children from the shame of the HIV diagnosis. While we encourage the family to include young children in sessions when it feels appropriate, the presence of children immediately raises the issue of secrecy. Parents may resist family therapy because they fear that the therapist will disclose the presence of HIV illness to children, while they wish to keep the issue a secret. Indeed, the therapist may feel that her hands are tied when a child seems to have heard the family whispering about what is going on, and his behavior confirms his upset, yet the family continues to deny the existence of illness.

It is important for children to understand what is happening to the family in as much detail as the family permits. Some parents feel comfortable talking to their children about a parent's or sibling's condition and in managing the secret in the outside world. Other parents deal with AIDS by discussing the illness under the name of one of the opportunistic infections, such as pneumonia, or as cancer. Still others may not have discussed HIV with their children themselves but will permit the therapist to get the child to speak honestly about what he knows.

While the therapist may feel that the truth is preferable to the fantasies a child may have, many families function well despite the fact that the children have not been told directly about the disease. The crucial issue is that parents feel empowered to handle the situation with confidence and in a planful rather than reactive way. For some parents, keeping secrecy about the nature of a child's or parent's death is a way of preserving necessary denial of their own potential illness. This denial permits them to conduct the tasks of everyday life and keep fears of illness and death at bay.

Yet all in all, most children are confused by the mixed messages they receive from family members and outsiders. While they may not have been told that a parent has AIDS, often they have overheard adult discussions. In sessions family members will talk to the therapist about the virus in front of the children and then deny that the children know that a parent has AIDS. Children are usually astute enough to signal that they know they shouldn't let on that they know. But because they are scared by information they are not supposed to have, or do not understand the social consequences of revealing it, they may blurt out the truth to teachers and schoolmates.

Overall, if the family can manage to tell the children about the disease, the children will be better able to address their own fears and contain the information. Most children can be taught the importance of protecting the family by keeping family secrets from outsiders. The mystery of a parent's illness and the apparent shame associated with it are bewildering to young children. Many, having little use of language or sensing that talking is dangerous, become symptomatic. Since secrets usually induce anxiety in the therapist, the therapist will have to be careful to take the time, in individual sessions with the parents, to explore the complex issues impeding revelation and to help the parent deal with the emotions she may face once the child knows. When the parent feels ready to discuss HIV infection, a therapy session is a safe place where the family can make sense of a child's behavior, develop strategies for dealing with it, be able to fully articulate what has happened, and allow the child to make sense out of the events.

CHAPTER 3
Creating a Systemic
Therapy Model

A SYSTEMS MODEL FOR HIV-infected people and their families normalizes illness and restores to the family its problem-solving and coping abilities. The professional's role is primarily as a consultant who encourages families to identify and change illness meanings, to define problem areas, and to effect solutions. The work is pragmatic and problem-focused, but it also must leave room for the ventilation of feelings elicited by the illness. For some periods of time the therapist's work may be only in witnessing the person's experience of illness.

EMPOWERING THE FAMILY

As we have experimented with using family therapy to help people with HIV infection, certain principles have emerged. The first is: *The therapist should empower the family to believe in its own capacities for problem solution and illness management.* Then, by carefully helping family members explore and define beliefs about illness and death, hopes for alleviation or cure, and skepticism about the limits of medical interventions, the therapist encourages them to resume control of their lives in relation to illness. By addressing the way in which a family's shared and individual beliefs are implicated in illness, the therapist helps the family gain the confidence to see illness as a deeply personal event rather than as an event belonging to the professionals involved. The family members are encouraged to handle illness in a way that honors their deepest beliefs and to defend their decisions even when those decisions are at variance with advice offered by medical professionals.

An African-American family with whom we worked had been relying on the decisions of medical professionals in caring for their daughter, who had suffered severe neurological damage during the course of AIDS. The daughter's illness had been contracted from a drug-using husband from whom she was estranged and who was now dying in a different city hospital. The physicians only saw a portion of the family picture: the patient's illness and the possibility of administering drugs that could prolong her life though not reverse the brain damage.

The family saw a picture that included the daughter as well as the effect of her lingering illness on her three children, whose lives were in limbo because they could neither leave their mother nor receive adequate care while they remained in her house. As the children's dysfunction increased from the continued stress of seeing their mother ill, the family sensed that the prolongation of their daughter's life was destructive to the people she loved the most. Yet the mother was too disoriented to understand her condition and make decisions.

Since African-Americans have traditionally found the strength to endure suffering through their connection with Black churches (Boyd-Franklin, 1989), the therapist asked about the role religion had played in their family. Family members agreed that their religious connections had been a source of strength at other times in their lives, but their sense of stigma had kept them from reaching out for the church's support. With the therapist's encouragement, the family sought guidance from the church pastor, who was compassionate and welcoming. As each member found spiritual consolation in the acceptance of death and the continuity of life through the care and healing of the children, they were able to muster the strength to refuse further medical intervention. The pastor was able to visit with the patient and the family and to help them comfort one another as they let her go.

NORMALIZING THE IMPACT
OF ILLNESS

The therapist should clarify and normalize the impact of illness on family life. A psychoeducational approach normalizes the family's illness experience

---

*The author was the therapist.

as it identifies psychological themes common to families dealing with AIDS. Gonzalez, Steinglass, and Reiss (1987) outline the following four areas that need to be addressed by those working with families in which there is a chronic illness:

1. Normative family needs are typically subordinated to the needs and requirements of illness [with the result that] the developmental, practical and emotional needs of other family members and of the patient are minimized or neglected with the build up of stress, frustration and poor communication within the family (p.1).

It is important for the patient's survival that attention be paid to needs of well family members who make up the caretaking system as well as to the patient's needs for care. If these two demand systems are not equally honored, patient and family may begin to distance from each other, to the detriment of care and patient survival. Reiss has hypothesized that this distancing may be a prelude to the death of the patient.

2. Within the family emotional coalitions and exclusions often develop in response to or are exacerbated by the illness. . . .This bond may conspic- uously exclude and isolate other family members and lead to divisive and destructive family interactions (p.2).

HIV infection, because it so often affects individuals who have already had difficult relationships with families of origin, may exacerbate old tensions. Consequently, we encounter the mother and father who war over their gay son or the parents of a drug user who battle to pull their daughter away from her drug-using spouse. Furthermore, as the work of Boscolo and Cecchin has shown, secrecy is a powerful promoter of coalitions (Boscolo, Cecchin, Hoffman, & Penn, 1987), and families with AIDS are frequently divided by who knows about the disease and who does not, a secret which is often kept beyond the death of the family member.

3. The family finds it difficult . . . to change the ways in which it handles illness even if the current coping strategies are dysfunctional, as if the family believes that any adjustments to the precarious strucure will bring the house down (p.2).

Peggy Penn (1983) has written of the taut, fragile skin that seems to hold family together during illness. The family's vulnerability must be respected by the therapist, the pace and content of the work adjusted to protect the family's defenses against too much change, even too much expression of emotion. Ironically, the work itself is often slow, as the therapist gently uncovers and recovers, despite the very real time pressures in the context of illness.

> 4. The rigidity of family coping style may be maintained by the family's relative isolation in coping with the demands of a chronic medical condition . . . . Even families with large kin and social networks tend to keep illness out of view in order to keep themselves as normal as possible (p.2).

The necessity of repeopling families that have been cut off from normal support systems by an illness as stigmatized as AIDS is obvious.

Psychoeducational models provide useful templates for helping families understand the universality of their experience when a chronic illness enters the family. Years of observation of the effect of illness on family functioning by family researchers is translated into concrete tasks that will make caregiving easier. Helping the family understand what illness does to all families facilitates attitudinal and emotional shifts in the family, from blaming and hostility to mutual support and problem-solving.

In a psychoeducational approach an important part of therapy is giving family members basic information about the interconnection of medical and psychological effects of illness and helping them understand that "negative" feelings are common to all families coping with disease (Anderson, Reiss, & Hogarty, 1986). The family is also helped to understand that, despite certain universals of illness experience, each family's illness response and management will be idiosyncratic to family belief systems, which have been shaped by the complex history of a family's collective experience (Reiss, 1987). As the therapist comes to understand the family experience and belief system, he or she emphasizes those elements that both promote coping with the illness and honoring the normative needs of the other family members.

REFRAMING FAMILY NARRATIVES

The therapist changes the problem-generating narrative about the patient, the family, and the disease itself. A fundamental principle of systemic therapy is that it provides an alternative paradigm to Western thought, which depends on practices of scientific classification and the objectification of individuals. Systemic therapists see behaviors not as fixed and classifiable, but as relative, flowing from the contexts which they in turn shape, subject to change as new information changes those contexts. Starting from the understanding that context is "all events in the surround that have actual or potential information or energy value for the target system" (Bloch, 1985, p. 42), the systems therapist looks at repetitive patterns of information or premises that rigidify certain behaviors. These patterns of information can be seen as dominant narratives; as such they shape the loop between the social system's view of an individual and the individual's perception of himself in the social system.

The knowledge that a person has AIDS immediately locates him within certain possible classifications, which then become dominant narratives, dictating how others perceive him and how he perceives himself. Such classifications include terminally ill, AIDS victim, drug addict, homosexual, sexually promiscuous. These classifications are in reality only constructed ideas that are accorded a truth status. As Michael White has said, "These truths are normalizing in the sense that they construct norms around which people are incited to shape or constitute their lives" (White & Epston, 1990, p.20), just as they also shape the information which the observer will observe.

The visibility of AIDS means that the infected person can no longer pass as "normal"; instead he must embrace a stigmatizing classification that reduces him "from a whole and usual person to a tainted and discounted one. . . breaking the claim that his usual attributes have on us" (Goffman, 1986, pp. 3, 5). If he once passed as "normal," he now experiences a denial of the respect people have usually accorded his uncontaminated identity. The stigmatized person now completes the recursive cycle by operating as if some of his own attributes warrant the stigma (Goffman, 1986). Stigma isolates the person with AIDS from surrounding systems and often extends to the family, as members become categorized, stigmatized, and isolated because of their association with him. The PWA Coalition's insistence on the use of the phrase "person with AIDS" (PWA) was a response to the dehumanizing terms "AIDS victim" and "AIDS patient," which subsumed the person's identity in his illness designation.

For most families, the prevailing narrative about the AIDS illness and the ill person generates challenging problems. Because of the association of AIDS with behavior considered to be socially deviant, the illness narrative may become fixed and rigid. Feelings about drug use or homosexuality are often linked to feelings about the person dying: "AIDS is a punishment for his choice to be gay. I will not turn him away now that he is dying, but I cannot condone his lifestyle." In this version the ill person is subsumed in the category "gayness"; attitudes are defined by his participation in the category "gay." Illness is seen as punishment and equated with death, and the family role is identified as compassionate attendance while he dies. The message to the patient is that family members can be loving toward him as long as he is dying, but if he lives they will have problems with his lifestyle. These messages are powerful and, in turn, may define the patient's attitude toward the meaning of his own illness and impending death.

In order to open possibilities for new and different interactions among family members, the therapist constructs alternative narratives about the AIDS patient, offering an opportunity to escape the rigid category of "drug addict" or "homosexual" that has dominated family members' relationship with him. For example, the therapist does not focus on the family divisions created by the client's homosexuality ("His gayness, which we can never accept, will always divide us"), but instead emphasizes other aspects of the family narrative. Asking a gay son, "Could you tell your father what you have learned from him?" elicits an affirmation of valued connections, creating what hypnotists have called a "yes set" in the father. If the father is to accept his son's affirmation of the positive qualities his son has learned by observing him, then he must say yes to the corollary, "I, as your son, am at least in part that which you have made me." The constructed narrative becomes one about the difficulties and successes of the father-son relationship. The message to father is clear: "What is most important here is your son's role as a son and your role as a father—not whether or not he is gay." Reframing is one way of introducing alternative constructions that disrupt the tedious regularity of the problem focus and allow other patterns to emerge.

Sometimes the family itself will create new, transforming narratives out of the experience of AIDS. Reiss's idea that families create paradigmatic change by constructing new narratives out of illness events is illustrated by description of a family for whom recognition and growth come through shared and explored experience.

CASE EXAMPLE*

Prior to the death of their son Michael from AIDS, this suburban Connecticut family's dominant narrative about itself was problem- satu-

*The author was the therapist.

rated. It was alcohol-ridden; there had been violence between the parents; the youngest son was in trouble, another gay and unhappy with his life. Three of the children were functioning well, although the doctor-son had a conflictual relationship with his sisters and was at odds with his family. Other stories were also present in the family's account of its history, a story of endurance and of the love that members of a large family can have for each other. The challenge of caring for an ill son during the last months of his life brought to the fore the stories of love and endurance. These ultimately replaced the problem-saturated narrative to become the family's dominant story about itself.

The experience of fully participating with their son and brother, Michael, in his dying bonded their sense of family, their pride in each other. It taught family members deep lessons about compassion and acceptance that they carried into their lives as his legacy. The father felt that he had fully guided his family through this event, lending the others strength and comfort. A sister who was a writer began to work out her experience of her brother's death in stories and poems; another sister became politically active. The brother who was a doctor found new meaning in his work as he became impassioned about the health care of minorities, including gay people. The youngest sibling, who had been in trouble, angry and confused, and perhaps on drugs, reexamined the meaning of his life. And the sister who was about to get married found in her brother's meager savings a very special wedding present. Both parents felt that their marriage and their sense of what really mattered had been strengthened by the family's ability to join together around Michael. This family was able to shift paradigms and use the illness as a transformational learning. In their own ways, the family members pay tribute to the transforming experience of attending Michael through his illness and death.

A crucial aspect of our work is attending to the flow of meanings each person in the family assigns to the disease itself. Illness meanings are generated at all system levels, from the societal to the familial to the personal. The prevailing social narrative defining our relationship with AIDS is its silent, omnipresent fatality. The infected person lives in a culture where AIDS equals DEATH. GMHC and the PWA Coalition have constructed an alternative narrative in which the experience of AIDS is one of constructing a meaningful life in the face of a sometimes painful, chronic condition. This fundamental reframing of the disease allows space for living and for making life decisions that might seem not to matter if the AIDS process were constructed only as preparation for death.

Within the family, the illness meaning may be intermingled with the family's view of the behavior that led to contracting the virus. For example, one mother felt despair at her son's illness. When he entered the session, he would have to lie down on a couch because of pain, and his mother would sit behind him, weeping, not unlike the Pietà. During his illness the mother contracted breast cancer. She felt that the cancer was a kind of equivalent suffering, although she knew, to her despair, that her prognosis was better than his. Both mother and son believed that the parents' bad marriage had led to his homosexuality and to his inability to have an intimate relationship. The son implied that if he had been able to sustain an intimate, homosexual relationship, he would not have been promiscuous and become ill.

For both mother and son, homosexuality was a disaster because it had ended in AIDS. The mother's failure as a mother had killed her son. Their narrative became increasingly fixed through their isolation: the son had few friends, and the mother refused to share her secret with other family members, believing that they would respond with hostility. This belief was so powerful that when she finally told a nephew and he showed dispassionate concern, she interpreted his behavior as confirming his basic inability to care for her—even though they had had little contact prior to the revelation of her son's illness.

Frequently the illness narrative dominates family life and obliterates the family's sense of itself as a surviving and functioning unit. Problems may loom so large that family members cannot see their capacity for resolving them. Often, the problem focus is so extensive that they cannot identify friends, relatives, or outsiders who could play a positive role in problem solution. The therapist works to enlarge the family's awareness of potential helpers, with the understanding that increasing the flow of information to the family and its sense of connectedness to a wider network will provide increased support and options.

IDENTIFYING FAMILY RESOURCES

The therapist should help the family identify resources both inside and outside of the family. One technique that informs the therapist of unexpected areas of strength and expands the family narrative is working with the family to create a family resource eco-map (Hartman & Laird, 1983). The eco-map resembles a genogram but broadens it to include family members both past and present, extended kin systems (with notations about the degree of involvement with the identified patient), significant friends, and a diagram of the client's involvement with larger systems (medical, welfare, child protection, volunteer agencies). The family or ill person is encouraged to analyze the interconnections of people in the system, to identify the positive effects of persons who might not be thought of as "family," to ascertain whether or not they represent potential resources for caregiving, and to pinpoint problematic interfaces between involved systems.

HIV diagnosis may mean that the family is separated from normal healing rituals, family gatherings, friendship groups, and church groups. Such isolation inevitably increases stress. The eco-map can identify systems which have been helpful to the family prior to diagnosis and with which reconnection would be healing. In addition, the eco-map identifies allied and conflicting systems, as well as workers who have entered the family's life post diagnosis and may be dominating family life in a detrimental manner.

The therapist can serve as an organizer and facilitator of meetings attended by representatives of the various systems with whom the family is involved. These systems may include health-care professionals, schools, child welfare, foster care, homemakers, and volunteers. Clarifying roles and developing a unified treatment plan in collaboration with the patient and the family can increase efficiency of care provision, just as such a meeting can be empowering and comforting to the family.

MOBILIZING EXTRAFAMILIAL SUPPORT

The therapist should encourage the family to become connected to community support systems, which can relieve AIDS isolation.

Aids isolates. The gay community responded to the epidemic by founding self-help organizations, which provided invaluable support networks for the ill and their caregivers, disseminated information, and empowered people to become active in decision-making about treatment. Political groups like ACT-UP converted despair into activism, while groups like the PWA Coalition and Body Positive helped people develop strategies for living positively with illness. Programs like ADAPT and the Montefiore Women's Center used community volunteers to develop networks of people who provided information and ongoing support to drug users and their families. Mothers' groups exist in many major hospitals, as well as voluntary agencies, and can alleviate the isolation that both HIV-infected mothers and their infected children experience. Support groups should be seen as an invaluable addition to family resources.

IMPARTING MEDICAL INFORMATION

The therapist should be able to impart medical information about the illness itself—etiology, symptoms, expected course, conditions conducive to optimal living, and environmental determinants of exacerbation.

Although therapists working with families often do not have a medical background, they should become familiar with the basic nature of the illness, the possible courses it takes, and the uses and side-effects of basic medications. Frequently, the initial contact with the therapist provides family members with their first opportunity to explore the medical questions that concern them. There are relatively few doctors specializing in infectious disease in the large cities where AIDS populations are concentrated, and many clients (particularly those from backgrounds of poverty) are fearful of pressing their doctors for information. As a result, they remain unaware of the potentially helpful protocols available to them: the use of the drug AZT, ddI or ddC or a combination of AZT and ddI as a general antiviral, or Bactrim or aerosolized Pentamidine to prevent recurrences of Pneumocystis carinii pneumonia (PCP). New vaccines currently in clinical trials may help HIV-positive people develop antibodies to some manifestations of the HIV virus.

Clients may need even the most basic information about the disease. For example, a common belief is that a diagnosis of AIDS means imminent death. In fact, one out of every ten people with AIDS lives for at least three years, and one out of 33 lives more than five. These figures include people with AIDS who do not receive adequate medical care; a person who receives good care has an even better chance of living for years with the disease. As both early diagnosis and medical treatment of opportunistic infections improve and more effective anti-virals are found, overall survival rates will improve. The client and his family may be far more frightened of contamination by means other than sex or blood products than they need be. The challenge to the clinician is to help the patient and family construct a more realistic picture of the disease and its means of transmission, as well as a more optimistic view of the possibilities for survival with the disease.

In addition, the therapist must attend to issues particular to HIV infection that may not be raised by clients. In essence, the therapist must take the lead in setting the agenda for therapy. Two such issues are safer sex information and future planning for children after a parent's death. For many people—particularly those from African-American, Latino, and African-Caribbean families—sexuality is an intensely private issue. Couples will avoid dealing with issues of sexual transmission because they are embarrassed to talk about sex, uncomfortable with condom use, and ashamed to acknowledge their discomfort. The therapist must be prepared to raise these issues with sensitivity and to keep them in the forefront of therapy until they are resolved. Often, the client reveals that many people in the family are at risk for infection and do not have access to HIV-prevention information. The family system then becomes a point of entry for introducing such information to a large number of people.

Because AIDS is an immunosuppressive disease, its progression from initial diagnosis of infection to death is highly variable. There is no predictable course of illness the patient will suffer. Medical crises may be frequent during the period of counseling, or the patient may appear to show no outward signs of disease. Most often, family members are the first to notice that the client is becoming more ill or is behaving oddly (a possible sign of neurological involvement), at which point they may bring their concerns to the AIDS team physician, who is their link to the medical system. Conversely, they may bring the AIDS patient for counseling, attributing symptoms of depression or anxiety to relationship issues or interpreting them as reactions to illness, when in fact a subtle process of neurological infection or reaction to medications is involved.

CASE EXAMPLE*

Friends and family of a distinguished older architect who was ill with AIDS referred him for counseling because of problems with his younger lover. They feared that the lover was draining his energy, not being sufficiently supportive, and only staying because he wanted his inheritance. The family and friends had become polarized around their dislike of the lover, who was from a different social and intellectual class than the architect, did not work, and had no discernible goals in life. They believed that the architect was depressed by the situation but too frightened of being alone to ask the lover to leave. When a physician knowledgeable about the neurological manifestations of AIDS began to work with the couple, he found that the lover's detailed report of the

---

*The therapist was John Patten.

architect's behavior supported more comprehensive neurological examinations than had previously been conducted. It was also clear to the physician that the lover, who was barely 20, was overwhelmed, both by the task of caring for a man who had played the role of his caretaker and mentor and by his own fears that he had become infected. Neurological examinations confirmed the physician's suspicion, and he was able to support the young lover through his partner's dying.

The interplay between psychological and medical factors in an immunodeficiency disease such as AIDS is never clear. Both the family therapist and the physician are always weighing the effects of stress and emotional upheaval on the medical course of illness, and the effects of illness on the person's psychological state. At times psychosomatic symptoms—an anxious cough or overwhelming fatigue—can mimic disease symptoms such as bronchial illness or debilitation. A person who feels himself to be in good health at testing may become ill shortly after a test reveals that he is positive; another may remain asymptomatic for more than ten years.

Did the stress generated by the positive test trigger an illness vulnerability in the first man? Did the client decide to be tested because he sensed subclinical signs indicating reason for concern? Was the onset of illness so soon after the test a mere coincidence? Or is there something about the life of the HIV-positive person who remains well that makes him less vulnerable to illness? Is it a matter of attitude, satisfaction about identity, fulfilling relationships? One PWA who largely ignored the fact that he had AIDS enjoyed many years of excellent health following the initial opportunistic infection. Although he was not given to psychologizing about his life, when he developed cancer he said that he felt that it had happened after the breakup of a love relationship because, "After I lost that, I became depressed, stopped fighting."

While the relationship among an optimistic attitude, positive interpersonal relationships, and better immune functioning is incompletely understood (Borysenko, 1989; Fox, 1989; Schmidt & Schmidt, 1989), preliminary studies in the field of psychoneuroimmunology indicate that these factors correlate with better survival outcome and suggest that behavioral factors "can alter immunity and disease susceptibility through direct central nervous system mechanisms or through endocrinological intermediaries" (Borysenko, 1989, p. 254). AIDS organizations, such as Body Positive, ACT-UP, and the PWA Coalition, are committed to creating a positive attitude towards illness, not just because this will improve PWAs' quality of life, but also because they believe that actual survival time will be extended. Psychotherapy should focus on life-affirming aspects of living with illness, work to improve the quality of family, friendship, and couple relationships, and actively encourage people to learn stress management techniques such as visualization and deep relaxation.

CASE EXAMPLE*

The following case underscores the complex relationship between mind and body and the power of familial and relationship patterns in determining the course of illness. A young couple, both ex-drug users, presented for psychotherapy because the wife was having difficulty adjusting to the husband's obsession with his health. Shortly before their marriage they had decided to get tested. After their honeymoon they received their test results: The wife tested negative, the husband positive. As they began counseling the husband started to manifest symptoms of anxiety and fatigue. Tests showed that his T-cell count was normal and there were no medically discernible signs of an active disease process. Yet he continued to feel worse. The wife became more and more enraged by his despairing attitude, his increasing inability to function, and his dependence on her.

Unlike his wife, the man had a pessimistic outlook and was helpless and dependent — qualities reflected in his drug use. His wife's drug use, by contrast, could be seen as a flight from the role she had played growing up as an overburdened caretaker of two alcoholic parents. As an adult, she had entered the helping professions and become involved with men who used drugs and alcohol; they viewed her as strong and caretaking. Having set her life in order, the diagnosis of her new husband as HIV-positive was a shock, since it meant that they could never have their own children. But she was willing to stick with the marriage if her husband would begin to act in a more adult manner. His dependency infuriated her because it forced her into replaying the caretaker role of her childhood. Her anger and withdrawal in turn increased her husband's depression and helplessness.

Counseling had some effect on their relationship and in small ways the husband became more active. Nonetheless, he remained convinced that he would become ill within a short time. Quite suddenly he developed toxoplasmosis and nearly died. The relationship improved after a defin-

*Ruth Mohr was the therapist.

itive diagnosis, as the wife dedicated herself to caring for a legitimately ill husband. As the wife accepted her husband's illness, thus fulfilling his most primitive needs, he became more mature and began working as an AIDS counselor to others.

MAPPING THE FAMILY ILLNESS STRUCTURE

The therapist maps the pre- and post-illness family structure in order to help the family return as much as possible to a pre-illness unit. In order to ascertain which problem behaviors occurred prior to diagnosis, the therapist takes a careful history of family development, exploring how family members have handled crises in the past and what options are open to them in the current crisis. "Circular questioning"—a technique developed by the early Milan team (Selvini Palazzoli, Boscolo, Cecchin, & Prata, 1980) to rapidly gather information about the structure and organization of a family without arousing resistance—forms the basis of the structured assessment interview. The questions induce family members into a method of systemic thinking in which they examine how beliefs influence behaviors. Thus, family members are able to identify illness-generated coping patterns and to seek a balance between illness needs and norma-tive family needs and functions. Pre- and post-illness functioning is usefully mapped in such areas as school, work, marital satisfaction, parent-child relationships, extended family relationships, and drug and alcohol use.

One aspect of understanding the family's pre-illness structure is the mapping of the development of family coalitions. Rigid coalitions can be seen as a response to the threat of family disorganization under the extraordinary stress of AIDS. In essence, family members hold onto and reiterate the known, almost as though it were a mantra, in the face of uncertainty and potential loss. In families with the greatest resistance to changing coalition patterns, we have discovered that these patterns were established during similar experiences of illness in the previous genera-tions. Only by addressing the past as it is reincarnated in the present have we been able to shift these dynamics (Sheinberg, 1983b; Walker, 1983). And only as family structure becomes more flexible and deeply felt and emotional needs of healthy family members find avenues for satis-faction, will illness meaning begin to change in the direction of allevi-ating psychological pain.

Because unlike other chronic illnesses, AIDS assaults the family's position in the community, often creating social isolation, internal conflicts between family members are exacerbated. The consolidation of coalitions to ward off fragmentation, as the normal supports and markers of pre-illness family identity fall away, may have an ugly side, in which scapegoating becomes the means to achieving temporary cohesion. As David Reiss writes:

> Blame, hatred, tyranny and exploitation rise and fall with staggering swiftness and according to unfathomable patterns. Each member feels as if the center of his life is loosening, that his unseen ties to others and to his past have become highly visible, vulnerable and finally torn. The family as a group loses its most precious possession: an extended and dependable repertoire of background understandings, shared assumptions, traditions and meaningful secrets which made it possible for them to function implicitly. (1981, pp. 177-178)

Reiss further hypothesizes that the family defends against disintegration by establishing increasingly rigid patterns of control. As family members lose confidence in their ability to function and provide care, they search for scapegoats—most often within the family itself. While the scapegoating process provides some opportunities for cohesion and improved functioning, as it focuses on the task of disciplining the person identified as the problem bearer, it does not provide any opportunity for growth and change.

CASE EXAMPLE*

An African-American family came to therapy because of problems with their ten-year-old son at home and at school. In the therapist's view, the boy's behavior seemed congruent with the extreme stress the family was undergoing, as his non-addicted mother was suffering a protracted and painful death from AIDS. Furthermore, the boy's father, a drug user whom the family saw as having killed his wife, was also dying. The family's reaction to the boy's problems seemed unbearably harsh. They mocked his bad behavior in school, predicted that he would be just like his father, and further attacked his father. The scapegoating process united the women, who felt defeated by the impossibility of their men ever escaping from drugs and alcohol and furious that their lives were destroyed by their men's addictions.

This coalition among the women was merely an exaggerated version of previous coalition patterns. The mother's death crystallized all the women's anger toward the men in the family. For reasons of history, tradition, economic reality, gendered learnings and compassion, the

*The author was the therapist.

women felt unable to abandon the men who oppressed them (Hines & Boyd-Franklin, 1982). As a result, the boy became a lightning rod for their anger.

Creating a family time line allowed us to explore pre- and post-illness family organization and functioning, as well as the crucial events underlying the belief system that defined family functioning around AIDS illness. It was clear that family members had managed to survive the failures of its men until the crisis of AIDS drove them beyond the limits of endurance. Some of the women had led successful and productive lives, despite abuse from the men. One son, who was away at college, seemed to have escaped the male tradition of failure.

AIDS had created a crisis that challenged the family's very survival. Threatened with public exposure and shame in the community, family members felt an increased sense of vulnerability and powerlessness. The successful son—seemingly pushed to carry out the family's deepest fears about the destructiveness of men—raped a college student. The little boy started stealing and exposing himself in school. As the women gradually identified the history of their beliefs about men in therapy, they began to understand how these beliefs could create a future map for the child that would trap him in the same cycle of abuse as his father and grandfather.

The rigid belief system softened when the therapist was able to identify a peripheral member of the family, a man with whom the aunt was involved in a romantic but conflictual relationship, who could represent a different possibility for both the family and the little boy's future. As he interacted with the child, with toughness and love, he helped the women challenge the rigid belief that they were powerless to change the future of their male children. Watching her man interact with the boy, as the therapist discussed family beliefs about men, may have helped the aunt see her lover in a more affirmative and trusting light. His emergence as a figure of male strength and kindness completed the women's evolving sense of the positive futures for their male children. After his mother's death the little boy went to live with his aunt and her new husband.

PLANNING FOR THE FUTURE

The therapist should help the family plan for its future while the ill person can participate. As family and therapist explore patterns of interaction, future-oriented questioning enables family members to anticipate problems and break negative response cycles by creating new narratives with different outcomes. Future-oriented questions may be of particular use with AIDS patients and their families because chronic or terminal illness introduces a sense of "frozen time"—a sense that change and evolution must stop in order to preserve the fragile structure the family has achieved (Penn, 1983, 1985). In answering such questions, the family is asked to challenge vicious, self-fulfilling cycles of response that are embedded in the prevailing narrative. The gradual introduction of a sense of future—even if it includes planning for the life after the ill person's death—is healing. In a sense, the "time-ice" begins to melt and the ill person and family members experience themselves once more as part of the changing flow of *living* systems. Asking the dying person to participate in planning an optimistic future for the people he or she will leave is an immensely healing experience.

CASE EXAMPLE

The following case illustrates the way in which a family's divided past can be healed by drawing on its strengths and connections. In this family the dying mother was able to do her most important mothering in the last months of her life. By planning with her children for their future she was able to heal the wounds of many years when she had not been a part of their growing up.

Carol O'Connor met the mother during her first interview as an intake worker at GMHC. Gloria was a tiny, lively woman who had two children in Puerto Rico. Her past history in New York was unclear, but it was likely that she had been involved at some time with drugs, which had made it impossible for her to mother her children, who had remained with her mother in Puerto Rico. AIDS had brought dramatic weight loss. She seemed disoriented and complained of problems in remembering. Because Gloria was without adequate housing, Carol arranged an appointment with an AIDS housing program as well as an immediate neurological evaluation. There was no further contact with Gloria until two years later, when quite by accident Carol interviewed a woman, Anita, and her 14-year-old niece Angelina, who turned out to be Gloria's sister and daughter. They were accompanied by a concerned social worker from the housing program to which Carol had referred Gloria.

Carol learned that Gloria was currently in the hospital. Anita thought Gloria was dying and had come to therapy because she wanted professional help in telling her niece. Shortly after the session began, Carol realized that the many social service agencies now involved with the family underestimated the family's capacity for managing the disclosure, for helping the daughter to prepare for her mother's death, and for planning for the children's future. Carol felt that the family members had a deep spiritual connection and strength that they could draw on to perform those tasks with minimal professional intervention.

Carol believed that the family's view of itself as strong and resilient had been undermined by the tragedy of the mother's illness. It had come to see itself as an AIDS family and possibly also as a family stigmatized by drug use. Also, family members' belief in their own competence had been undermined by their involvement in professional helping systems, which they credited with possessing greater wisdom than they had.

Carol's first task was to encourage Anita to take charge of her family. When Anita resisted, Carol began to explore what Angelina knew. In order to protect the girl (and herself) from becoming overwhelmed by the grief that was just below the surface, Carol asked Angelina to stop her whenever she felt they were going too fast. They moved close to the issue of death, drifted a distance, then ventured nearer and nearer until the word could be spoken. It emerged that Angelina knew everything, and indeed had a clear sense of the direction her family must take.

As Angelina spoke movingly and wisely of her mother, of her resentment for the past because her mother had left her, of her forgiveness and love of her mother in the present, and of her hope for her future with her mother, no matter how brief, Anita became increasingly unemotional and silent. Carol tried again to put her in charge of her family and again she resisted. As Anita resisted Carol's invitation and fought her emotions, it became clear that she did not want to cry in front of Angelina. Carol suggested that if Anita could let herself cry, she would give her niece permission to cry. At that point Anita was able to embrace her niece and share her grief with her.

The gentle encouragement to cry together challenged the family myth that "You don't want to break down and cry in front of your family . . . . We all have problems." This family, primarily headed by women, believed that confronting pain with others might increase the pain and ultimately make survival more difficult. In the second and last session Anita addressed that belief. She said that she had learned that sharing her grief with her niece was comforting and strengthening to both of them, a better way than the isolation of pain not shared.

The first session ended with the family making plans for bringing Angelina's little brother to New York to be with his mother, plans that the family made without any input from the professionals.

Angelina decided to defer the next session until her mother was well enough to attend. She wanted to demonstrate that, despite illness, her family had healed the past, with her mother restored to her rightful place. When the session occurred, it focused on Gloria's wishes for her children's future. The three women joined together to face their tomorrows with grace, courage and strength.

Here Gloria, through tears, is able to discuss her illness and her fears. She passes her dreams and her simple wisdom to her teenage children as she begins to say goodbye: "I'm afraid. I don't know where I get strength, but it really hurts to think that I'm not going to be around for my family, for my children. When I'm dead, they will know how much I loved them anyway. I tell my daughter what to do—when I'm not here, she has to be strong and pretty soon she will be bigger and work for herself and not depend on nobody." Gloria goes on to plan with her sister and her daughter—practical things, where they will live when she is gone, how her daughter will care for her little brother since she does not want her children separated, where her daughter will finish school, her wish that she will go to college.

Gloria lived for six months after that session, with her sister and children. She died peacefully in her sister's arms, her work of reconciliation and planning for her family's future completed.

CREATING A CONTEXT FOR ONGOING THERAPY

The therapist should frame therapy as an ongoing process. The Ackerman Clinic is located at some distance from most of the families we serve. Nonetheless, many families have stayed with us over the long course of infection. Therapy often takes the form of intensive initial work, with follow-up sessions as illness or social events disrupt family functioning. A man, for example, will see us together with his lover during the lover's illness and then return alone after the bereavement period, when he is considering a new relationship or when his health undergoes a crisis. Recently we have realized that it is important to actively encourage families to return even after the period of reorganization, when AIDS has disappeared as an active presence in the family.

Because of the trauma of AIDS and often because the events leading up to HIV infection have also traumatized the family, many of these families are highly vulnerable to destabilization following some relatively minor crisis or dislocation. In one family, the birth of a baby to adoptive parents created a crisis for an orphaned child, which the family could not handle alone. After several years of good functioning, the boy's behavior so deteriorated that the family considered placement. During a follow-up telephone call, the adoptive parents made it clear that they had not connected this crisis with events related to AIDS. AIDS was a closed chapter in their lives.

Nancy Boyd-Franklin (1989) has suggested that therapy be framed as an ongoing process. In this model, during the "termination" process which closes each piece of work, the family is helped to understand that it is normal for crises to occur. They are sensitized to identify events that call for therapeutic help and encouraged to return. Follow-up telephone calls are an important way of defining our ongoing commitment to the family's well-being.

PUTTING THE PRINCIPLES TO WORK: A CASE EXAMPLE

The following case example demonstrates the application of the principles outlined in this chapter for structuring the first session of therapy with an HIV-infected person.

Juan and his wife Nereida came to therapy because of the deterioration in their relationship following Juan's diagnosis as being HIV-positive. Juan made the initial phone call. He seemed extremely upset, admitting that his first instinct after diagnosis was to commit suicide. He still thought about suicide as a solution to his and his family's problems. As a security officer, Juan was licensed to use a gun. The intake worker viewed the threat as serious and scheduled a session for the following Monday.

For a while, Juan had kept his diagnosis a secret, but as the anxiety had receded he decided to tell his wife because he knew she needed to be tested for the virus. As a sort of trial run, he called his ex-wife, the mother of his son, and told her about his diagnosis. Fortified by her supportive response, he then told Nereida. While showing little upset or surprise at the diagnosis, she was furious when she learned he had told his ex-wife first.

In the session Nereida, a dark-haired, fiery beauty in her thirties, appeared to be a strong Latina woman who held a realistic though fatalistic view of "the life": "Juan always did what he wanted. He womanized, he hung out with the boys, he had a good time and he never thought about the consequences. That is the sort of man he is." Nevertheless, she was extremely touchy about her rights in relation to her husband's former wife.

Juan presented as an attractive man, with dark appealing eyes. He and Nereida had been married for five years and were together two years previous to marriage. Both have children from their first marriages.

Nereida stated that she had come to therapy because Juan needed to talk about his problems. While she expressed feeling angry at him for "the hurts he gave me," she did not seem likely to leave, nor was she overtly concerned about the infection adversely affecting their feelings for each other. She said she lived "a day at a time," and that they were managing well with what she termed their "little problem"—except that Juan seemed to be very upset.

As Juan began to relate the history of his diagnosis, he was breathing heavily; indeed, his affect throughout the session mirrored absolute terror. His large body shook with anxiety, and he was almost in tears a number of times. He had gone for the HIV test after noticing an inexplicable weight loss. He was then given a battery of tests, including the HIV test. When the doctor told him that he was positive for HIV, he was shocked and horrified. He had never thought that AIDS could be an issue in his life. Feeling terrified and out of control, he immediately thought of suicide; suicide, at least, was a way of taking charge.

Since his initial diagnosis, Juan has had very intense periods of fear and loneliness. He is frightened that Nereida is angry enough to leave him. He is afraid of the future. We entertained a number of hypotheses as we observed behind the mirror. First, we wondered whether Juan's anxiety was due to inadequate medical information about his condition. Today, people who are HIV-positive can expect to remain symptom-free for a lengthy period of time. What had the doctor told Juan and what had Juan asked about the disease? As a Latino from the inner city, Juan would not necessarily feel comfortable talking to a physician about his fears and worries. Therefore, we asked the therapist to discover how much he knew about his situation.

Juan said that his T-cell count was very low, 180, and he was afraid he would die immediately. Before he received his T-cell results, his doctor had recommended that he go to Body Positive, a self-help group for HIV-positive people. In the group, Juan learned that average T-cell counts ran between 500 and 1,500 and that anything below 500 was considered abnormal. Thus, his fear was intensified rather than abated by his group participation. To arrest HIV replication and protect him against pneumocystis, the doctor put him on AZT and Bactrim. His next

T-cell count showed a gain of 100 T-cells. Even though his immune system seemed to be improving, and he had additional information about the disease, Juan's anxiety had shown little decrease since initial diagnosis.

When asked about his terror, the most that Juan could express was that he was afraid Nereida would turn on her heel and leave one day. After he mentioned this fear, he randomly commented about various friends who had committed suicide: He had a friend who had committed suicide last June—perhaps he was HIV-infected; his ex-girlfriend had attempted suicide in his house with Nereida present when the girlfriend learned he was going to leave her—maybe she was HIV-positive, too. At one time, he had even told Nereida that he was thinking about arranging his death in such a way that she would be able to collect his life insurance premium. Now he felt better, he stated, and didn't think about such things. When the therapist pursued, asking Juan if he still had suicidal thoughts, he immediately denied it. But the issue hovered in the air as cloud of overwhelming anxiety.

We wondered to what degree guilt played a role in his intense feelings of anxiety, terror, and despair. As we listened to Juan, we heard him continually refer to a sense of terror, which his whole body seemed to express. He said the terror was with him constantly. When we asked him what he did with his night terrors—whether he told Nereida that he was frightened—he said evasively, "Oh, I've told a number of people about my infection. I told my brother and two of my best friends from the security agency." But he avoided the question of whether or not he spoke to Nereida or sought her comfort when he was the most frightened.

As we attempted to pursue this question of whether he could talk to Nereida about his fears, Nereida became more distant and withdrawn. Watching her carefully, Juan said, "I don't want to upset her by talking about these things. I feel so guilty. I have done so many bad things and I've made her life so miserable. I don't see why she would stay with me. I think one day she'll just walk out."

In group consultations, we put together several clues. Juan kept referring to his weight loss. At the moment, however, he seemed rather overweight—a short man weighing around 185-190 pounds. Before diagnosis, he weighed between 30 and 50 pounds more. Weight loss, in his case, would seem positive. What did weight mean to him? We hypothesized that weight had something to do with largeness, with strength, with being "a big man." Perhaps the issue for Juan was not so much the HIV infection itself, but what it had done to him as a person.

We speculated that neither Nereida's retaliation for his past life nor his guilt about it terrified him. Rather, we felt his fear came from the fact that HIV weakened him, making him emotionally vulnerable and dependent. His frequent proclamation, "I've never been physically sick," and his fear that Nereida would leave seemed linked to his terror of losing his identity as a strong man by becoming a sick man riddled with fears.

Nereida was asked if she, in fact, had withdrawn from Juan. She evaded the question and spoke about how they were managing on a daily basis. Juan jumped in: "You're withdrawing from me because you're angry with all the things I've done. You couldn't possibly love me. You're going to leave me!" Nereida said that his accusation was unfair and hurt her deeply. She enumerated some of his actions that had made her angry, asserting that she had a right to her feelings. She shouldn't have to keep them to herself after all the years of difficulty, but she still had no intention of leaving him. Juan immediately confirmed her accusations, adding a long confessional speech about his bad behavior.

Listening carefully, we felt that Nereida was more upset by Juan's statement that she didn't love him than by his past activities. We wondered if Nereida was upset about the change in the relationship, Juan's vulnerability, and her newfound voice of anger. Carol O'Conner posed a crucial question, believing that a fundamental shift had occurred in the relationship after Juan's diagnosis—a shift that neither partner could tolerate. Her question, a circular one, was addressed to Nereida.

"Nereida, do you think that Juan believes you could love him if he were not the macho man you fell in love with, but if he were weak or sick?"

Nereida thought about the question for a while and tried to say, "He's not weak, he's strong." Then she said, "No, that's a good question. There's some truth in that. I don't think he believes that I could love him if he is not strong."

Nereida avoided answering whether she herself would love Juan if he were not strong, and if she could tolerate taking care of a sick man.

The therapist followed her question to Nereida by asking Juan what he thought about Nereida's response. He answered immediately: "I've had to be strong all my life. I've never been afraid of anything. I don't know if she can love me if I'm weak and afraid."

The therapist asked again if he had ever talked about his fears with Nereida. He said, "No, she doesn't want to hear. She goes away."

Nereida added quickly, "He's not always weak. He does have a very good attitude. He is trying to be strong. He is trying to fight it." Nereida kept reiterating her version of what Juan should be: the strong man with the optimistic attitude who was going to beat the disease. By contrast, what we saw before us was a rather childlike, anxiety-ridden, weeping man, who was still enormously upset three months after the diagnosis.

We wondered whether Nereida actually turned her back on Juan each time she saw that he was afraid, or whether Juan was so afraid of his own vulnerability that he would not share that part of himself with her. Probably, both were true. We now had an organizing hypothesis which explained Juan's anxiety. In exploring the pre- and post-illness organization of their relationship, we had discovered a major transformation. Juan and Nereida had had a traditional and successful Latino marriage. Although Juan was typically "macho" and hurt his wife by his many infidelities, he was good to her children and good to her, sexually and financially. Because he was able to care for her in those ways, and because he was successful and ambitious for himself and his family, Nereida was comfortable with her marriage. She probably even enjoyed his rather fiery sexuality. The diagnosis of HIV infection had shifted the balance, stripping Juan of his macho strength and making him feel overwhelmed with guilt and fear. For Nereida, there was something frightening about the needs of this man whom she had loved.

However, the intensity of feeling in both members still seemed to exceed the challenge of their shift in roles. The team asked the therapist to generate two problem-focused genograms. We wanted to ask Nereida about the men in her life and in her family and to ask Juan about the patterns of illness and loss in his family. We needed to understand why this particular kind of macho man was so important to Nereida and why illness was so terrifying to Juan.

The therapist asked Nereida if the men in her life had been as macho as Juan. She spoke admiringly of her father and added that she'd wanted a husband who was like him, although she did not wish to be as "submissive" as her mother was. She married her first husband when she was young. He was weak, not like her father, and his weakness led to abuse. Nereida believed that if a man were outgoing, forceful, confident in his masculinity, and satisfied sexually – both by his wife and by other women if he so chose – he could be good to her in fundamental ways, just as her father had been good to her mother.

Juan's illness and vulnerability shattered Nereida's belief. Her first marriage had taught her that a weak man is abusive. She became afraid, perhaps not only of the weakness she saw in her husband, but of his underlying destructiveness embodied by the HIV infection he bore. While the couple still enjoyed safer sex, we assumed that Nereida secretly harbored fears of infection, which she would not voice to her husband. At the moment, she was behaving as the good Hispanic wife who has sex with her husband when he wants it, voicing none of her misgivings.

We surmised that while Juan's response to illness could be seen as appropriate to the gravity of HIV infection, it was out of character with this man who had "rolled with all the punches," who was strong enough to take on anything. Our question to Juan concerned the role of illness in his family.

Juan was one of four boys. Two had already died: One had had cancer and the youngest brother had committed suicide at the age of 17. As he mentioned the deaths of his brothers, Juan started to weep.

"We were a big family. My father has passed away, too. How could Tony [his remaining brother] live if I were to die? When I told Tony I had HIV infection, he threatened to commit suicide. I kept saying to him, 'Tony, you have a child to live for. How could you die?' I was scared that if I killed myself, Tony would be alone. I've always looked out for Tony."

We asked Juan why he had decided to tell Tony, knowing how vulnerable he was, and Nereida answered, "It was *I* who told him. I thought it was time he helped Juan. Juan is always taking care of him. I thought it was time Tony grew up." Clearly, these major tragedies in Juan's family had become connected to his experience of disease. For Juan, the impact of multiple tragedies had resulted in the formation of a strong, protective bond with his younger brother. We did not know much about Nereida' history, but we did know that strength—both her own and Juan's—was deeply important to her. Her brave front was her first line of defense against her fears that the tragedies which ravaged Juan family could just as easily ravage hers.

At the end of the session we had enough knowledge of central themes to formulate a treatment plan. Certainly, Tony would be asked to join the sessions, and we would work with Nereida's feelings at a number of levels. For now, we offered only a quiet observation. Juan had always been the strong member of his family who kept everything together. In revealing his illness to Tony, Nereida was giving Tony a chance to support his brother, to be the strong one for him. Nereida was also wise to know Juan deeply loved and valued his family. Perhaps strength also had another side: the strength to tell people, as Juan had done, that he was human and afraid and to allow them to comfort him.

Carol's hypothesis and the supporting information about past history seemed to greatly relieve the couple. At the end of the session both appeared relaxed as they joked affectionately. Clarification of illness meaning in relation to their complex feelings about the change in their relationship seemed to set the stage for a reorganization that would permit new relationship patterns to evolve.

PART II

The Illness Journey

CHAPTER 4

The Biopsychosocial Origins
of an Epidemic

B ECAUSE WORK WITH PEOPLE who are HIV-infected constantly refers back to the social context in which it exists, the history of its spread is important. The acronym *AIDS* stands for "Acquired Immune Deficiency Syndrome," a term developed by the Centers for Disease Control (CDC) to denote the epidemic first observed in the United States among gay men and IV drug users in the early 1980s. The term AIDS was used when the cause of the syndrome, the HIV retrovirus, was still unknown. While the first cases were reported to the CDC during May and June of 1981, there is evidence that HIV may have been present in the United States as far back as 1959. The rapid spread of HIV infection from a few cases buried in the population to an epidemic can be attributed to the tragic but elegant fit between the virus, its modes of transmission, and certain populations—specifically, hemophiliacs, gay men, and intravenous drug users. This fit created an ecological niche that promoted the spread of the virus (Bateson & Goldsby, 1988).

HEMOPHILIACS

Economic, technological and cultural changes in the last three decades sensitized three key American populations to the rapid spread of a virus transmitted by the sharing of blood or blood products and/or sexual contact. For hemophiliacs during the 1970s, technological advances made it possible to replace cumbersome hospital-based transfusions of plasma with portable infusions of concentrated clotting factor. However, the production of each infusion required as many as a thousand blood donors, thus vastly increasing the likelihood of receiving blood from an infected donor. Although the risk to hemophiliacs was known, both the American Hemophilia Association and the CDC drastically underestimated the threat of receiving contaminated blood, as well as the rate of conversion from infection to actual illness. Hemophiliacs were advised to infuse "as usual" by the doctors they trusted to propitiously direct their medical lives.

THE BETRAYAL OF "GAY PRIDE"

At the same time that technology was inadvertently making blood products an ideal vehicle for the spread of AIDS, various sociocultural changes were increasing the likelihood of its transmission through sexual activity. Among the cultural changes of the 1960s was the loosening of sexual restrictions. In the long-closeted gay community, the open expression of sexuality following the Stonewall riots was a reaction to decades of repression. It was also a statement of determination to claim the right to gay sexual identity. "Gay pride" activists began to define this population as an oppressed minority and to organize the fight against discrimination stemming from a pervasive national homophobia. For gay men who had felt isolated and different, the language of sex became a language of human connection and solidarity. Gay bars and baths served as community meeting-places as well as environments for sexual encounters. Ironically, it was precisely during this period that the AIDS virus began to spread through gay urban populations.

AIDS represented betrayal for the gay man, just as technology had betrayed the hemophiliacs. To claim one's identity as a gay person in the face of culturally instituted homophobia had been a monumental accomplishment. The gay pride movement had proferred a different set of values, including the open celebration of sexuality. But a fatal and disfiguring disease that was spread sexually raised for many the specter of internalized teachings they had tried so courageously to erase. Illness as God's punishment for deviance, a sense of inherent badness or contamination, a rejection of sexuality in favor of cleansing celibacy, and self-loathing were old emotional experiences that had to be faced anew.

IV DRUG USERS

In the 1970s and 1980s the third major risk population, the IV drug community, was rapidly expanding, largely due to two factors: Cocaine became widely available as an alternative to the predominant use of heroin, and poverty, hopelessness and despair increased in the inner cities due to the drastic cutbacks in social programs during the Nixon and Reagan administrations. Furthermore, the government's failure to create an effective strategy of interdiction, coupled with the lack of a cocaine equivalent to methadone to block craving, fostered an unchecked spread of IV cocaine use. Most frightening was the proliferation of "crack houses" and "shooting galleries," where hundreds of customers traded sex for drugs or shared the same needle or syringe (Drucker, 1989a). The popularity of crack merely increased the risk of sexual transmission by stimulating hyper-sexual behavior with multiple partners (Rosecan, Spitz, & Gross, 1987), and crack users often used IV heroin to medicate the "crash" that followed crack euphoria. The extent of the crack epidemic, as well as the frequency with which infected crack users traded sex for drugs, provided a channel for the eventual flow of the HIV infection into the heterosexual, non-drug-using community.

INNER CITIES: GOVERNMENT NEGLECT

In the face of government neglect, the more affluent and organized gay community financed its own often effective prevention programs, reducing the infection rate dramatically in San Francisco and New York. But in the drug-ravaged inner cities, cutbacks of social programs—the closing of community health centers, afterschool programs, and outpatient centers where prevention programs might have taken place—forced workers to stand by as more and more adults became infected and more children became ill or were orphaned. For this third population of non-addicted sexual partners and their children, the failure of government to provide adequate care was less a betrayal than a policy of "business as usual"—a sad fact of life for disenfranchised African-American and Latino populations. "All my friends got AIDS," one woman told me. "But I don't worry about it. It's just another thing you gotta deal with."

In the 1990s, a decade after the identification of the epidemic, there are few prevention programs—despite the fact that AIDS is spreading rapidly in the inner cities to non-addicted sexual partners of drug users and their children. As a result of the lack of effective AIDS information and education programs, the statistics of those infected with HIV, those currently ill, and those who have died from the disease are appalling. By

1994 396,299 cases of AIDS had been reported in the United States (Center For Disease Control, 1995). Approximately two-thirds of these have died. Originally, HIV infection was a disease of gay men and intravenous male drug users; today the number of infected women has grown to 64,357 women, 14 percent of the total number of people infected (CDC, 1993). Men and women of color are disproportionately affected. Forty-five percent of men diagnosed with AIDS are non-white, but 75 percent of women are non-white. The current reservoir of infection is enormous and deadly: Between I and 1.5 million Americans are thought to be currently infected (Needle, Leach, & Graham-Tomasi, 1989). The majority are sexually active and not aware of their infection. Recent studies underscore an additional current of threat: People outside the gay community tend to deny the possibility of risk and any need for active prevention.

The IV-drug-using community is largely heterosexual and will continue to have children at risk for infection. Currently, the women most at risk for AIDS are poor, urban, minority women. The CDC identified 48 percent of those women infected to be IV drug users; 27 percent were infected through sexual contact, and 10 percent through blood transfusion. To date, 52 percent of the women and female children infected with AIDS are African-American. Current statistics may not accurately reflect the gravity of the epidemic because of the long incubation period between infection with HIV, symptomatic AIDS-Related Complex (ARC), or the full onset of AIDS (Lifson, Ancelle-Park, Brunet, & Curran, 1986). In women, the first wave of infection was among IV drug users; the growing number of women infected through sexual contact with HIV-carrying drug users represents the second wave of the inner-city epidemic. The third generation will be comprised of sexual partners of individuals who have been infected through sexual contact themselves.

Given these statistics, the potential medical and social disaster of the AIDS epidemic is enormous. Any psychosocial intervention must focus on prevention as well as counseling those infected in ways of managing their illness. Most prevention programs focus on the individual. Women, for example, are urged to use condoms in the family planning or maternal care clinics they visit, but there is no similar outreach to men or couples. The power of families and kin networks to function as caretakers of the ill and their children as well as conductors of information and counseling to other family members has been largely ignored. Adequate family counseling about HIV infection, the development of prevention strategies with leading family members, and the provision of services to family networks ravaged by the disease would allow families to maintain their integrity in the face of illness and, perhaps, to save the lives of other family members.

The location of AIDS in two non-traditional groups—the gay community and the IV-drug-using community—tempts us to invoke the concept of *otherness* to deal with our terrors about the proximity of this disease. The challenge to family therapists is always to underscore the ill person's *ordinariness rather than otherness*. For example, it is easy to view the drug user in terms of the otherness of his drug-using behavior rather than empathize with what it feels like to die before one's children are even grown or to have harmed the person loved most. Therapists must learn to find ways of focusing on whatever part of a person's life is positive, strong, and effective. Seeing even the most hardened drug user in this way not only creates a bond that is therapeutic for the client, but also forces the therapist to face the intensity of emotions engendered by working with AIDS patients and their families.

We must become familiar with the mores, beliefs, traditions and sexual practices of groups different from our own if we are to work successfully with AIDS patients and their families. Family systems thinking tends to *homogenize* human relationships; despite its claims to objectivity and neutrality, it has implicit beliefs about *normative* family structure. The very principles we apply with most of our clients, however, are challenged by the core issues generated from the AIDS epidemic and seen to be limiting and unsuitable.

CHAPTER 5
Confronting HIV Infection

INITIAL HIV INFECTION takes place most frequently without the person's awareness. For the majority of the infected, there are no discernible symptoms (Mayer, 1989). As a result, it is hard to know that one has been infected at all or to date the probable onset of infection.

The "worried well" are a growing population of people who perceive themselves to be at risk for HIV infection but have not been identified as actually carrying the virus. Since the latency period between infection and development of symptoms is of uncertain length, people search their sexual or drug-using histories for evidence of potential infection. Some know they have engaged in high-risk behaviors; others are young adults who fear they have been exposed to the virus through sexual involvement with high-risk partners. Others worry about brief periods of adolescent experimentation with IV drugs or sexual encounters with partners whose sexual history was unknown to them. A large number of the "worried well" could be said to have developed AIDS anxiety from ignorance of its actual transmission routes and epidemiology. It may alleviate paralyzing anxiety to know that the virus is not as easily transmitted as is popularly believed. For example, the risk of infection in heterosexual couples is less than 1 percent for a single act of intercourse, and for couples with regular sexual contact over extended periods it is less than 50 percent (Bartlett & Finkbeiner 1993). However, such statistics should not be used to encourage denial of risk.

If the "worried well" worry too much about exposure, others who are clearly at risk deny the possibility that they have been infected. Public perception of the disease and the descriptions of AIDS as a "gay lifestyle disease" in early scientific reports have created an indelible association with stigmatized groups. Many infected individuals do not perceive themselves to be at risk because they view AIDS as a disease of immorality, or of an alien sexual group, or of a lower social class, or as affecting only males.

Until 1985, four years into the epidemic, evidence from Africa that AIDS affects men *and* women equally was overlooked (Mayer, 1989). As a result, women have become the invisible group of people with AIDS. The symptoms in women that differ from those in men include reproductive tract infections, and neoplasias associated with the human papilloma virus (HPV). The risk to women has been downplayed by government propaganda, which emphases monogamy, implying that the monogamous woman is safer than the promiscuous woman. Yet, monogamous women living in the drug-infested inner city are actually at far greater risk than women with many sexual partners who are members of low-risk populations. Many women of poverty are also highly vulnerable; AIDS is not a top priority when issues of survival, housing, and violence threaten their everyday lives.

CASE EXAMPLE*

Althea is a passionate, feisty, smart, and politically committed woman. An African-American woman in her early thirties, she has fought her way from a difficult childhood in poverty to the top of her profession. She comes to see me about work issues. She runs a youth center and suffers the stresses of tackling city bureaucracy, fighting for kids who, just when you think they are safe, get into serious trouble—the trouble of racism, urban poverty, underlying anomie and despair. We talk about these children who are at risk for drugs, crime, AIDS.

In the first session with Althea alone, she told me she was worried about her husband, who was having a hard time. Was he using drugs? Her husband had been an IV drug user at one point in his young adult life, but he was now drug-free and involved with a challenging career. I asked her if she was worried about HIV infection. As best she knew, she had been his sole sexual partner for many years. Even though he shot cocaine during the period when HIV infection was possible, she was convinced that neither he nor she was infected. And no, they did not use condoms. I asked whether her husband had shared needles. She became angry, offended by my stereotype of black men. "He's not that kind of

*The author was the therapist.

street person," she answered firmly, closing the discussion. I asked her to bring him in. I was worried.

In the couples session I risked Althea's anger and her protectiveness of her husband by asking Ronald directly if he had ever shared needles. He hesitated and then, almost relieved, almost shyly, admitted that not only had he shared needles but he had used IV drugs and shared a needle fairly recently. Althea was stunned. When I explored why he had not used a condom knowing that he might be infected, he admitted that he had difficulty using one. Both partners were shy about condom use, and they had had several experiences of failure because they were not using them correctly.

Later that day I observed a session with a middle-class Hispanic woman recently divorced from an IV drug user. She had recently suffered from a painful case of shingles in her right eye, which her doctor suspected might indicate underlying HIV infection. She had been tested at her doctor's insistence, but she had not gone back for her test results.

"I am sure I'm not sick. How could I be? I was married to him. I never went around. I'm not that kind of person." Since immorality and con-- tracting AIDS were inextricably associated for her, she used her sense of herself as a moral person to deny her risk for infection.

"AT RISK" FACTORS FOR HIV INFECTION

Clients who have had the following experiences should be considered at risk for HIV infection. Testing should be recommended and, if they are sexually active, they should be counseled to practice safer sex:

- Men and women who have had unprotected sexual contact with multiple male or female partners during the past 15 years. Monogamous men and women who live in areas where high-risk populations are concentrated and who do not know their partners HIV status should also regard themselves as at risk. (Thus, people living in communities characterized by a high rate of IV drug use and needle exchange are likely to come into contact with someone who has used drugs or has been the sexual partner of a drug user. San Francisco, for example, has a high rate of drug use but a much lower rate of drug-use infection than New York City, probably because needle-sharing habits differ.)

- Gay and bisexual men, a result of the high rate of sexual contact during the 1970s, when multiple partners were common.
- Drug users who have shared needles within the last 15 years.
- Women who suspect that their male partners have had same-sex relationships or have been IV drug-users. Women who have had sex with drug-using women or with women who have had sex with bisexual men should also consider themselves at risk. While lesbian women have traditionally thought themselves to be at lowest risk for HIV, there is increasing evidence that a number of lesbian women may have been infected from sexual activity with lesbian partners who have been bisexual or used IV drugs (Stuntzner-Gibson, 1991).
- People with hemophilia or other diseases or disorders of blood coagulation, who have received large quantities of blood or blood products by transfusion before 1985, when the blood supply was first tested for HIV.
- People who have received blood transfusions, blood products, donor sperm for artificial insemination, and other donor tissues or organs from persons who were at risk for HIV infection.
- Children of women who are/were at risk for HIV during pregnancy or breast-feeding. (While there have been reported cases of HIV infection transmitted to the baby through breast-feeding from a mother who was infected after birth from a transfusion, the great majority of these children were born to IV drug users or their infected partners.) It was commonly thought that if a child was truly HIV-infected (as opposed to passively carrying the mother's antibodies), he or she would become ill before the age of two. Recently children as old as 11 are showing their first symptoms, although it is clear that they, too, were infected perinatally.
- Children who have been sexually molested by parents, family members, and strangers at risk for HIV infection and/or who have been abused by needles. Since some studies (Kaufman & Kaufmann, 1979b) have reported that up to 90 percent of all female heroin users have been sexually molested in childhood, and that the majority of these women come from families in which there was substance abuse, it is clear that incest and sexual molestation of children is a potentially significant transmission route. Furthermore, children as young as eight and nine years old

may be initiated into drug use and therefore become at risk for infection from drug use or from prostituting themselves to support drug use habits.

- To date only a small number of health-care workers are known to have been infected in the course of their work. However over time, as the number of infected people grows, the risk to front line workers such as those manning emergency rooms, trauma and paramedic units, and operating rooms, will increase in highly impacted areas. Unless other workers, who come in contact with blood products in the course of their work—including school personnel, police and sanitation workers—routinely take precautions those infection routes may increase.

CLINICAL ISSUES IN TREATING THE WORRIED WELL

Dilemmas of Disclosure: Heterosexual Affairs

As clinicians, a large number of our clients will fall into the category of the "worried well"—people who are at risk for the disease, or who have irrational fears about their risk status due to ignorance about transmission routes, guilt about past sexual activities, or because they tend to catastrophize potential risk factors. Often, dealing with the possible need for disclosure *if* test results are positive becomes a focal point of the therapeutic work. A married woman who has had an affair may feel that AIDS is her punishment for sexual betrayal, even though her partner did not seem to be in a high-risk category. Her immediate turmoil revolves around whether or not to disclose the possibility of her infection of her husband.

CASE EXAMPLE

John Patten tells me of his work with Viola, aged 28 and married for seven years, who came to therapy because she was worried she had become infected during a brief, hidden, extramarital affair many years ago. Viola had no symptoms, her partner had not been a member of a high-risk group, but her guilt about the affair haunted her—particularly now that she and her husband were deciding to start a family. Viola feels that her silence violates the deep contract she shares with her husband. At the same time, she fears that the knowledge of her infidelity would deeply hurt him and perhaps jeopardize their marriage. Viola has been tested, but she does not know the results. If she waits until she knows that she is negative, she may never have the courage to disclose her secret. If she is told that she is positive, she will not have chosen to tell her husband but be forced into it.

"One of the reasons I want to talk to him before I have the test results is because, if it were the other way around, I would feel very left out if I knew that he had been tremendously worried about something and had talked to other people but not to me. I mean, obviously there's a difference because of the relationship. I'm just so frightened that it's going to be positive. I think I would like to tell him that I had an affair a number of years ago."

Brief therapy supported Viola's decision to tell her husband of her affair before she received the test results. Her admission led to an opening up of buried marital conflicts, which were later addressed in couples therapy. Not surprisingly, Viola tested negative.

Dilemmas of Disclosure: Bisexual Affairs

Bisexuality is more widespread than most of us choose to recognize. Since the prohibitions against same-sex relationships are so powerful, a man who defines himself as heterosexual but finds himself compelled to have same-sex relationships is bewildered by his own feelings and driven to secrecy. When AIDS enters the picture, revelation becomes even more terrifying. Furthermore, in Latin American and Mediterranean cultures, where patterns of gender division are accentuated, men who have sex with other men do not identify themselves as bisexual unless they allow receptive sex. If they are the insertive partner, they see themselves as heterosexual and ignore messages aimed at homosexuals. If they are the receptive partner, they are considered to be a woman in man's body – a condition which is shameful and must be hidden in a macho culture (Carrier, 1976).

Clinicians must explore their own feelings toward bisexuality to be able to understand and to sensitively address the client's fears of revelation before the decision to be tested is made. If a client tests positive, the clinician must find a way of helping him to disclose his bisexuality and his infection to his heterosexual partner, as well as to anticipate that for the bisexual man suicide may feel preferable to exposure. If he tests negative, he may need help to protect himself from further exposure to the virus.

A bisexual man who fears that he is sero-positive has to face the implications of his sexual attractions and deal with the issue of revealing his homosexual experiences to his wife. Overwhelming anxiety can result in psychosomatic symptoms which mimic AIDS/ARC symptoms, leading the person to conclude that he is infected without even being tested. These symptoms range from unexplained weight loss to night sweats, fatigue, and lethargy (Millar, 1986). In the following case, a bisexual man had so many symptoms that his physician suggested testing to confirm an almost certain infection.

CASE EXAMPLE

Andrew speaks haltingly of his devastation as repeated inexplicable symptoms lead him and his physician to believe that he will test positive for the HIV. Andrew is married and is socially and financially successful. He represents the world of finance and law, the quietly respectable old-fashioned kind – working hard, summering in Maine or the north shore of Boston – not the fast-moving world of leveraged deals and arbitrage.

Andrew feels that he has just begun to realize his carefully constructed plans for his life. While he was bewildered by his compulsion to periodically seek out sexual encounters with men, he kept this part of his life in a comfortably secret compartment, almost forgetting it in the flow of his marriage, fatherhood, social life and work. As the press swelled with graphically detailed symptoms of people who had become infected, Andrew found himself observing every cough and fever – and *wondering*.

Therapist: How long have you been having bisexual affairs?

Andrew: It happened maybe a half dozen times. How do I go back and tell my wife that her whole life is over? Everything she's worked for, especially in the last seven years, is over! That in three months, she will likely deliver a child that will die, and that she herself, in a couple years, will die? And that her loving spouse is dying? And that, potentially, her son has been infected?

Therapist: How old is your son?

Andrew: He's going to be four in August.

Therapist: What's his name?

Andrew: Alexander. [*He sobs.*] Yesterday we were in the park all day. What's the incentive to take care of me for what I have done? I cheated on her and then turned around and infected her. I don't see what her incentive is but to leave me.

Therapist: But she has a right to make that choice, too.

Andrew: Oh, I'm not saying it's not her choice. No. I'm not suggesting that . . .

Therapist: You're not suggesting that you would make that choice for her?

Andrew: I can't.

Therapist: By leaving her or . . . killing yourself . . . or . . .

Andrew: Well, see, killing myself only comes to mind because then I don't have to draw out an illness that will shave off five years from my mother's life.

Andrew's experience raised difficult issues for the therapist and the consultant, both married women. Andrew's bisexuality and the figure of his wife's pregnancy elicited emotions in the clinicians that mirrored his own. The intensity of feelings that his situation generated was not clear until the next day. Since the therapist, Ruth Mohr, took Andrew's suicidal preoccupation seriously, the day after this session she accompanied him to his appointment to receive his test results. His surprising negative diagnosis was an enormous relief to Andrew and to Ruth; however, as she returned to the office she found herself overwhelmed by feelings of irrational anger toward Andrew. It was as though, in order to do her work and to master her fear for Andrew, his wife, and her unborn child, she had buried her anger at Andrew for the behaviors which had placed them all in jeopardy. As Ruth told me of her experience, I realized that I shared much of her emotion. While I believed that I accepted Andrew's bisexuality as a part of normal sexual desire, the images – the wife full with a soon-to-be-born child, the son who might have died – brought forth archaic fears of bisexuality as a violation of a morally ordered world. Anger and fear were our responses. The emotions were fleeting but instructive.

COUNTERTRANSFERENCE ISSUES

Because we share our clients' fears for their own mortality as well as for the vulnerabilities of their family members, the specter of AIDS frightens us in a way that most other diseases do not. In reviewing a tape of a consultation that a colleague had sought from another therapist, I realized just how difficult countertransference may make it for a clinician to raise (and face) the issues of a client's possible HIV infection. My colleague – an experienced therapist – had worked for several years with an individual patient, seeing her through a slow recovery from a childhood filled with painful loss. She had sought consultation when the therapy seemed bogged down by her patients obsessional ambivalence about marring her fiancé. In mid therapy the young woman fell in love with a worthy young man who was a hemophiliac and who was subsequently discovered to be HIV-positive. As therapy continued, the therapist and client had many sessions about the client's attachment to the young man, her ambivalence about marrying him, her family's and friends' attitudes toward marrying someone who could become ill. Oddly enough, none of these sessions focused on the issue of the woman's possible infection and her fears for her own safety. It was as if the stark reality of AIDS had been subsumed by more therapeutically manageable issues: the obsessive nature of the woman's thinking and her chronic ambivalence. Clearly, neither therapist nor patient was prepared to deal with the presence of this terrifyingly unwelcome "guest," who perhaps threatened the young woman's very life and certainly dramatically changed her future plans, which therapist and client had constructed in collaboration. So powerful are the fears elicited by AIDS, so complex are the moral issues raised by its presence, that the consultant focused on the safe area of the client's obsessional thinking, thus carefully avoiding recognizing the unwelcome guest, AIDS, who surely stood at the heart of the therapeutic impasse.

Because of the overwhelming nature of HIV infection and its impact on a person's life, the clinician may share the client's denial that infection could present. What does one say to a young woman with whom one has worked and come to care for, when she finds that she cannot have the children she longed for and may even face a shortened life? To a mother for whom a test result may mean that her children will be orphaned? To an ex-drug user who has pulled himself out of the ghetto and is beginning family and professional life at the same time he begins to feel bouts of tiredness and intermittent fevers? Or to a young gay man whom one has supported during the painful process of "coming out" and who now looks drawn and thin?

Family therapists have learned to be efficient problem-solvers, to have an illusion that strategic intervention can substantially improve life for their clients. Events including illness have meaning and can be shaped and controlled. The overwhelming nature of AIDS, its arbitrariness, forces us to face our own helplessness in the face of human situations that appear to have no answers and no apparent meanings.

The helplessness of AIDS is an unpleasant feeling for the helper—one which may make us eager to avoid the subject altogether. But in these times AIDS must become a part of the thinking of everyday practice. The clinician must be able to raise issues of possible HIV infection with clients as a normal part of therapy, rather than hoping a client is not at risk. In order to do so, the clinician must become aware of the complex feelings that AIDS arouses in all of us: our own vulnerability and the vulnerability of people we love, our fears for a client to whom we have become attached, our anxiety about introducing issues that provoke feelings of anxiety and powerlessness. Joan Gilbert, a therapist on the Ackerman AIDS project, has spoken of the calm place she finds in herself when she is open to experiencing the most troubling feelings that a client's pain elicits. She feels that her willingness to travel those dark currents with the client brings them both to a peaceful and calming shore. If she defends herself against her own feelings, the session remains anxious and unresolved (Gilbert, 1990).

Discussion of AIDS-related issues demands that the clinician feel comfortable discussing issues of sexuality: gay sexual practices, demonstrating correct condom use, issues with people for whom sex is a taboo area of discussion. The therapist may end up providing life-saving information the client has been afraid to seek from other professionals. As with the middle-class couple described above who were uncomfortable with condom use, a therapy session may be the one place where people can discuss these delicate issues frankly and informatively.

CHAPTER 6

Testing: Political, Medical, and Psychological Repercussions

A GAY COUPLE, ONE OF whom was diagnosed as HIV-positive, questioned whether the other partner should be tested. Their questions and concerns poignantly illustrate the many difficult issues surrounding the dilemma of testing.

"Isn't it better to maintain hope that at least one of us will survive?" They wonder whether not knowing the HIV status of one partner has affected their ability to regain the sexuality that had been a very important part of their long and faithful relationship. Their presenting problem: "We don't have sex anymore." Yet neither felt much anxiety about the lack of sex.

"If we were both sero-positive, would we have sex?" one ventured. The untested partner answered, "I don't think I am positive. But I don't think I could handle the anxiety if I were."

They describe their relationship as closer, more intimate, and even more physically affectionate than in the past. Sometimes, when they are holding each other, one partner will think about sex—but now there is something forbidden about permitting the expression of their old passion.

Oddly, they had not even noticed the change.

"We seem to make important decisions about our relationship without knowing that we are doing so," one partner noted. As we talked, they described the passage of a very hard year. Several close friends had died the past summer, and their world is one of continual loss and mourning.

Do they fear sexual intimacy as a painful reminder of potential loss and of all their friends who have died? Would testing change that? If the untested partner tested positive, would that not bring more grief and fear to this couple? Their initial question, "Isn't it better to maintain hope that one of us will survive?" hovered over the session.

Later I asked a colleague about his experience with other gay couples. He affirmed the prevalence of decreased sexual intimacy after one partner is diagnosed as HIV-infected. Safer sex is logical, but the deep, inextricable linkage of sex with disease, contamination, and loss cannot be addressed with logic. This couple had spoken of their relationship as being more playful and childlike than it was before the diagnosis, noting that non-genital play is comforting; they feel like small children protecting each other against the storm. We talked of a world in which the young are dying outside, falling like soldiers on the battlefield. The need for male comfort is enormous, but it is often separated from sexual need. The couple reaffirmed that "we don't even notice the absence of sex. It doesn't seem to matter anymore."

THE POLITICS OF TESTING

In the politics of AIDS, the question of conducting mass HIV testing has been a subject of ongoing and heated controversy. In the early days of the epidemic, testing did not lead to the use of effective medications to arrest the illness. Since psychosocial concerns often outweighed any tangible benefits of testing in terms of improved health, many gay activists argued against testing and in favor of changing high-risk behaviors, whether or not one knew one was HIV-infected. While testing was widely available, it was not widely used by people in high-risk groups.

The argument in favor of mass testing was mounted by epidemiologists, who contended that it was necessary to obtain a more accurate picture of the spread of the disease and develop strategies to protect the public from HIV infection. Government officials rode the wave of AIDS hysteria by promoting costly programs for the mandatory testing of low-risk groups: applicants for marriage licenses, immigrants, or unpopular captive audiences such as prisoners or inmates of mental hospitals. Health-care workers argued that they needed medical information, both to better treat patients who were suspected to be HIV-infected and to protect themselves from the risk of infection.

Civil libertarians raised crucial issues as they opposed the call for mass involuntary testing. They argued that mass testing in the absence of anti-discrimination legislation and in the current climate of AIDS anxiety would make people vulnerable to discriminatory practices. They contested the popular belief that mass testing would be the golden road to AIDS prevention with studies showing that knowledge of one's antibody status did not correlate with positive behavioral change. They worried that testing would lead to contact tracing and to calls for quarantine of those who did not cooperate with safer sex or drug-use guidelines.

It was clear to most knowledgeable people that AIDS testing was not the magic bullet that would end the epidemic. In fact, there was much concern that coercive mass testing would drive the epidemic underground, thus actually inhibiting people from learning their antibody status, revealing it to others, and changing their behavior. Only voluntary testing, with competent pre- and post-test counseling and absolute assurances of confidentiality, would encourage individuals to come forward to learn their antibody status and receive the counseling that might help them change.

Civil libertarians and others also argued that scarce funds would be better spent on AIDS education, developing strategies for reaching people at risk for infection and helping them change their behaviors, than on increasing expensive testing programs for people who might not be at risk at all. Furthermore, since the worlds of sexual courtship and drug usage do not encourage truthfulness, encouraging people to rely on another person's statements that he or she has tested negative could have disastrous consequences. Promoting safer sex and cleansing of drug works were considered more effective public-health strategies than testing.

As the epidemic progressed, the belief that new medications could arrest viral spread in the early, nonsymptomatic phase of HIV infection tilted the equation towards greater reliance on testing. For example, for low-risk pregnant women, testing could lead to medicating with AZT which substantially reduces the risk that the baby will be infected (Altman, 1994). Early identification of infection leads to monitoring of immune functioning and appropriate medical intervention if CD4 cells fall substantially, including the use of reverse transcriptase and protease inhibitors (e.g., AZT and ABT-538) and prophylactic medications against some specific opportunistic infections. Because the medical and public health benefits of testing people suspected of being at risk are now so obvious, counselors may overlook a client's psychosocial and civil rights concerns.

THE PERSONAL EXPERIENCE OF
TESTING

To consider being tested is to face a crisis in one's life, the magnitude of which cannot be underestimated. When a client is weighing the question of testing, it is important for the clinician to explore several key areas: why the client has decided to be tested now; whether the client understands the medical meaning of a test result; how positive or negative results would be received emotionally; what the client understands about strategies for protecting himself and others from exposure to the virus; whether having a definitive diagnosis of HIV status would be likely to increase the clients willingness to adopt such strategies; and what impact a test result is likely to have on a client's significant relationships. Studies have shown that support is crucial in managing test results. If a client has a partner or spouse, it is often helpful to include him or her in the process of pre- and post-test counseling. One program, the Women's Center at Montefiore Hospital, which is aimed at providing counseling for drug-using women, places clients in peer support groups comprised of drug users (many of whom are HIV-infected) before the person is tested (Eric et al., 1989). With the media focus on the fatal aspects of AIDS, people are confused about the difference between a positive diagnosis of HIV infection and the actual AIDS illness. Therefore, it can be extremely helpful to women who decide to be tested to see other women who are sero-positive leading productive lives. In addition, those who have been through the testing process are better able to counsel people to be tested than professionals who are not living the complex emotional turmoil triggered by the testing process.

THE SCIENCE OF TESTING

HIV is a retrovirus which infects certain types of white blood cells, most particularly CD4 cells and macrophage-type cells of the immune system, disrupting their functioning. Because HIV possesses a special enzyme, reverse transcriptase, it makes a DNA copy of viral RNA, which is then integrated into the genetic material of the host cell (Hamburg & Fauci, 1989). "Unlike other known pathogens, HIV infects the very cells of the immune system that are intended to direct the immune system's attack against such invaders" (Hamburg & Fauci, 1989, p. 28). HIV may also infect bone marrow precursor cells, as well as monocyte and macrophage cells which circulate through the body and can spread HIV to the brain.

Infectiousness varies over the course of the disease. It is thought that infectiousness may be elevated in the early phase of infection and again when opportunistic infection signifying the onset of full-blown AIDS occurs. At other times infectiousness may remain low (Turner, Miller, & Moses, 1989).

This variation of infectiousness may in part explain why some clients have had years of sexual contact with an infected partner and remained uninfected, while others are infected after one or two contacts.

Until 1985, there was no way to determine whether one had become infected with the then unidentified virus that caused AIDS. When Luc Montagnier of the Pasteur Institute identified the previously undescribed T-lymphotropic virus (LAV) in 1983 (a finding replicated by Robert Gallo of the National Institutes of Health), it was possible to develop a test to determine whether or not the person was actually infected with the virus which was later named HIV (Hamburg & Fauci, 1989). In the spring of 1985 a blood test called ELISA (Enzyme Linked Immune Absorbent Assay) was made available. When HIV enters the body, viral antigens signal the immune system to produce antibodies to combat the virus. ELISA detects these antibodies, though not the presence of the virus itself or infection with other, rarer forms of HIV. Various physical conditions (pregnancy, some forms of cancer, lupus, rheumatoid arthritis, hepatitis, and alcohol-related conditions) produce large amounts of antibodies that can cross-react with antigens used in HIV tests, giving a positive result even if the person has not been exposed to HIV (Gross, 1989). For a typical screen of two ELISAs, the actual number of false positives is less than 1 percent in an unselected population, 6 percent in dialysis patients, and 1–10 percent in pregnant women. In low-risk populations (blood donors, for example), the percentage of false positives is somewhat higher. Taking into account the devastating consequences of a false positive, the counselor should make sure that the client who has tested positive on two ELISAs is given a confirmatory Western Blot, a more sensitive (and more expensive) test. It should be noted that in rare cases even the Western Blot may not identify a false positive (Gross, 1989). Some laboratories confirm a positive ELISA with tests such as IFA (immunofluorescence assay) or RIPA (radio immunoprecipative assay).

A positive result on all three tests—two ELISAs and a Western Blot—is considered to be a true positive. A negative on the ELISA is not usually followed by a confirmatory test; it is considered to be a true negative, which means either that the person is not infected or that the

person may be infected but has not begun to produce antibodies to combat the virus. HIV tests that test for antibodies will be negative at the
time of infection although the virus is rapidly reproducing in the body
and lodging undetectable reserves of virus in the bone marrow and macrophage cells. It takes at least 3 to 10 weeks for the body to develop
antibodies to HIV and 6 to 12 weeks for there to be enough present in
the bloodstream for a reliable test result (Bartlett & Finkbeiner, 1993).
For this reason, a client who believes he could have been exposed recently to the virus should be encouraged to retake the test one or more
times at three- to six-month intervals. There have been rare cases in
which no antibody was discernible for as long as three years (Gross,
1989). Many people who test negative once dangerouly presuppose that
they are free from the virus—whereas, in fact, the virus may have entered their system but not yet have produced detectable antibodies. Safer
sex clubs, where people present negative test results to their partners, are
a dangerous outcome of this wishful thinking.

If a person tests positive, it merely informs him that he has been
exposed to the virus. Neither test indicates that the person currently has
AIDS or will necessarily contract the disease. Since transmission patterns are not well understood, there is no way to predict the infectiousness of the person who tests positive or the susceptibility of his or her
partner to infection. We have seen a case in which a young woman was
infected as a result of two instances of unprotected intercourse with a
high-risk by asymptomatic partner, and other cases in which women
engaged in unprotected sex with infected partners for as long as seven
years, yet tested negative. It is clear, though, that anyone who tests
positive should assume that he or she *can* infect others.

MEDICAL ADVANTAGES OF TESTING

Adult Patients

While therapists need to review with the client the decision to be tested
from a psychological and behavioral perspective, recent advances in
medication make it advisable to know one's HIV status and immune
system functioning. Monitoring of immune functioning indicates when a
patient should consider medications designed to inhibit the replication
of HIV (AZT, ddI, ddC or the newer protease inhibiting drugs) and
when the patient needs prophylaxis against opportunistic infections.

Once the client knows his immune status is compromised, he is faced
with decisions about how to proceed for treatment, forcing him into an

unfamiliar world of medical uncertainty. For example, the usefulness over any length of time of commonly used drugs such as AZT, ddC, and ddL is uncertain and even politically controversial since these drugs have potentially serious side-effects and have not yet been proven to prolong life (Federal study, 1991). While standard practice encourages asymptomatic HIV-infected individuals with a T-cell count below 500 to use low dosage AZT to inhibit viral replication and opportunistic infections, the recent discovery of the potential for the HIV virus to rapidly develop strains resistant to these drugs has encouraged the use of drug combinations, which the virus has less chance of escaping.

Controversy remains about at what stage in the immune system's battle with HIV such drugs should be administered. Some researchers have argued that long-term use of these drugs impairs the person's potential for fighting the disease with holistic interventions. A client's skepticism should be welcomed as a valuable component of the decision-making process, and he should be advised about how to obtain information about new protocols that are being developed almost monthly, which may provide less toxic alternatives to those medications used currently. Empowering the client to learn about the disease and to make informed decisions compatible with his beliefs provides a counterbalance to the helplessness that dependance on medical systems engenders.

Newborns

Since perinatal administration of AZT has been shown to reduce the chances of an HIV-infected mother giving birth to an infected child from approximately 25 percent to 8 percent, pregnant women who are thought to be at risk are encouraged to seek testing (Altman, 1994). For approximately the first 15 months in the life of a baby born to an infected mother, the baby will carry maternal antibodies to HIV, but as the baby's own immune system develops, between the ages of 18 months and 2 years, maternal antibodies disappear. From age 15 months onward, HIV testing is repeated every 3 months until a definitive positive diagnosis is made or until the baby has two negative tests (Mallory & Allan, 1993).

However, a small percentage of babies may fail to mount an antibody response to HIV if they have been infected since birth, so a number of negatives may ultimately prove to be false and the baby may show symptoms later (Gross, 1989). A more accurate but expensive test is a genetic screening for viral DNA (Polymerase Chain Reaction, PCR) which can be given at two months. Fifty percent of babies who test positive will show symptoms by the age of three, but others will remain healthy. In fact, an increasing number of school-age children are only now becoming symptomatic.

The medical advantages of knowing if a baby is HIV-positive are clear. Since many babies will become seriously ill and die before they are two, constant vigilance for the onset of symptoms is essential. A mother who has been helped to understand the effects of HIV infection may be able to respond more sensitively to her baby's needs. Children with HIV infection often need immune boosters to prevent life-threatening exposure to chicken pox and require different vaccines than children whose immune systems are normal.

Medical prophylaxis against advancement of the disease in pediatric cases is still in its early stages. Intravenous gamma globulin treatment as a way of boosting immune system effectiveness in battling the virus is standard for children and is administered at designated clinics. The administration of low dosage AZT used to be standard treatment for children with HIV (one argument for testing was that knowing a child's HIV status allowed early intervention with antivirals). Many parents, however, worried about the drug's long-term effects and efficacy and resisted the administration of AZT to healthy HIV infected children. Recent studies (Altman, 1995c) confirmed parents' worries, demonstrating that children on AZT alone were in fact showing more rapid rates of disease progression, the appearance of AIDS-related infections, side effects such as abnormal bleeding and neurological impairment, and death. It is still unknown whether protocols such as AZT given in combination with ddI, or ddI alone, show any more effective outcome.

TESTING FROM A PSYCHOLOGICAL PERSPECTIVE

When a client is considering testing, we jointly explore the client's possible reactions to a sero-positive and a sero-negative test result and assess what benefit he expects from the process. If the client appears to be overwhelmingly frightened and unable to handle the possibility of a positive result, it may be clinically advisable to postpone testing, perhaps indefinitely. The clinician is then faced with finding other strategies for obtaining proper health care to monitor the client's immune system functioning. For example, in the Montefiore Methadone Program, one client was so frightened of his test result that, although he consented to testing, under no conditions did he want to know whether he had been tested or what his results were. However, he was willing to have an immune system work-up, to learn that he was immuno-compromised, and to go on low-dosage AZT without ever actually being told his test result.

Clients often avoid testing because they believe that denial offers the best insurance of their continued functioning. In addition, they may wish to avoid the complex and painful task of informing others of a positive result. The clinician needs to work out strategies that initially protect the denial process, while working with the client to define underlying issues that psychologically "overcharge" the issues of *knowing* and of *revealing*. Maintaining the slow, careful pace of investigating a client's psychological issues when social repercussions of carrying and spreading HIV virus are so vivid can be difficult for the clinician.

Understanding the meaning of disclosing a positive HIV status, both in the family's perception of the client and the clients perception of himself, often illuminates the difficulties and points to strategies for intervention. The client's prevailing story about himself may be that he is a person who cannot handle stress, or he may believe that his wife will not be able to handle the result and that she will leave him or become desperate herself. Introducing alternative narratives about the client and his family that emphasize positive outcomes and coping abilities demonstrated in managing past stressful situations, together with hypnotherapeutic suggestions for stress reduction, can be helpful here. It should be noted that many clients learn of their HIV status and handle this information responsibly. Perhaps more frequently than in other diseases, many people have used a sero-positive diagnosis as a catalyst for redefining their goals and making positive life changes.

Testing and Drug Use

Drug users will often resist HIV testing because denial is so much a part of their *modus operandi*. Drug users are frequently fatalistic; upon discovering that they have a fatal disease, many simply go about "business as usual" or medicate their anxiety with increased drug use and sexual acting-out. In the street culture, distinctions between being HIV-infected, having AIDS, and being in imminent danger of death are seldom made. The drug user needs repeated clarifications about the meaning of the test. Once the medical meaning of the test result is made clear, identifying the drug user's prevailing narrative about himself can be useful in altering self-destructive behavioral patterns.

As mentioned previously, one strategy that has been found helpful in the Montefiore Methadone Maintenance Women's Center has been to involve clients at high risk for HIV infection in support groups prior to testing (Eric et al., 1989). These groups de-emphasize drug use while supporting women's coping skills and their aspirations for themselves and their children. Because the groups are nonjudgmental, view addiction as a disease rather than as a character flaw, and take women's concerns seriously, attendance is surprisingly high. Many of the women have used HIV infection as a catalyst to get off drugs, to seek proper health care, education, or job training, and/or to focus on the care of their children.

Pediatric and Maternal Testing

Recent advances in the use of medication to reduce the infection rate of babies born to HIV-infected mothers offer compelling reasons for women at risk for HIV who are pregnant or contemplating pregnancy to be tested.

A woman who is HIV-positive and lives in an urban ghetto, where the infant mortality rate was high prior to the AIDS epidemic, may find the odds that she will bear an infected baby acceptable. For many of these women, identity and meaning are predicated on childbearing, and life without children seems inconceivable. As a result, most studies show that knowledge of a sero-positive status has little effect on a woman's decision to become pregnant, carry her pregnancy to term, or abort. There is no difference in the reproductive rate of sero-negative and sero-positive women, even after the sero-positive women have received fairly intense counseling (Pivnick, Jacobsen, Eric, Hsu, & Drucker, 1990).

For drug-using women, pregnancy has often been the only indication that life itself has enough importance to enable them to give up drugs. This is particularly true when drug use has separated women from other children they have borne; the need to create a replacement child to fill these early losses can be a powerful incentive to risk all in childbearing (Pivnick et al., 1990). Even if she understands that though there are fairly good odds that she will bear a healthy child, the odds that she will survive to see her child grow up are extremely low, many drug-using women have learned to rely on extended family to help them with child-rearing. Others are too impulsive to make coherent plans for their children's future. The emphasis in counseling should be on respecting the woman's cultural values while, at the same time helping her plan for her family's future by guiding her to testing, prenatal and HIV care, and necessary social services. Above all, a woman's right to reproductive choice *should be respected.*

A mother who suspects she has HIV but did not elect to be tested before the baby's birth may refuse to have him tested after birth. Quite apart from her guilt that she may have borne an ill child, she may fear that, if the child tests positive, both the child and her family will suffer the painful social consequences already discussed (ostracism by other adults in the community, loss of housing, ostracism of her other children at school). If the mother is a substance abuser, she knows that if she is incapacitated by drugs, illness, or death, it is likely that her child would be raised by other family members. However, if the baby were revealed to be HIV-positive, temporary placement with other family members might be threatened. And she may also understand that if her child tests positive, her confidentiality cannot be guaranteed. There are too many ways in which the secret could be revealed. For example, one mother had kept secret from all outsiders her sero-positivity, in addition to the fact that her husband had died of AIDS, not cancer, and that it was suspected that her newborn had died of AIDS. She told no one in her family except her mother, who had visited her in the hospital when she had to undergo minor surgery and had seen the precaution sign on her daughter's door. Some time after her husband's death, this woman realized that a member of her church congregation was a nurse who worked in the same hospital where her husband had died, and she began to live in terror that the nurse would reveal her husband's disease to church members. There was a very real danger, she thought, that she and her children would be shunned by her church, which was the strongest community support group for her family; the church had provided recreation programs for the children, as well as friendship and support for her as a widow of a man everyone thought had died of cancer. Perhaps her belief that people did not already know was an illusion, but for her—a woman who took great pride in the family's middle-class respectability and economic stability—the terror of revelation and public humiliation was of the deepest importance.

REACTIONS TO TEST RESULTS

It is important for clinicians to understand that reactions to a test result will vary from person to person and over time. For most people, receiving a test result is an overwhelming experience, and in the jumble of emotions following the announcement of the test result little information is absorbed. For this reason it is extremely important that testing programs have careful pre-test as well as post-test counseling.

Reactions to a Sero-negative Test Result

Those whose results are sero-negative and who do not seek subsequent counseling can be given risk prevention strategies and helped to antici-pate reactions ranging from euphoria and omnipotence to sorrow or guilt. Any of these reactions can lead to risk-producing behaviors. While a negative test result invariably relieves anxiety, it can also pro-vide a false sense of security—a sense of omnipotence that, despite dan-gerous sex, "I have not become infected" (Fox, Odaka, & Polk, 1986). Some studies have shown that an individual's lack of anxiety diminishes self-protective behavior. Gross (1989) reported that people who find re-lief in testing negative are less able to maintain risk-reduction behavior over time. They then resort to repeated testing as a way of monitoring whether they had become infected in the interim. It is clear that a client's reactions to a negative test result should be explored and followed by consistent, risk-reduction counseling.

Negative test results may be accompanied by feelings of "survivor guilt," which can also lead to conscious or unconscious strategies for becoming infected. One client described feelings of overwhelming grief as he realized that he would survive the people he loved who were dying. Another decided that he wanted to die with his HIV-infected partner. Another found himself struggling with heterosexual impulses, wondering if he were merely reacting to the epidemic or if heterosex-uality was a legitimate choice for him.

Reactions to Sero-positive Test Results

While studies are contradictory in predicting whether knowing one's an-tibody status will cause beneficial changes in behavior, it seems clear that knowing one is HIV-positive will have adverse effects on psycho-logical functioning. A recent cohort study of 270 homosexual men from Boston found depression present in 94 percent of the sero-positive sub-jects who were aware of their antibody status at six months after noti-fication of their rest results (McCluster, Stoddard, Mayer, Zapka, Mor-rison, & Saltzman, 1988). Beeson, Zones, and Nye's (1986) survey of a San Francisco cohort of sero-positive men and women showed that psy-chological reactions to a positive test result can be psychologically devastating, as did a study of gay and bisexual men (Lyter, Valdessari, Kingsley, Amoroso, & Rimaldo, 1987). Positive diagnosis may result in increased psychiatric symptoms, such as anxiety, panic attacks, difficulty in concentrating, depression, and inhibition of sexual desire, as well as psychosomatic symptoms mimicking ARC, such as headaches, fevers, coughs, and diarrhea.

As the meaning of the test results become clear, the individual may try out various strategies for handling the information. Bargaining with God by determining to abstain from sex is one strategy. However, if the person has previously had an active sex life, attempts at sexual abstinence are unlikely to work and may be followed by sexual bingeing behavior. Or a positive result may actually precipitate sexual acting-out. The self-hatred that follows can turn into reckless anger at others or reignite a compulsive need to return to addictive behaviors that in the past have served to allay anxiety.

Depression and isolation are other strategies. Believing that they will die shortly, some become paralyzed by their anxiety. Others seek help in dealing with the strong emotions generated by a sero-positive diagnosis and develop methods of coping with the exigencies of infection by joining sero-positive support groups.

On the other hand, a positive result, as noted previously, may act as a catalyst for positive changes on many different levels. Many gay men who have tested sero-positive have helped each other treat the diagnosis as a challenge. In their affirmative view, HIV infection can change sexual relationships for the better, increasing intimacy and forcing people to be more open, honest, and caring about their partners. Clients have said that knowledge of possible illness and death has focused their lives and given them greater meaning.

Few people make a satisfactory psychological adjustment without long-term counseling and a wide, supportive network of friends (Beeson et al., 1986). Individual counseling, couples counseling, multifamily and peer support groups are all valuable modalities to provide support as the person deals with his roller coaster of emotions. Counseling also helps him address the behavioral tasks that follow from knowing that he is sero-positive. He may need to role play disclosure to sexual partners, practice with his partner safer-sex techniques that are erotic and pleasurable (Palacios-Jimenez & Shernoff, 1986), make connections with health-care systems that can manage the course of his infection, and decide whether to inform other family members.

CASE EXAMPLE*

It is two years since Simon's lover Martin died. Now Simon is edging toward a new relationship, placing his life with Martin behind him. He wonders whether he should be tested. The following exchange starkly illustrates the enormous pressure felt by a person who is sero-positive, thoughtful, and responsible whenever a new relationship is contemplated.

Simon: I think testing would be very disastrous for me emotionally. On the other hand, my new lover, David, said to me, "Simon, do you think you're positive?" I said, "Yes, I do." He said, "Well, what have you really got to lose? What are your chances of being negative?" I said, "Maybe 20 or 30 percent." I think it would just add a whole new dimension to everything. After all, I may die. I mean, I really may die.

Therapist: When you say *disaster*, what does it mean to you?

Simon: Right now I've been having very safe sex. The question is, every time I meet a man who wants to be intimate with me, then it becomes a moral thing. Am I morally bound to say, "By the way, I took the test and I'm positive. Let's be very safe." I mean, what should I do? On the other hand, maybe I shouldn't have to say that and just be safe.

Therapist: Would you expect a potential sexual partner to tell you whether or not he had taken the test and what the results were?

Simon: If I brought him home and he had taken the test, honestly, I would not expect him to say anything. Being in a high-risk group, Joan, we all have to act and assume that everyone is positive. That is the only way to combat this disease.

Therapist: So, when you are with a sexual partner, you assume that he is positive?

Simon: To protect myself, yes. It limits what I do sexually.

Therapist: That's a very kind of subtle thing—what is spoken and what is not spoken. If you assume that your partner is positive and you use safe sex, what would be the difference if he were to tell you he's positive? Would that change things?

Simon: [*Long pause*] Yeah. Number one, I would say, it would tell me positive things about the person—he is very up-front and honest,

*Joan Gilbert was the therapist.

and I would appreciate that. But, on the other hand, I probably would not want to do anything with him – even safe things. I would probably just take a deep breath and lose everything, lose any passion that I was feeling.

The decision of a non-infected partner to be tested or not is complicated by many familial and relationship issues. While medical prudence makes knowing one's HIV status advisable, people are only too willing to put off the frightening moment when they have to face the probability that they are infected. The following case illustrates the complexity of the issues and some strategies for intervention.

CASE EXAMPLE

The subject of my session with Serena and Abe was Serena's decision not to be tested. Serena and Abe are an odd couple: He is melancholic, a scholar, and a dreamer; she is pert, attractive, but simple and uneducated. They married in early middle age after many years of loneliness as single people. Both came from families in which there was tragic loss and violence between family members. Abe's mother was killed in a violent physical fight with her second husband. Abe grieved that, after a boyhood of deep pain struggling to protect his mother from his violent father, he could not protect his mother from his stepfather. Serena's family was quite mad. She was the good girl who didn't marry because her job was to take care of everyone. No one had ever cared for her as much as Abe, and she was grateful for his love and protectiveness.

Shortly after they married Abe contracted a life-threatening chronic illness, which required the use of blood products. In remission, he was routinely tested for HIV and was found to be positive. When Abe and Serena married Serena knew that Abe had also been bisexual. Since there were no known health consequences at the time for being bisexual, and she was satisfied that they had an excellent sexual relationship, she viewed the bisexuality a passing phase in her husband's life. When Abe tested sero-positive, Serena was upset and frightened; still, she chose to view the use of blood products as the source of infection. Abe had complicated feelings about his bisexuality and tended to think of his infection as God's punishment. He was frightened that he had infected Serena, but she refused to talk about it. She felt well and was content not to be tested.

Because Serena refused to be tested, both partners chose to believe she was negative. This belief, however, adversely affected their sex life, because while Serena wanted to have sex, Abe was literally terrified that he would kill her with his sperm – even if he used a condom. Their lack of sex was a source of great suffering to her, as she believed their precious intimacy was slipping away. She could not be satisfied with sex without intercourse, because for her the incompleteness of the act was a reminder of her husband's illness. Gradually, they came to avoid the physical expression of love that had been central to their relationship. Although this couple appeared to function well, given Abe's illness, each felt secretly lonely and sad. No intervention succeeded in dislodging their sexual arrangement, and for a while the couple coped with their decision not to learn Serena's serology status.

Abe's physician then urged Serena to be tested because the medical picture had changed. Still, she resisted. No, her decision not to be tested was not about fear of how she would handle a positive result; she was a fighter, Abe said. She would deal with the test result. She wouldn't become morbidly depressed as he had. Serena volunteered that her greatest fear was that, if she were positive, she would become overwhelmed with anger at her husband. After further questioning she agreed that the anger would be short-lived because, ultimately, her love for him and her knowledge that he would never intentionally harm her would win out.

Thinking further, she almost blurted out: "What I am really afraid is that if I tested positive, I would burden him with guilt. He feels so guilty already. He has had to suffer so much. He is so vulnerable from the illness and the HIV. I might lose him. I love him so much and he loves me. I don't want to lose him." There were tears in her eyes as she took his hand.

Abe acknowledged with his usual gloom that his guilt would be unbearable if he knew he had infected her. Drawing on my knowledge of his mother's death and his wish that he could have protected her, I asked him whether it was better to run the risk of feeling guilty in the short run, but to have taken steps to protect Serena. She was facing the sudden possible occurrence of an opportunistic infection. Did he want to gamble on this unwanted possibility by allowing her to protect him from guilt while potentially jeopardizing her health? Abe thought for a moment, turned red, and then said that because he felt protective of his wife, he would manage any emotions she directed towards him; his own feelings of guilt were not important in the larger picture of protecting her health.

They then discussed where she would be tested. The couple had entered into a pact of love that put Serena at risk, and from which only Abe could absolve her. As they left, I knew the decision was medically wise but I wondered if they could manage the emotional turmoil in the event of a positive test. The fragile skin that protected Abe's survival and hers was already drawn so thin.

Abe and Serena were able to plan for Serena's test together. In the following case, we see how one partner's impulsive decision to be tested triggers unforeseen effects on the relationship.

CASE EXAMPLE*

Daniel works as an AIDS counselor in a New York City hospital. He is active in gay- and AIDS-related causes. As part of his work, he counsels people about testing. Quite suddenly, without telling his partner, Adam, he decided to be tested.

"I felt I had to know what people went through when they were tested. I wasn't worried at first, until I got the result that I was positive. Then everything changed."

Adam was furious when he found out that Daniel had been tested. He was not angry that Daniel was positive—he suspected that they both might be positive. He felt betrayed because Daniel had not told him about his decision, and because Daniel's reaction to the test drastically changed their relationship.

Adam was a passionate, happy-go-lucky person. He had grown up as a caretaking child to a divorced mother whom he saw as depressed and distant. Freed from the oppressive atmosphere of his childhood, he wanted to enjoy life. Daniel had grown up in a family where there was alcoholism and violence and also felt liberated in Adam's presence.

During late adolescence, Daniel had considered a religious vocation, but as he came to accept his sexual orientation, he decided to direct his idealism through working with people who had AIDS. Both Daniel and Adam said that their relationship gave them great pleasure and that they were very much in love. However, at some level Daniel must have been haunted by a sense that, in abandoning the tenets of his religious background, he had committed some sin for which he would have to pay.

After receiving his positive test result, Daniel became profoundly depressed. Adam felt that he was back home again, caring for a depressed, uncommunicative mother. Despite their knowledge that Adam would probably test positive, Daniel's test results had spun the couple

*The author was the therapist.

into different time zones. Adam refused to be tested. He had had enough of childhood's depression and wanted to continue to dream that he was just beginning a long and joyful life. But for Daniel, the play and exploration of young adulthood's summer were over; he felt he had to retrieve what time he had left. He needed to put his house in order for the coming winter of illness and death. He began to think seriously about resuming his religious vocation and dedicating himself to the service of others. While it was agonizing for Daniel to think of leaving Adam, the test result reactivated all his previous doubts about living a secular, gay life.

Daniel's decision to be tested left the future of his relationship with Adam in doubt. This consequence, though painful, might ultimately be in the best interest of each partner.

CHAPTER 7

On Becoming HIV
Sero-positive

THIS CHAPTER ADDRESSES several crucial issues that confront the patient and family once a sero-positive status is confirmed. These include basic medical issues, diagnosis, transmission, response to medical treatment, the process of disclosure, and repercussions in ongoing relationships.

BASIC MEDICAL ISSUES

Upon receiving a diagnosis of HIV infection, the person enters a world of constant uncertainty as to the meaning of physical symptoms. Normal symptoms of everyday life, such as fever and fatigue, are now scrutinized as possible harbingers of more serious HIV disease. As noted, people often equate a diagnosis of HIV infection—which may remain asymptomatic for ten years and more—with an AIDS diagnosis. Though they are asymptomatic, the media's presentation of AIDS fills their minds with terrifying images of cadaverous people in the terminal stages of the disease. Even the actual onset of AIDS may take the form of relatively mild symptoms and long periods of good health. Helping the client understand the distinction between HIV infection and HIV disease is critical in establishing a hopeful attitude toward the situation. Hope is a critical ingredient in marshaling the energy to take the necessary steps for maintaining good health and in foregoing activities that will spread the virus. Hopelessness frequently leads to performing dangerous behav-

iors which may lead to re-infection with new forms of the virus. Depression is also known to negatively affect immune functioning.

While there is no way to estimate the length of time between initial
infection and actual illness manifestations—and there is even some evidence that some people will never become symptomatic (Altman,
1995a)—the knowledge that one has HIV infection makes it hard to
perceive oneself as a healthy person. Adding to the uncertainty, the
statistical predictions of how many people can expect to become ill
change monthly. First it was said that people with HIV had a 10 percent
chance of becoming ill with ARC or AIDS symptoms. Later the statistics began to creep upward. Today it is believed that half of those infected with HIV will develop AIDS within 10 years; 25 percent will
develop symptoms indicating progression to AIDS, 15 percent will experience only minor symptoms, and 10 percent will be nonprogressors, that
is, will not show any signs of disease (Altman, 1995a). While the causes
of nonprogression are not as yet known, but may include differences in
the virulence of the virus, viral mutations, and genetics, most nonprogressors attribute their wellness to their own determination to live,
personal action regarding health care, and determination to lead a
healthy life style (Remier & Wagner, 1995). Informing clients that
a number of people with HIV do not become ill, and that many live
asymptomatically for more than 10 years postinfection, can help the
client develop a positive attitude in the face of societal pessimism about
the outcome of HIV infection.

There are other anomalies: those few who, diagnosed with HIV infection, no longer show antibodies to the virus and are asymptomatic;
others who are symptomatic but show no trace of the virus; still others
who have Kaposi's sarcoma, once thought to be a certain sign of AIDS,
but do not show HIV infection. Kaposi's sarcoma has been shown to be
a sexually transmitted herpes virus (Cohen 1995) that is spread at the
same time as HIV. Perhaps the presence of HIV, which compromises the
immune system, causes an increased vulnerability to contracting and
spreading Kaposi's sarcoma.

The period of time between infection and the onset of symptoms
varies from person to person. The mean time between infection and the
appearance of disease symptoms now appears to be between 7 and 11
years for gay men (Lifson, Rutherford, & Jaffe, 1988). However, some
become symptomatic within weeks of diagnosis and within months of
infection. Those who contracted the disease from blood transfusions
seem to have a shorter symptom-free time (approximately two to three

years) than people who contracted the disease through sexual contact; on the other hand, hemophiliacs seem to develop symptoms at a somewhat slower rate than infected gay men (Lifson et al., 1988).

Nevertheless, increasing knowledge of the disease is resulting in better treatment and longer survival time. It is probable that HIV will eventually become a manageable chronic illness with indefinite survival time. After testing, people who have access to the most up-to-date medical care can choose to undergo a series of blood tests, called lymphocyte subtest studies. These tests should include a T-cell panel, which will indicate the strength of the immune system as it battles the virus, and tests that determine the amount of virus in the bloodstream and level of viral activity. If T-cell counts remain above 500 there is little risk of developing life-threatening opportunistic infections, with the exception of tuberculosis. During this "asymptomatic" period many people experience enlarged lymph nodes, a sign that the immune system is fighting HIV and that the lymph nodes are sites where HIV is reproducing. Symptoms which may herald the onset of the early symptomatic phase may include oral thrush, shingles, some weight loss, diarrhea, night sweats, and fevers. Diseases in women have been underreported and often missed as evidence of possible HIV infection. These diseases of the reproductive tract include candida vaginitis, vaginal warts, cervical disease, pelvic inflammatory disease, and genital ulcers.

If T-cell counts fall below 500 many physicians recommend initiating anti-viral prophylaxis. These tests should be repeated at regular intervals and are best done in conjunction with a physical examination by a physician well-versed in detecting signs of the various opportunistic infections. It must be remembered that T-cell counts or percentages are only statistical predictors of the likelihood that a person will become ill; a relatively normal number of T-cells in an HIV-infected person does not guarantee freedom from the sudden onset of an opportunistic infection. Some infected patients with almost no T-cells are alive and well, whereas others whose immune systems do not appear to be compromised unexpectedly become ill. Since the immune system has to perform a continuous battle against viral replication from the moment of infection, keeping as healthy as possible may be a factor in long-term survival. Patients should avoid behaviors known to compromise immune functioning. For example, it is known that frequent inhalation, ingestion, or injection of licit or illicit drugs may suppress the immune system, as does extensive use of alcohol; volatile nitrates or "poppers" have been epidemiologically associated with Kaposi's sarcoma in persons with AIDS.

Reinfection with other strains of HIV may increase the virus's ability to evade drugs. The patient who is positive must still use protection while having sex with a positive partner. Patients should seek healthful life styles that involve stress reduction, good nutrition, and getting adequate rest while focusing on leading a fulfilling life.

Once one has established sero-positivity and the relative functioning of the immune system, a number of medical treatment options are available. The most common anti-virals, low dosage AZT, ddC, ddI, and the newer protease inhibitors, were discussed in the previous chapter.

TRANSMISSION

The person who becomes HIV-infected must become informed about the transmission of the HIV virus. HIV is transmitted by any practice that results in direct bloodstream contact with an infected partner's blood or semen. HIV has been found in breast milk and can be passed from mother to baby through breast-feeding. Small amounts of HIV are also found in urine and mucous membranes as well as anal excretion. Although tiny amounts of HIV have been identified in saliva and tears of people with AIDS, these fluids are not considered to be likely vehicles of transmission. In fact recent studies have shown that saliva may have protective factor which neutralizes the virus (Altman, 1995b).

However, deep mouth-to-mouth kissing involving repeated ingestion of the infected partner's saliva poses a potential though low risk of infection if the person has bleeding gums or open sores or has vomited blood. Recently, a few cases of infection through fellatio have been reported. Until now oral sex, fellatio, and cunnilingus have not been considered to be documented high-risk activities.

Early research emphasized anal intercourse as the primary sexual means of HIV transmission and despite overwhelming evidence from Africa of heterosexual transmission, the CDC initially regarded sexual transmission of the disease as primarily limited to gay men. The virus was thought to be transmitted into the bloodstream through small tears in the tissue of the rectum—tissue that is particularly vulnerable to fissures. More recent studies show not only that HIV can be transmitted directly into the cells of the colon, but that it may directly infect the cells of the inner lining of the vagina and the cervix. At the same time, the presence of sexually transmitted diseases (including herpes) creates small sores through which the virus can enter the bloodstream in either males or females. Overall, the male-to-female transmission rate is around 20 percent (Curran, Jaffe, Hardy, Morgan, Selik, & Dondero, 1988), but it rises to almost 50 percent for female partners of IV drug users, who tend to come from communities of poverty characterized by higher rates of untreated sexually transmitted diseases.

Anomalies appear in the number of sexual contacts necessary for a woman to be infected. In a study published in the *New England Journal of Medicine*, of 19 women without apparent risk factors for HIV infection who had sex with an infected African male, 11 were infected—in two cases, through a single act of intercourse. Similar experiences, which may be the exception rather than the norm, have been reported in California and Sweden (Clumek, 1989). It may be that the HIV-infected person is more infectious at certain times during the disease process, or that he carries a more virulent form of the virus, or perhaps the woman is vulnerable because she is carrying a venereal infection. Herpes, a relatively common, recurring infection for which there is as yet no permanent treatment, may provide a suitable niche for entrance of HIV. Female-to-male transmission may be more difficult than male-to-female, but the presence of sexually transmitted diseases in either partner makes transmission more likely. The uncertainty of how or when HIV can be transmitted underscores the need for safer sex.

People who are diagnosed as sero-positive are often humiliated by myths that the disease can be spread through casual tactile contact or by using the same linen or tableware. HIV is (ironically) a fragile virus, and it is important to underscore the fact that there is no evidence of AIDS being spread by insects or by casual or household contact—even in families in which members share toothbrushes and other intimate articles. To be absolutely safe, however, latex gloves are advisable when handling bodily fluids, including changing the diapers of an infected baby. A simple solution of diluted chlorine bleach can be used to sterilize all surfaces and kill the virus. However, certain opportunistic infections such as TB are highly contagious and require taking precautions against infection.

INDIVIDUAL DIFFERENCES IN
RESPONSE TO MEDICAL TREATMENT

If clients do not choose to conform to state-of-the-art medical treatment, clinicians may find themselves using covert coercion to gain compliance and becoming secretly angry if clients choose not to do so. As a result, clinicians may put themselves in conflict with clients' beliefs about illness, medical care, and the nature of healing. In a world of high technology medicine it is easy to objectify the disease by separating it from the person who suffers. But this is also a world of medical uncertainty and desperation, where fortunes can be made from the successful drug of the moment, where information that the newest savior drug, AZT, is highly toxic at the initially recommended high dosage is made public only by an activist group, ACT-UP. It is not surprising that many clients set their own medical course. If the disease truly belongs to the patients, then the treatments they elect will be congruent with their own beliefs and lifestyles, but may not reflect prevailing medical wisdom. Trusting and respecting these choices is a challenge faced by all clinicians in this field. The following is a very personal report of my own experience with this challenge.

Case Example

I like Brad so much and it is all I can do to sit on my hands and tell myself to respect his odd way of handling his illness. Because I like and admire him, because his wry Southern wit makes me laugh during our sessions, I want him around. So, I think, if only he would take his AZT or go on the protocol his doctor suggested. Not that Brad has been sick since his original bout of pneumocystis three years ago. Since that time he has rearranged his life, quit a job he hated, gotten out of a bad relationship, into a somewhat better one, out of that one, and finally traveled to Venice—a city he had always dreamed of visiting. Brad has a dangerously low T-cell count, and takes AZT and Dapsone irregularly, at best. When his physician encourages him to be more regular in his use of the medications, he says that "it doesn't feel right." When pressed for an elaboration of this decision, he creates any number of plausible explanations. One centers on self-hatred and internalized homophobia leading to self-destructive behaviors; another that he is lazy or just a Southern "bad boy" who never does what he is told; still another is that the medication reminds him of his illness and that he may die soon, despite the fact he is just beginning to do what he has always dreamed of doing. Then he adds in a puzzled way: "I guess it's just that my body tells me not to take the AZT. I am more ambivalent about the Dapsone." He grins and adds: "I think I take them sometimes because I don't want my physician to be mad at me. After all, if I get sick, I need him to be on my side. He's a good doctor, one of the best. But if I followed my instinct, I wouldn't be taking anything."

As a clinician I am steeped in the tradition of American medicine that emphasizes aggressive treatment and obedience to doctor's orders. AIDS is a disease for which "aggressive treatment" is recommended on the basis of statistical probability (Payer, 1988) even before physical symptoms appear. As a result, I feel uncomfortable with a patient who feels that as long as his body feels well and he is functioning well, he wants to do less than is medically advised. I suppose I also tend to look at the death of a patient who tried holistic remedies as being his own fault, while I excuse the death of a patient on AZT as a tragic event due to the power of the disease. Yet who is to say that my client does not know his body better than anyone else – and that not reminding himself that he is sick, and not using the standard dosage of AZT (which is now considered to be too high) has been responsible for his continued good health?

THE EXPERIENCE OF DISCLOSURE

Issues of disclosure preoccupy the HIV-infected person, and it is at this time that many seek professional counseling. *How can I tell my beloved spouse (or lifetime partner)? How can I tell my sexual partners? Will they leave? Will they keep the secret? Can friends be trusted? Should my family be told? How do I deal with a new date? How will my wife manage a disclosure of bisexuality?* These are a few of the questions confronting the HIV-infected person.

The foreboding sense of bearing a hidden stigma that eventually may be exposed arrives with the receipt of testing results. Those who need to be told at this point are limited to people actually at risk for contamination through sexual activity or the sharing of blood products, although the infected person may want to tell family or trusted friends. The most crucial issue for clinicians at this stage of counseling is to help the sero-positive person come to terms with the need to disclose the infection to actual and potential sexual partners. Shame, guilt, fear of loss and of abandonment are powerful emotions which must be identified and worked through. The person who must reveal his status in order to protect his partner takes a great risk of losing a deeply important relationship. Yet, not to do so is to live with intolerable guilt, which ultimately takes many forms, including self-destructive behaviors – as though hastening death would be the only way of making the situation tolerable. A partner's forgiveness and testament of love in the face of anxiety about his or her own status may awaken additional, intolerable feelings of guilt and an intense need for self-punishment.

Because bisexuality is a shameful secret in most social groups, men who act upon strong sexual attractions to other men usually keep these activities a discreet and separate part of their lives. Revelation would bring not only consequences to the heterosexual relationship, but also the likelihood of social ostracism. While their female sexual partners might have sensed a problem, they frequently kept their suspicions to themselves. They might be afraid of the social repercussions of revealing a partner's bisexuality or of the stigma to their children in a culture where bisexuality is terribly misunderstood. They may have a deep love for their partner and not wish to endanger the relationship. Because bisexuality is often falsely constructed by society as a woman's failure to be "woman enough," female partners may have difficulty in dealing with their own sense of failure. Or, finally, they simply may not know that their partner has another sexual life.

The client may decide to inform his sexual partner but to conceal the actual behaviors that led to infection. Bisexuality and drug use are less acceptable in most "heterosexual" cultures than the idea that a man is seeing female prostitutes or having an affair with a woman. As a result, an HIV-infected man may choose to identify his risk source as heterosexual sex when, in fact, he has also been having sex with men or is secretly using IV drugs. For example, the most common explanation of HIV infection for Latino men who are not drug users is one of "messing around" with women, without mentioning that their extramarital affairs also may have included some sexual contacts with men. While a small number may have been infected through sexual contact with prostitutes, studies show that the infection rate of men whose only risk behavior is using female prostitutes is relatively low (Wallace, 1988)—despite the high rate of sero-positivity in prostitutes who live in cities where prostitution and IV drug use are linked. A difficult problem in therapy is deciding whether or not to accept an explanation that does not seem to accurately describe the behaviors leading to transmission.

When the family learns that a family member is sero-positive, the need to preserve important relationships may motivate them to find a relatively benign explanation for the infection. For example, in one case a blood transfusion recipient and his wife elected to identify the transfusions as the route of infection, even though he had also had bisexual experiences. To deal with the issues raised by bisexuality—which, in theory at least, had occurred prior to the marriage—would disrupt a relationship that was extremely precious to both partners. In another family a mother accepted the blame for her infection and attributed it to an affair she had during a period of time when her husband was absent from the family. While there was considerable evidence that her husband was involved in IV drug use, he was the father of her eight children, held a steady job, and therefore, was crucial to the family's sense of its identity. He decided not to be tested and his wife was content with that decision.

A less obvious form of disclosure—but one which can be quite painful—is disclosure to health-care professionals such as dentists and gynecologists, who may be at risk or who need to know the client's HIV status for medical reasons. Negative experiences with these more secondary revelations can influence how the client deals with family, partner, and friends.

CASE EXAMPLE

In the following excerpt, one client graphically describes her experience with disclosure. Note how critical it is for her to reestablish herself as a person and how she uses healthy anger to counter shame and to educate the treating physicians.

Bernice: I told the people I needed to tell—my doctor and my dentist. [*Beginning to cry*] I hate the way they treated me. I thought I was over the crying part [*fighting back tears*]. I've known my dentist for years. I'm particular, and I didn't want to switch. When I went to see him after I was diagnosed, he was all excited to see me and to tell me about his practice.

'How are you? How are the kids?' he asked enthusiastically. I said, 'Doctor, I have to talk to you.' When I told him the news, it was as if someone pulled a shade over him. He'd been so concerned when my daughter was ill. But now the curtain had come down. I tried to talk to him. 'Don't you realize how hard it was for me to tell you? Look at all the people who don't know, or who know but *don't* tell you. I was in here two months ago. I had it, but I didn't know—and you did not treat me the way you are treating me now.'

After a while he began to treat me like a person again. He stopped putting on the goggles and the three robes and the ten pairs of gloves!

When her internist washed his hands throughout her appointment, she challenged him.

Bernice: You didn't used to wash the stethoscope after you put it on my chest. It's fine that you wash your hands before you examine me.

You should be careful—the last person you saw before me could have had the virus and *not* told you, so I want you to be careful and treat everybody the same. But stop your constant hand washing on my time! You are just touching my skin, not handling secretions or blood.

Her attempt at education was once again successful: She now receives thorough examinations—minus the overly thorough ablutions.

RELATIONSHIP ISSUES

HIV infection confronts people with difficult relationship issues. Parents who test positive often fear for the lives of their recently born children, who now also must be tested, and worry about the future of their well children: How long will they have parents? For couples, confronting the reality of HIV infection can catalyze a period of stormy questioning and accusations. Should they stay together or part? What will the future be like if one or both of them dies? If a partner of a HIV-infected person tests negative, he or she may not wish to stay in the relationship. Conversely, the person who has tested positive may do everything possible to push the well partner out of the relationship, out of deep feelings of guilt, shame, and protectiveness.

CASE EXAMPLE *
When Samantha's baby was born, Samantha's new life fell apart. After a turbulent adolescence she had pulled her life together, gone back to school and begun to pursue her dream of becoming a nurse. Giving birth at the age of 20, along with the tragic death of her most beloved brother, had made her think about her life. It was as if her brother's "good spirit" finally gave her the guidance she needed. She met a young man who resembled him in his gentleness and dark, handsome features. He was sweet and slow and only wanted to be with her, to have a baby, and to provide for his family.

Then, to her shock and horror, her baby was diagnosed with AIDS. She was healthy and had never suspected that she could have been infected by the man with whom she had previously been involved. Seeing her husband's hurt and the little baby's suffering was unbearable. When he picked up Jessie with his large dark hand, which could almost cradle the baby's whole body, and gazed at her with love and sadness, Samantha had to turn away. She knew her husband was sero-negative

*The therapist was Lauren Kaplan (1988).

and she wanted him to have a different life—one with a woman who was not infected, and who could bear him healthy children.

Each time he made love to her, she was afraid the condom would break and he too would die. She couldn't get those thoughts out of her mind, so she began to provoke him by staying out until 3:00 A.M. without telling him where she was. Predictably, he would become furious. As the fights grew worse, he feared that he would become violent with her—if he did, he would leave, he thought. He had watched other men's violence toward women and he did not want to become one of those men. The stress of the baby's illness, his wife's behaviors, and the fighting was unbearable.

In the first session with Samantha and her husband, a ritual was used to clarify the meaning of her provocative behaviors in relation to the guilt she felt about what had happened. She was asked to notice for herself all the ways she would incite Thomas to fight with her during the upcoming week and to jot them down on a piece of paper. Then, either during or after the fight she was instructed to say to herself: "I'm doing this so that I can punish myself and protect Thomas...I'm doing this so that I can punish myself and protect Thomas...I'm doing this so that I can punish myself and protect Thomas."

The husband was also given the task of helping his wife forgive herself by finding ways of consoling her for the baby's illness when she seemed most tense and upset.

The ritual seemed to break the tension in the couple by providing an explanation for what was happening. At a later session Samantha's mother was asked to join the therapy so that the family could construct a different meaning for Samantha's adolescent behavior, which had led to infection. Once the behavior was seen as "troubled" rather than "bad," resulting from a sensitive young girl's reaction to family losses, both mother and daughter began to develop more positive perspectives. The disease was then reframed as being a normal though tragic loss. The therapist linked the young woman's potential loss of her own child to AIDS to her mother's loss of her son. Guilt and self-blame were identified as normal tactics used in an attempt to explain the tragic and inexplicable. Finally, a religious meaning was attached to illness and death, as mother and infected daughter were asked to turn for guidance to the memory of a wise and religious grandmother, whom they had loved, and who had been able to accept her own death as part of the mysterious order of things.

CHAPTER 8
Issues of Secrecy

S EVERAL ISSUES ARE of immediate concern to clinicians once the person has decided to be tested, especially as new treatments for early stages of the disease become available. What are the clinician's legal and ethical responsibilities concerning the reporting of a person's sero-positive status to sexual partners or to persons with whom the patient may have shared needles? To what extent should the client be advised to maintain secrecy within his kin, social, and health-care networks? What are the pros and cons of revealing pediatric infection to health-care, child-care, and other workers or social contacts who are in contact with an infected child?

CONFIDENTIALITY AND AIDS:
AN OVERVIEW

The issue of the limits of confidentiality is confusing for clinicians as well as epidemiologists, whose task is to ascertain the "larger picture" of the epidemic and devise strategies for its control. Overemphasizing confidentiality for the sero-positive client may abrogate the rights of those already or potentially infected, while contact tracing and mandatory testing could drive the epidemic underground. In the absence of firm policy guidelines, clinicians have to weigh the rights of their patients against the rights of persons they may have infected or may infect. Is the construction of a supportive environment that encourages people to volunteer for testing and/or counseling the most effective way to manage the epidemic and empower people at risk to act responsibly?

The clinician's dilemma over "duty to warn" versus confidentiality cannot be separated from larger questions about the role of confidentiality in preserving public health. Early in the epidemic, when there was little treatment available to people in the early stages of infection, public health guidelines in most states encouraged anonymous testing accompanied by pre- and post-test counseling. The goals were to identify infected persons and, through counseling, to encourage them to use safer sex and clean needles to avoid spreading infection. Those identified as sero-negative but at risk were instructed to take precautions in order to avoid becoming infected. To encourage people to come forward for testing, strict confidentiality was maintained and punitive measures such as contact tracing or isolation of persons believed to be engaging in unsafe activities were avoided. It seemed sensible to spend money on educational programs aimed at changing people's sexual behaviors, even if they chose not to learn their serological status.

In the gay community, AIDS activists developed and funded a non-coercive approach emphasizing education of all community members and safer sex practices. Since medical intervention in the early stages of the disease process was not available, testing was not considered essential. Those who elected to be tested and received positive results were encouraged to insist on protection of their confidentiality. In the majority of cases, sero-positive men either notified partners or adopted safer sex. The underlying premise of the gay community was that all men should consider themselves to be at risk or infected and should act accordingly. Educational programs dealt straightforwardly with the reality of sexual desire and practice. As a result, the combination of community networks and education programs was successful in making safer sex the norm.

Ten years into the epidemic, while safer sex has dramatically reduced the rate of new infection among gay men, there is evidence that some gay men who have practiced safer sex are beginning to engage once again in risky practices, particularly if they are in committed relationships. These findings indicate that reinforcing "safer sex" practices is an ongoing process. The clinician should not be lulled into believing that, once the issue of sexual practice has been discussed with a client, it can be dropped from therapeutic discourse.

The gay community created model educational programs that in effect changed the sexual mores of a community. Because the government refused to be involved in what happened to gay men, these programs, paid for by the community, could reflect the reality of gay sexual life and operate in a language relevant to gay sexuality. The belief that every sexually active gay man was potentially at risk, or infected, circumvented the issue of whether or not sero-status must be disclosed by professionals to sexual partners. The gay press made it clear that it was each person's obligation to protect himself and that it was irresponsible by community standards to engage in unsafe sex.

By contrast, the development of educational programs for heterosexual populations was dependent on government funding and government guidelines. This dependency forced such programs into the political arena and made them subject to the ongoing debate between conservatives/fundamentalists and liberals that characterized the political scene in the eighties. Fierce debates took place about the morality of educating teenagers and school children about safer-sexual practices as opposed to advocating abstinence. For example, condom distribution in the New York City high schools initially was bitterly opposed by parents and politicians alike, despite the overwhelming evidence that the majority of teenagers in the public schools was sexually active and from highly impacted communities.

The result of these debates was that, while testing remained confidential and easily available, comprehensive educational programs for non-gay populations were sorely lacking. Unlike in the gay community, where the press and leadership always made available the latest information on HIV infection, in the urban ghettos the extent of HIV infection remained shrouded in secrecy. The lethal combination of secrecy, lack of comprehensive education in an environment of poverty, drugs, and impermanent relationships fostered the unchecked spread of the epidemic to non-drug-using inner-city populations. As a result, many heterosexuals remained ignorant of the risks they were taking. In this environment the clinician's responsibility to warn the sexual partners of infected persons, who may have no reason to know that they are at risk, becomes more compelling.

As the epidemic threatened to spread from urban ghettos to more middle-class populations, an increased sense of failure propelled cries for harsher interventions, including mandatory testing, contact tracing, and isolation of people known to be sero-positive. These attempts at harsher legislation, while usually not successful, only served to drive the epidemic further underground, as they fueled a climate of discrimination against the infected. Furthermore, the futility of such approaches as a means of halting the epidemic and protecting the uninfected becomes obvious in the light of the needle-sharing patterns of drug users and the client turnover of those who prostitute for drugs.

As with syphilis, mandatory testing, reporting, and contact tracing will only make sense when an effective preventive vaccine or a cure for infection has been developed. Until that time, HIV education addressing the complex web of social attitudes and conditions that promote disease spread is the only sensible means of prevention. In our clinical experience, as our gay clients gained self-esteem, accepted their sexual orientation as legitimate, and learned to value other aspects of their lives, they found the strength to change high-risk behaviors. The punitive interventions of contact tracing or premature disclosure often have negative consequences that actually promote the spread of infection, as the client feels betrayed, coerced, disempowered and devalued.

Similarly, understanding that drug use does not define the totality of the drug user's existence may also contribute to the person's ability to shift the direction of his life. The AIDS epidemic in the inner-city communities would look very different if it were attacked through social interventions aimed at changing some of the conditions of poverty that promote unprotected sexuality and drug use. Education and job opportunities, adequate housing, and the restoration of public services in the urban ghettos would have more effect on breaking the twin cycle of addiction and HIV infection than any amount of money spent on partner identification.

ISSUES FOR CLINICIANS: CONFIDENTIALITY AND THE DUTY TO WARN

Near the end of 1990, medications were introduced that to some extent arrest the progress of the disease when they are administered in the nonsymptomatic phase of infection. As a result, the issues of a clinician's duty to warn sexual and drug-using partners and the public-health mandate for contact tracing have become more complex. Compounding this complexity for the clinician is the fact that different states have different policies regarding the protection of confidentiality and the enforcement of mandatory contact tracing. While in some states HIV tracing by public-health officials is mandatory, in others the decision to warn persons at risk is left to the clinician's judgment and his option to warn is protected.

As a clinician considers the serious decision to warn a partner in the absence of the client's permission, he or she must be aware of the influence of personal value systems. The clinician is a part of the society he treats and his values play a part in his approach to this disease. A "straight" clinician, for example, may identify emotionally with a bi-sexual client's spouse. In his haste to protect her, he may also underesti-mate his client's ability to change behaviors or to notify his spouse on his own within a reasonable time. It is difficult to manage the uncertainty that a current sexual partner may actually become infected during the time that one is doing counseling. It is also difficult to feel comfortable with the knowledge that the client's partner may be infected already and is not receiving adequate treatment. On the other hand, if a client does not have the opportunity to work through his own feelings about revealing an issue as sensitive and delicate as bisexuality, the clinician-turned-informant may be unable to salvage either the therapeutic or the marital relationship. The betrayal may force the client out of therapy, and without a holding environment, he may well act out his anger in other sexual arenas.

For many clients struggling with HIV – a disease that elicits powerful emotions of anger, rage, and even vengefulness – the preservation of the counseling relationship is a crucial source of support for responsible behavior. Optimally, when they are ready to inform their partners, clients should feel enough trust in the counseling relationship to be able to invite their partners into the therapy process.

In making a decision to inform a sexual partner who may be at risk, clinicians must remember that, while the confidentiality of the client-patient relationship is privileged, it is not absolute. Sisella Bok, in her eloquent book, *Secrets: On the Ethics of Concealment and Revelation*, analyzes four premises that demarcate the limits of confidentiality. The clinician should consider the implications of each of these premises when making decisions about breaking confidentiality.

For Bok the first and fundamental premise "is that of individual autonomy over personal information but of course this control should only be partial. Matters such as contagious disease place individual autonomy in conflict with the rights of others" (1983, p. 120). This conflict of rights is, of course, the clinician's dilemma, which has been described above.

Bok's second premise "presupposes the legitimacy not only of having personal secrets but of sharing them and assumes respect for relation-ships among human beings and their intimacy" (p. 120). Without the loyalty and trust represented by the respect shown for the other person's need for privacy, the social bonds between people, which are at the heart of a democratic society, would be weakened greatly, as George Orwell's *1984* vividly illustrates. Orwell's society was terrifying precisely because there was no place for secrecy. As the state intruded on each private thought of the citizen and prohibited the sharing of secrets, it effectively prevented any meaningful social relationships from forming. The gay community's insistence on preserving the right to manage information within the limits of responsibility may stem from its historical knowledge of what is at stake when the right to privacy can be infringed or summarily overridden.

Bok's first two premises lay the groundwork for the privileging of the therapeutic relationship but contain the caveat of its limits when it conflicts with the rights of others. In her description of a third premise we see how the contract of confidentiality compromises one's freedom to reveal:

> The third premise holds that a pledge of silence creates an obligation beyond the respect due to persons and to existing relationships. Once we promise someone secrecy, we can no longer start from scratch in weighing the moral factors of the dilemma . . . . promises of secrecy . . . agree to perform some action that will guard the secret—to keep silent, at least, and perhaps more. Just what action is promised and at what cost are questions that go to the heart of the conflicts over confidentiality. To invoke a promise, therefore, is not to close the debate over pledges of secrecy. (pp. 120–1)

Bok argues that the therapist must make a series of decisions. Is it ethically acceptable to make the pledge in the first place? Is the pledge binding? Are there circumstances which might justify overriding it? If it is binding, what circumstances might justify overriding it? If clinicians are timid about defining these limits from the outset, they will forfeit certain freedoms of action and judgment. Clarification of possible contingencies is a crucial aspect of forging the initial contract with HIV-infected clients.

Bok's fourth premise brings us to the complex issue of the duty to warn:

> The fourth premise assigns weight beyond ordinary loyalty to professional confidentiality, because of its utility to persons and to society. As a result professionals grant secrecy to their clients even when they would otherwise have reason to speak out. According to this premise individuals benefit from this confidentiality because it allows them to seek help that they might otherwise fear to ask for . . . . Society therefore gains in turn from allowing such professional refuge, the argument holds, in spite of

undoubted risks of not learning about certain dangers to the community; and everyone is better off and professionals can probe for secrets that will make them more capable of providing the needed help. (p. 122)

Against this pledge of confidentiality is balanced the duty to warn potential victims to whom serious harm is likely to occur. While it has been established in cases like Tarasoff (Stone, 1976) that a therapist has a clear duty to warn when he or she has knowledge that a client threatens violence to another person, the issue is less clear-cut when the issue is the *possible* transmission of a *potentially* fatal disease to another person. While unprotected sex or shared needle use with an infected person is always risky, the vagaries of transmission are such that it is hard to estimate the degree of danger to the other person. Some clients have sex over a long period of time with an infected person and test negative; others are infected through one or two sexual contacts. Statutes vary from state to state. In New York, for example, a physician is protected if he reveals a person's HIV status to a sexual partner whom he *has reason to believe* is at risk, but it is not clear whether he has a duty to warn those he *only suspects* are being put at risk by his client. Nor is it clear what liability he would incur, if any, if he failed to warn a sexual partner who later was infected by his patient.

Nancy Dubler (1987), a lawyer and medical ethicist at Montefiore Hospital, summarizes the current dilemma. She argues that requiring that an individual physician determine where there is an endangered third party and requiring that the physician warn that party may (1) discourage early testing for serology status, (2) lessen the vigilance of third parties who assume that they will be warned if endangered, and (3) erode the trust necessary to an effective physician/outpatient collaboration. In the climate of AIDS, people pay a price for disclosure, in terms of social stigma and economic loss. The promise of confidentiality protects against such penalties and encourages clients to get help. Loosening these guidelines by requiring therapists to routinely warn all those with whom the person is thought to have had sex or needle contact (even if such warning were feasible) is tantamount to inscribing a red cross on the sealed door of the plague-infected. As Defoe recounts in his classic *Journal of the Plague Year*, which describes the 1667 plague of London, all that happened as a result of such attempts at identification and containment was that citizens so identified and contained left their houses through back windows and vanished into the streets, thus spreading the plague wherever they went.

But while coercive measures may in fact spread the epidemic, the clinician's dilemma remains. There are unknowing victims of the disease, especially those who acquire the disease from heterosexual partners, who have a moral claim to assistance. Dubler argues for a balance between the physician's judgment and legal requirements:

> These innocent third parties must not be abandoned to the vagaries of contagion which will determine their fate. Therefore whereas society has not, and I argue should not impose on physicians a duty to warn, I think it must also especially protect those physicians and healthcare workers who may opt to warn. (1987, p. 8)

All things considered, if contact tracing were to be mandated, it would be better left in the hands of public-health officials than located within a privileged relationship—the purpose of which is to provide support for crucial behavioral changes, as well as to engender the courage to inform partners who may be at risk. But since, to date, the ethical (and perhaps legal) obligation to warn is, in many states, left to health-care professionals, we have translated the debate concerning the balance of confidentiality and the responsibility to warn into the following guidelines for therapy:

1. The therapeutic contract must include an initial discussion of the issues involved in the preservation of confidentiality. The client must understand the realistic limits of confidentiality as well as trust the therapist's intent to protect the client from the social consequences of disclosure. We stress the importance of an honest therapeutic relationship that defines its limitations in terms of morals and ethics rather than compensatory protectiveness. We believe that this differentiation is respectful of the client's strengths.
2. Clients should be informed that we are willing to work with them so that *they* will be able to inform their partners within a reasonable period of time. We tell them that we believe that the fear generated by diagnosis and illness robs clients of their sense of control over their lives. Regaining control over such crucial aspects as disclosure is an empowering experience, which will better enable persons to handle an illness that will often place them in positions of helplessness.
3. If, however, we feel, after working with the client, that the client is placing an unknowing partner at risk and is not willing to

reveal a positive HIV status, we will observe our ethical obligation to warn. In a few cases we have had to present an ultima-
tum: if a client has not been able to inform his sexual partner by
a certain date, the clinician will have no other moral option than
to do so for him. In no case have we been unable to persuade the
client that it is better for him to be the person notifying his
partner—always, if at the last moment, the client has found the
courage to do so.

4. We construct the decision to come to therapy as a courageous
   decision to act morally and responsibly and to confront the
   painful issues that HIV has raised. We also understand entering
   therapy as a wish to protect the partner, since it is obvious that
   no therapist could condone a decision to continue to place
   another at risk. We let the client know that we understand that
   disclosure of a positive HIV status, and possibly the revelation of
   concealed behaviors that led to infection, will be one of the most
   stressful events of his life. We reassure him that we will take time
   to work through the issues involved. Most clients can come up
   with strategies for keeping their partner safe during this phase of
   the work, even if they are not yet willing to disclose.

5. We construct with the client a narrative of courage and morality, identifying times in his or her life when he or she has made
   difficult and costly moral decisions. We ask the client to talk
   about the way he felt about himself during those times and how
   others perceived him. For example, one client, facing disclosure
   to a new lover, was able to identify the value his father placed on
   honesty. As he talked about his father he realized that honesty
   was a value that had shaped many of the critical decisions he had
   made about his own life. Until this exploration he had thought
   about himself primarily as a "bad boy," someone who had led a
   superficial, somewhat irresponsible life. As he began to think
   about himself in this new way, he realized that his internalized
   negative feelings about being gay had shaped his self-image. As
   he constructed a far more positive self-image, deep feelings
   emerged about his experience as a gay man, about the dreams he
   had abandoned when he understood that he was gay, and about
   the loss of closeness with some family members whom he
   "protected" by not discussing his sexual orientation. Even
   though he and his new lover practiced safer sex, he was able to
   tell the lover that he was infected, much to the lover's relief, as he
   too was infected. After this revelation he had the courage to

discuss his sexual orientation with homophobic family members, a task that he saw as critically important to complete in the months before he died.

6. To handle our anxieties about the rapidity of notification, we remind ourselves that a client in a stable relationship is likely to have already infected his/her partner. Most clients who come to us already know their test results, have informed their partners, and are seeking counseling as a way of dealing with the fallout of notification and living with the threat of ARC and AIDS. Others come to us for help in handling the diagnosis and the process of disclosure. While not immediately prepared to notify their partners, these clients often find ways of avoiding sex or having safe sex until they are able to disclose their sero-positive status. Clinicians who handle their own anxieties about the sexual partner who is to be notified are able to establish an atmosphere of trust, caring, and protectiveness that promotes the client's willingness to bring his partner in for counseling.

CASE EXAMPLE*

Joshua was a young man who had learned early in life that survival depended on controlling as much of his environment as possible. This included anticipating the behaviors of those around him so that he could behave in self-protective ways. He learned to control his emotions and to be the dominant partner in relationships; he was the one who initiated — and the one who left. A sero-positive test disrupted his way of ordering his life by triggering a vulnerability long buried with his childhood. Feeling out of control in his own life, he described his attempts to control his lover's response.

Therapist: How aware is your lover of the risk of being infected?
Joshua: Very aware.
Therapist: You've talked about it with him?
Joshua: Yes.
Therapist: You said he asked you once if you were sero-positive?
Joshua: Right. The first time we ever met, he asked me if I'd been tested. I told him yes, but that was it.
Therapist: Uh-huh. What do you think he understood that to mean?
Joshua: I don't know. [*Pause*]

*Joseph Rosenthal was the therapist.

Therapist: What a dilemma for you. If you tell him when he comes back from his trip home, and he's real angry, he might say, "What! I came all the way from Paris to the United States to be your lover, and now you tell me *this?*"

Joshua: But that's stupid, because all he has to do is to get right back on the plane and go home.

Therapist: Aren't you thinking about visiting him? What if he asks you while you're over there?

Joshua: I don't know if I'll tell him.

Therapist: Well, what if he asks you point blank, "Are you sero-positive?"—not just, "Have you been tested?"

Joshua: Maybe I would lie.

Therapist: What would you think about that?

The therapist knows Joshua is a decent person. The issue is: How will he take charge of the situation so that his responses are not guilty defenses to his lover's queries?

Joshua: I haven't told him because of the way I am. But I know the cards are on the table for me to tell him, not for him to ask.

Therapist: When you think about the issue of giving someone the freedom to respond versus your being in control, how does that link up?

Joshua: [*Pause*] I don't know. I mean, I don't think about those scenarios.

Therapist: I think you do. And I think that it really comes down to how much you or I or anyone can control events, as much as we'd like to.

The therapist challenges the client's ideas about control in order to help him take the risk to let go, despite his fears. The client will gain a sense of personal control by taking charge of the decision to initiate disclosure and by accepting his own ability to weather the reaction of his lover. Joshua decided to go to Paris to disclose his sero-status to his lover. The next session was immediately after his return.

Therapist: When did you get back?

Joshua: Last night.

Therapist: Ah, so, you had a great week in Paris?

Joshua: Yeah, but the question you should have asked is, "When did *we* get back?"

Therapist: So he did come back with you?

Joshua: Yeah.

Therapist: So it all worked out?

Joshua: Um-hum. He knows everything—I'm in a state of euphoria
about it all.

Therapist: What makes you most euphoric?

Joshua: Well, you know, I think he loves me for who I am—not for the
image that I let him see.

Not only did Joshua find strength in his honesty with his partner, but
he was able to discover a new story about himself: "I am someone who
does not need to be in charge of the way the other person sees me in order
to be loved."

HELPING THE CLIENT
UNDERSTAND THE LIMITS OF
CONFIDENTIALITY

When a person decides to be tested, he faces the reality that information
about his HIV status may be revealed. All public officials involved with
testing agree that confidentiality of test results cannot be guaranteed.
Even if the client uses an anonymous test site and results are identified
only by number, in the emotional crisis of receiving a positive test result
the person may inadvertently reveal his secret to someone else. Furthermore, blood is sometimes tested without consent in hospitals before
procedures are performed or with consent as a prerequisite to a surgical
procedure. However, if a positive test result is to have any benefit, then
diagnosis has to be revealed through a medical system that can provide
follow-up and treatment. While there are standards governing confidentiality of medical records, anyone who works in this field knows clients
whose rights to privacy have been violated. As a part of the pre- and
post-test counseling, clients should be advised of the social and political
consequences of revelation, as well as the emotional and physical consequences of enforced secrecy.

The freedom to change jobs or make a drastic career change can be
crucial to a newly diagnosed client who is determined to give meaning to
his illness by using it as an opportunity to explore more fulfilling
vocational paths. Such aspirations, unfortunately, can be difficult to
actualize. Despite anti-discrimination statutes, employers who have access to insurance records often find reasons to discharge the client. The
Justice Department's infamous ruling that people could be discharged
from employment because of *fear* of contagion rather than the actual

possibility of contagion further jeopardizes the economic well-being of those who choose to be tested.

Clinicians must help clients grasp the precarious nature of confidentiality when counseling about the advisability of testing. Physicians and other health-care professionals may falsely imply that HIV status can be limited to a few intimates in order to reassure the client and thus preserve the doctor/patient relationship. The promise of confidentiality to a person whose civil liberties are in continual jeopardy is often the helping person's way of building an illusion of shelter that seduces the client into testing and medical follow-up. Sensing the vulnerability of these clients in a hostile social system, feeling helpless to protect them from the harsh reality of their diagnosis, we may wish to offer them some modicum of hope that, at least, they are protected by us.

SECRECY IN THE FAMILY

Secrecy is as indispensable to human beings as fire and is greatly feared. Both enhance and protect life, yet both can stifle, lay waste, spread out of all control. Both may be used to guard intimacy or to invade it, to nurture or to consume. And each can be turned against itself; barriers of secrecy are set up to guard against secret plots and surreptitious prying, just as fire is used to fight fire. (Bok, 1983, p. 18)

Bok describes the "conflicted ambivalent experience of secrecy" (1983, p.18), reminding us that we must always keep in mind that secrecy contains both aspects, the protective and the harmful. In this section we will look at some of the effects of secrecy maintained in the family and its intimate networks.

Therapy with a family in which a person has AIDS cannot be divorced from the politics of AIDS. The secrecy enforced by family members reflects the attitudes of the larger culture toward the disease they harbor. Families are extremely vulnerable to the social consequences of revelation. As mentioned, they can and do lose housing if the disease is detected; even uninfected children are ostracized at school or forced to leave by parents as well as by teachers who are too frightened and uninformed to deal courageously with parental pressure. Keeping HIV infection a secret within the family and from children who may reveal it can be seen as an attempt to protect the family from outside harm.

Even if family members believe their secret is secure, rumors fly— children overhear whispered truths and inadvertently reveal what they have heard to a friendly teacher or playmate. A child dealing with the grief of family illness or loss—a grief that cannot be fully processed for fear of revealing the secret—may develop behavioral problems in school as he withstands the taunts of other children who have heard the rumor. A parent who decides to reveal the secret to the guidance counselor may add the constraint that it not be revealed to the teacher. Thus, the teacher does not have the information needed to help the child with the behavioral problems. As the teacher feels increasingly ineffective, the child misbehaves even more and the negative cycle escalates until the child is removed from the school. A secret begun as an act of protection becomes another source of shame and failure for the family.

Let us continue this generalized profile of a family's struggle with "the secret." As the child's behavior becomes unmanageable, the mother, who is now ill herself, must deal with her fears for her own future as well as the futures of the children who will survive her. As she loses control over her child, she feels a loss of control over the future—a haunting sense of her own mortality, with "business" left undone. The child's behavior profoundly affects her, stressing her to the point of exhaustion that, in turn, exacerbates her disease process. But she cannot turn to professionals in her community to help, because she fears the consequences of revelation. Even the guidance counselor—the only person to whom she has entrusted the secret—is murmuring that AIDS is beyond her ability to handle. Meanwhile, the child's mourning process is frozen and inaccessible, as he attempts to cope with a bewildering array of emotions in a home environment that silently but clearly warns him to monitor what he says. He has heard the word *virus* or *AIDS* but he has heard it in whispered tones, and he *knows* not to ask questions.

CASE EXAMPLE*

When Wilma lost her new baby to a mysterious disease, she became pregnant shortly thereafter with a replacement child. At the same time, her husband was diagnosed as having AIDS. Wilma tested positive and had an abortion.

It had never occurred to her that her husband could be infected. She began to fight with him wildly, furious that his infection, transmitted to her, had killed their baby; furious that illness brought not a decrease of drugs but an increase to subdue his fear and pain. Her husband's habit

*The therapist was Ruth Mohr.

had destroyed her life, leaving her HIV-positive. Worse, he continued to demand unprotected sex.

Because the family was proud of its stability in the community, the husband's drug use had never been discussed with the children; it had only been an issue for the parents. Like many drug users, Wilma's husband supported the family well, and from the children's perspective he was experienced as a beloved parent attentive to their needs, playful and affectionate, a good teacher of survival skills in a prejudiced world. Bewildered, the children watched their mother rage at their father. Her anger made no sense to them, especially because he was sick now; before the illness she seemed to love him. The husband became angry and bitter. Because Wilma wished to preserve secrecy, she gave her children no coherent explanation. Frightened and confused, the daughter drew closer to her father, nursing him devotedly. How can young children understand or forgive their mother's actions? Yet, these children sensed their mother's pain, too, and censored their own confusion and anger accordingly. Not surprisingly, after the father died the son developed symptoms of encopresis, uncontrollable crying outside the home, and beating up little girls.

Wilma never told the children "the secret." Were she to tell them, the issue of her own infection might arise. Perhaps they would suspect that the baby had died of AIDS, as the father had. She told her children that both had died of cancer. For Wilma, *not* telling the secret was a source of strength. She was able to enforce her own denial, put the illness in the background, and go about her business of raising the children. But it seemed unlikely that the children did not know. Their grandmother had discovered Wilma's HIV infection when she had visited her daughter in the hospital following an operation and seen the HIV precaution sign on the door. Because another uncle had died of AIDS, she knew what the sign meant. Grandmother was known as central switchboard, sharing her gossip with all family members. Wilma had taught her children to keep their counsel, so as to avoid revealing her family secrets to grandmother, so they knew not to ask questions or verbalize their fears.

Wilma moved into her mother's house. The new stability of her family—the meals they shared together, the homework she helped with, her stable job, and her growing sense of confidence—all gave her son strength and his behavior steadily improved. In therapy she learned to identify her fear that he would end up like his father. Gradually, she began to distinguish her son in all his promise and uniqueness from her long-dreaded self-fulfilling prophecy.

Wilma felt that her life was in order. In keeping "the secret" she had protected her family and put the past behind her. She wore brilliant-colored clothes for the session in which she decided to take a break from therapy.

But suddenly her daughter began to fail in school. A teacher intercepted a letter from the daughter to a friend wherein the daughter accused her father of sexual abuse during the time he was home sick with AIDS. Wilma learned from the letter that her daughter had been truant from school to stay home and nurse him. School records confirmed this truancy. Horrified by the allegations of sexual abuse, Wilma spoke to her pediatrician, requesting an HIV test for her daughter. Since she could not bring herself to tell him about her daughter's letter, he must have thought that she was worried because her baby had been infected. Since her daughter was now 12 and in good health, he dismissed her concern and refused to test her daughter.

Although strangely relieved by her pediatrician's casual response, Wilma confronted her daughter again, who now denied the abuse. Wilma became so enraged that she hit her daughter. Realizing that she needed further help, she came back to therapy. Now Wilma's daughter is carrying the secret of whether her father abused her, just as Wilma is carrying a secret about the father's illness and death from AIDS. The therapist worked carefully with Wilma to understand how secrets had been processed in the previous generation. She learned that Wilma's mother had humiliated her daughter publicly by revealing the "secret" of her first menstruation at a family gathering. Wilma believed that any revelation of her secret would lead to public humiliation for her family. She could not believe that information of this nature could be managed. A secret revealed had been the fire that damaged her relationship with her mother, a secret concealed became the fire which laid waste to the relationship between mother and daughter.

While Wilma began to understand that her secret must be revealed to determine whether or not her daughter was abused, she was still reluctant to reveal the story of her husband's drug use, AIDS, and her own infection. When the therapist asked her if she had any experience that the revelation of a shameful secret could be beneficial, she remembered her recent trip with her family to the drug program where she had worked and where she had first met her husband. It was family day. People were partying and awards were being given. A young man rose up to receive a reward for his father who had died, saying, "By telling me about his drug use openly and honestly, my father helped me choose a different path."

For a moment, as if in a vision, Wilma saw her own son standing there on that stage, knowing the truth and being stronger for it. She told herself, *perhaps it could be like that.* Weaving this vision with the limited truths she had been able to share with her children, Wilma began to believe that she could build a new narrative—to let air and light into the closed and secret world of the family.

But shortly after she began to move toward revelation, she had two humiliating experiences with physicians who "treated me like a leper" when she revealed her HIV infection. The balance again tilted toward maintaining secrecy. A year later, she still debates whether secrecy protects her children or harms them. She has come to believe that her daughter was not abused. After all, the children are again doing well and she is feeling all right. So why reveal?

CASE EXAMPLE*

Contrast this family with another family where Carmelita, the mother, carefully discusses with her two older sons the fact that their youngest brother has AIDS. They know that the baby's father died of AIDS and that she, Carmelita, is infected. She gives them all the medical information about AIDS they need and instructs them as to who they can tell and who they cannot. The school must not know, outsiders must not know. The boys guard their secret well, but what cannot be discussed is the boy's fears about their mother's possible death and her own deep feelings about her infection.

These forbidden topics become an emotional secret that organizes the family. Claudio, the oldest boy, becomes almost too good, the quiet protector of his mother, while Ricky, his younger brother, acts up whenever he senses his mother is weakening or depressed. Carmelita continually tells the boys that she wants them to grow up fast and do well, but in her anxiety her behavior changes subtly. As she feels the pressure of foreshortened time, worry about the boys' future causes her to lose her old firmness, upon which they have come to rely. Ricky realizes that if he grows up and does well, she may die. His school failure is reinforced because it seems to keep his mother active and engaged.

In the session Carmelita is at last able to talk about her feelings about HIV infection.

*The therapist was Ruth Mohr.

Therapist: You want to build in the boys a foundation so that they will be able to take care of themselves through education and knowing how to be in the world . . .

Carmelita: Exactly. I want them to understand, so they will know how to function and be a part of society.

Therapist: OK. Now this is different from the way you acted before your diagnosis, when you just told them what to do without any explanation.

Carmelita: Yes . . . I don't know how long I'm going to be around, so they have to understand that this is very important. I guess before, I took it for granted. I didn't have to explain.

Therapist: But since your diagnosis, . . . what has changed is that you're trying to kind of telescope the process . . . to teach them quicker. You explain to them, "You've got to do this because you've got to stand on your own two feet and you have to be able to take care of yourselves." Claudio receives this one way and Ricky receives it another way and perhaps even gets a little angry because he wants you to be around a long, long time. But he may think that, if he doesn't learn how to stand on his own two feet, maybe you will have to stay around.

Carmelita: [*Crying*] I know what my concern is. My concern is that I won't be around. I mean, should they get in trouble, I won't be here. It's really difficult for me, and I don't express that feeling too much because I don't want to burden them, but I think about them not having a father, and then when I think of them not having a mother, you know, being really alone, I know there's nothing that can take the place of mother. It's like I wish there was something I could do to assure them they're gonna be healthy emotionally as well as physically so that they could do the right thing. So that they could be productive and lead happy lives. I've been through quite a bit and I don't want them to have to go through that. [*Each boy, including the baby, tries to comfort her.*]

Therapist: Are the boys used to seeing you cry? Or was this something unusual? You don't cry much.

Carmelita: I don't like for them to see me cry.

This moment opened the secret of the mother's feelings about her foreshortened future and the boys' anxiety, which they had been afraid to express directly. It also led to an open examination of how the diagnosis had changed the pre-illness family structure. The therapist notes that before diagnosis the boys had relied on Carmelita's confident firmness to guide them through the dangers of inner-city life; now they worry about her unsureness and anxiety. Since they sense the unspoken rule that these changes cannot be discussed, their behaviors (Ricky's regressive acting-out, Claudio's adult-like overresponsibility) are strategies for mastering their anxiety. The initial work of therapy involved two tasks: the boys needed to understand the emotional issues that lay behind the changes in their mother, and Carmelita had to identify her old ways of handling her sons, so that under her guidance the family could return in some measure to its pre-illness identity.

WORKING WITH SECRECY: A THERAPIST'S EXPERIENCE

In general, therapists believe that healing involves bringing matters into the open, decoding mysteries, finding solutions to puzzles. However, in the context of AIDS, the issue is seldom clear-cut.

The following case generates questions about ethics, the benefits and harm of secrecy, and the limitations of therapy in the face of insoluble human dilemmas.

I am supervising a couple whose two-year-old child was diagnosed as having contracted AIDS from a transfusion given during an operation in infancy. They tell no one, but they are haunted by fears for the people who have intimate contact with their child—babysitters, preschool personnel, other family members, nieces and nephews. How will all of these people know to protect themselves if he bleeds? Yet the parents remain adamant that if they were to tell anyone, a river of disclosure would surely burst forth and the child would be shunned.

Now four years old, their son is chubby, active, dark-eyed and merry. He has experienced a few terrifying hospitalizations for lung disorders, but he has recovered. A few weeks ago, I was in the playground with my daughter and happened to see him playing with his father. (His father doesn't know me—I am the invisible supervisor behind the one-way mirror.) I stood watching while my child and his crawled through the tunnel to the castle. Secrecy permits the child to have as normal a life as possible. But secrecy also torments the wife, who worries about the inevitable ostracism if the child's illness were revealed; who worries that someone could become infected because he or she was not informed. Secrecy also binds the couple together, strengthening a fragile alliance, placing boundaries between them and their families of origin, to whom they are both deeply attached.

Ironically, both parents were professionals in their forties when they decided on marriage and childbearing to honor their parents' wishes. The wife's ill mother still longed for the grandchild her daughter had been unready to bear; the husband's father, a Holocaust survivor, viewed the birth of this child as a symbolic reparation. Neither grandparent was told that the child was ill.

When the wife's mother dies, she feels a sense of freedom. She begins to wonder why so much of her life has been given over to providing the grandchild for her mother, after years of avoiding motherhood. She realizes that in fulfilling this task she has abandoned the other areas of her life that give her sustenance and define her adult identity. She questions her marriage, the continuance of which has become predicated on this reparative act of raising a child with an illness that she secretly knows will be progressive and fatal. This knowledge introduces an additional layer of secrecy, which she must keep even from her spouse. While she is aware of loving her son deeply, she now allows herself to feel a surge of resentment at the infinite ways in which AIDS dominates her life. She wants to reveal her secret to break her isolation and her dependence on her husband; she wants a more normal life, where friendship and intimacy also exist outside the marriage.

When the husband's father dies, he responds to his grief by clinging to his child and beginning to drink. As his wife pushes for more openness, he becomes even more adamantly opposed to revealing their secret. For the husband, revelation seems to have many meanings. Keeping the secret protects the child from stigma; in this act of protection, he renews his reparative link with his father. Secrecy is also the "wedding ring" that binds their marriage, and revelation could threaten their precarious bond. When denial no longer subdues his fears for the child's future, he begins to drink to medicate his anxiety—to keep "the secret" from awareness. As the marriage cracks under the strain of illness and secrecy, no family therapy guidelines emerge to give comfort, no solutions appear to resolve the terrible ambiguity of the secret's many meanings.

For us, supervision becomes a series of debates about the politics and ethics of secret-keeping. There is no doubt that family dynamics become intertwined with the politics of the AIDS epidemic as it is experienced in the larger culture. For this particular family, understanding the inner and outer dynamics that brought the parents together, as well as the events that culminated in a child with AIDS, only makes the clinicians and the parents more aware of the prison created by the politics of AIDS in the larger culture. The family's ambivalence about secrecy cannot be understood merely as a drama of family dynamics. Instead it must be recognized as being isomorphic to political and social structures that determine how AIDS is viewed in our society.

In rereading family therapy texts, I have noticed how infrequently the larger political context is included in understanding the internal politics of the family, and how frequently we draw a boundary around the family not unlike the 19th-century boundary shaped by the proverb, "One's home is one's castle." We stand in the doorway of the castle looking in, analyzing what we see *inside* but not understanding the larger location of the castle. Surely the interaction of the castle's inmates with the outside world illuminates what occurs within the castle as clearly as the elaborate, multigenerational genograms we draw so carefully. The issues of AIDS secrecy, of confidentiality and the duty to warn, bring into sharp focus the poignant if unacknowledged interplay between the political and the familial in clinical decision-making. Ultimately, the larger political context binds and weds the secret to the family in a painful unity of disgrace and denial.

CHAPTER 9

Sexuality in the Context
of HIV Infection

DAVID AND SONDRA, AN African-American couple, are ex-drug users in their early twenties who have been together six months. Sondra was physically abused in her last serious relationship, and a year ago she was badly injured in a violent rape. While men seemed frightening to her, her need for love was strong enough to let a man into her heart. She met David, a "cool," handsome young man, who was just completing a drug-treatment program.

"He's my best friend" she says, giggling shyly. "I can tell him anything."

He nods. "I can tell her anything, too—things I could never tell my male friends. She understands me. Sometimes we just talk."

Sondra has a two-year-old son by her abusive partner who lives part-time with her and part-time with her mother. Both women are comfortable with the situation.

As the session gets underway the therapist, Sippio Small, gently asks if he can ask a very personal question. He knows from David, who has brought Sondra to therapy for the first time, that he told her that he was HIV-positive. What does she think about that? Sondra looks at David with melting eyes and says nothing. The therapist tries another approach. "When you are intimate, do you think about any risk?"

Sondra looks at him. "He knows," she says, nodding at David silently. The therapist asks David to fill in Sondra's sentence. As we observe behind the mirror, we are touched by the sweetness of this couple, their tenderness for each other, but we all want to rush in and shout, "Stop! You are killing her! Stop!" Yet we also know that the therapist has to move slowly or Sondra will never come back. He is already on dangerous ground. All the work he has done with David on the need for safer sex is not as useful as sessions in which the couple can confront the issue together.

David says that both he and Sondra dislike rubbers. Sondra adds, "When it's a choice between the feelings and thinking about the infection, you choose the feelings." Delicately the therapist suggests that they have made a choice not to use safer sex. He again attempts to elicit Sondra's degree of information about David's infection. After a few moments of silence she answers, "You see, I don't want to think about it. I always had a dream of a house and two children – a son and a daughter – and a car and a man I loved. I don't want to think I can't have that dream."

The therapist asks if she has been tested. Yes, she has been tested three times: twice just after the rape and once recently.

The first two tests were negative; the last test was inconclusive and it was suggested that she be tested again. However, she doesn't want to know with certainty because if she were positive, then she probably would have another abortion if she were to become pregnant. She has been pregnant twice by David – the first time she had an abortion and the second time she miscarried. She wanted the child she miscarried. No, she doesn't want to know. The therapist holds his feelings in check, making no move to persuade them to use safer sex. He strives simply and gently to connect with her, to build a rapport, so that she will feel safe enough to return.

When the dreams a person has held for a lifetime are at stake, it is only human to deny and go on dreaming.

SOCIAL, CULTURAL, AND PSYCHOLOGICAL IMPEDIMENTS TO SAFER SEX

At present the use of safer sex is the only way to prevent infection and arrest the AIDS epidemic. Although this need is clear and most people have access to information about safer sex, changing sexual practices is a psychologically complex. Erotic experience is infused with multiple meanings derived from political, cultural, familial, and individual history. Furthermore, the meaning of sexuality changes as the adult ages and experiences different psychological and social needs (Gagnon, 1989).

As mentioned, the politics of poverty and race give childbearing enormous weight for both partners. Job opportunities are slim for David as a young African-American male. Lack of access to power and respectability jeopardizes his sense of masculine identity, and also makes him vulnerable to continued drug use. With Sondra, he can feel like a man; like Sondra, he dreams of children who will love, respect, and validate him. Since his future always seems to hang in jeopardy (the statistics on early death for young African-American males were disproportionately high before HIV infection), he tends to focus on the present and its immediate fulfillment of desire. Even if he decided to use safer sex to protect Sondra, his vulnerability to drug use would impair the judgment and planning needed to follow through on his decision. The virus is invisible; pleasures of the moment are tangible and may not come again. The dream of children with their promise of a future remains more compelling than the possibility of infection for Sondra and her unborn child.

Culturally conditioned gender premises also shape fundamental beliefs about the relationship between sexual behavior and the construction of socially appropriated gender identity. For example, in many traditional cultures the woman may need to be submissive to her man in bed in order to feel deeply feminine and sexually appealing. Denying her own needs in the interests of becoming a pleasing object for her man's desire, receiving pleasure by seeing herself reflected in his delight, may be as profoundly important to her as the experiences of dominance and conquest are to him. As a result, the negotiation necessary to ensure safer-sex practice assumes a sexual assertiveness that flies in the face of her traditional values, just as negotiation for the man symbolizes a vulnerability that is at odds with his culturally prescribed macho power.

In traditional cultures reproduction tends to be inexorably tied to sexuality. In the African-American culture children embody the hope of a future that was denied the parent and represent community survival. Condom use both violates the sexual intimacy of the relationship and suggests an immorality that is at odds with the couple's mythology about their sexual encounters. The more committed the relationship, the more the partners may deny the risk that infection—an outside, invisible element—could contaminate the closeness they share and value deeply.

In the Latino culture discussion of sexuality between men and women is also inappropriate. As a result, men and women may not be aware of each other's sexual past and women are certainly not aware that their men may engage in same-sex sexual activity (Stuntzner-Gibson, 1991). A Latino man who has recreational sex with men but is the insertive partner may not define himself as "homosexual" and so not perceive that he is at risk. *Machismo*, which is connected to heterosexuality, is as important for men as *marianismo* is for women. Worth and Rodriguez (1987) have written that Latino culture equates purity and sexual inexperience in women with attractiveness. "Men are seen as seducers of the inexperienced (sexually uneducated) women. A woman prepared for sex (e.g., carrying condoms) is perceived to be experienced, loose and therefore unattractive" (p. 6). By the same token, if men propose condom use women may perceive them as wanting sex for pleasure and not for marriage and childbearing (Stuntzner-Gibson, 1991; Worth & Rodriguez, 1987). If the partners are in a committed relationship, the request for condom use constitutes an implication of sexual betrayal, of "messing around" outside the relationship.

Family history and individual experience also define the meaning a couple gives to their erotic life. Both Sondra and David were sexually abused as children—David by an uncle; Sondra by her stepfather. Sondra was also physically abused by her son's father. David's mother committed suicide when he was ten, driven to it by his boxer father's physical abuse. After her death the father abandoned the family, and David and his half-brother were raised by his maternal grandmother. Since David's brother was psychotic, he absorbed all his grandmother's attention and attachment. David first turned to his uncle for affection, who returned it with the added ingredient of sexual abuse. When David was 15, he ran off with a woman who would have been approximately his mother's age, had she lived. When that relationship failed, he turned to male prostitution as a way of obtaining food and shelter.

David attributes his HIV infection to this period in his life. Male prostitution was a complex experience for David. On the one hand, the men he slept with often gave him the affection and caring he craved. On the other hand, the very pleasure he experienced filled him with shame. The stigma of same-sex experiences in his culture made him question his very masculinity. While David may be truly bisexual, he must hide same-sex attractions and relationships from others and even from himself. For David, infection signifies "punishment" for his past sexual deviances and continuously reminds him of stigmatized sexual experiences. In the world that David inhabits—the therapeutic community of ex-addicts and the street community of drug users—homosexuality is stigmatized, despite the fact that many, like David, have had experiences as male prostitutes. For these reason, David finds it is critical to show to himself and others that he is a man in the traditional heterosexual sense—and what better way than to impregnate his partner?

Additional family factors probably influenced David's attraction to Sondra. He fell in love with her shortly after the violent rape, and his gentleness with her could be seen as a fulfillment of the rescue he did not achieve for his mother against his violent father. Moreover, since David has lost touch with his young son, as his father did with him, he yearns to father a child with whom he vows to be close. Yet if Sondra has unprotected sex with him in the interests of becoming pregnant, he may destroy her life as his father did his mother's. These irreconcilable needs create enormous tension, which pushes him toward drug use—and drug use makes it less likely that he will have the foresight or restraint to protect Sondra by using safer sex.

Sondra has to deal with the fallout of sexual abuse: shame and a poor self-image. Abusive adult relationships and drug use are common outcomes of child sexual abuse. Denying the reality of abuse is another common strategy for dealing with it without losing the relationship. Drugs dulled the pain of Sondra's childhood and allowed her to manage her previous abusive relationship. When she entered the relationship with David, she was drug-free and full of hope. As a result she overvalued David's seeming gentleness, ignoring the danger signs of his continual slips into cocaine use and the way he "messes with her feelings" (David's words) by dating other women and refusing to use condoms.

MORALISM AND SAFER SEX

The historical location of the AIDS epidemic in a conservative era following a period of sexual experimentation for both homosexuals and heterosexuals must be well understood in relation to the negative cultural and political meanings attributed to HIV infection and the sexuality which is its cause. Therapists who focus on safer sex must address these meanings, understanding that safer sex is not about changing people's private sense of sexual morality or what satisfies them in the area of relationships. It is merely about finding the most effective means of preventing the spread of a virus while preserving the possibility of a satisfying, intimate, and erotic life.

For many people the association of sexual behavior that was previously celebrated with disease and death suddenly questioned their right to take pleasure in any sex outside monogamous relationships. It was easy to view HIV infection as the wages of sin or a warning to abandon "promiscuity" in favor of monogamy. One result of such questioning has been the "sexual addiction" movement, as Dennis Altman (1987) has noted in his excellent book, *AIDS in the Minds of America.* This recent movement, which often gets attached to safer sex counseling, is a conservative ideological reaction to the sexual permissiveness of the sixties and seventies. Its basic premise is that multiple sexual conquests are powerful addictions similar to alcohol and drugs, a substitute for real intimacy, sharing, and a committed relationship. It assumes that those who have multiple sexual partners are in the grip of an uncontrollable force, which demands a 12-step program for correction. Many gay men, impelled by the AIDS epidemic to renounce sexual practices associated with HIV infection, joined this movement (Altman, 1987). That many therapists have lent a quasi-scientific authenticity to what is essentially a political and moral movement should be viewed with alarm by clinicians who are counseling people about safer sex.

In terms of preventing the spread of a sexually transmitted viral infection, the introduction of moralism, in fact, can be bad for one's health when monogamy or even heterosexual sex becomes equated with protection against infection. "I lived a clean life," women tell us, not realizing that their monogamous partners have been living other lives. Protected by virtue, they do not think to take precautionary steps. Moralism also leads to shame about past behaviors, which is not useful unless those behaviors have been intentionally harmful to others. As noted, for gay men such shame has often led to making "bargains with God" in return for health—those vows of celibacy that frequently are doomed to end in risky, bingeing behavior.

In terms of counseling it is easier to help people change behaviors in the direction of safety if they can construct a positive rather than a shameful story about their past sexual experiences. David's shame about his past homosexual experiences shapes his current relationship with Sondra. In a culture more accepting of diversity and fluidity of erotic experience, David might feel more at ease with incorporating same- and opposite-sex experiences into a more positive view of himself. Perhaps the overall success of safer sex education workshops in gay communities reflects a political evolution that effectively counters the homophobic rhetoric of the larger culture with a pride in community and a determination to survive. As a result, an extraordinary number of gay men have been able to modify their sexual practices by utilizing community support groups, safer-sex workshops, education programs, or simply networks of gay friends promoting the ethos of personal and community survival.

Dennis Altman (1987) wisely cautions that the gay community is by no means monolithic: many men who engage in homosexual acts are actively hostile to gay men and to the idea of a gay community or gay leadership. One such group, which has been extremely hard to reach, are gay and bisexual men in the African-American and Latino communities. For these men, like David, the primary identity is ethnic and community mores impose strong prohibitions against a homosexual self-definition.

CLINICAL CONSIDERATIONS OF
SAFER SEX

Ideally, issues of safer sex are best introduced in the flow of the therapeutic conversation. However, therapists must be willing to take the lead in raising the issue whenever they think it is necessary. Often, clients and therapists collude in avoiding a detailed discussion of sexual practice in any therapy, much less discussing as loaded an issue as HIV infection. Such avoidance could cost clients their lives. Simply offering information about safer sex is also not sufficient. Rather, an interventive stance is recommended.

Some safe-sex advocates have argued that people should practice *absolutely* safe sex: sex that does not permit penetration even with a condom and avoids deep kissing. If we understand that there is no moment in our lives when we are free from risk, then we will balance our needs for pleasure and intimacy with an evaluation of *acceptable* risk. Obviously, the incorporation of safer sex into everyday life will be more successful if it is satisfying physically and emotionally, even if these sexual practices do not meet the most rigid criteria of safety.

The goal of discussing safer sex in therapy is to make sure that clients are protected and protective as well as comfortable. An English gay man has summarized the ideal of learned safer-sex behaviors (Rampton, 1989):

> I found myself looking at what I was doing, asking if I was liking it, and finding out how I could continue to enjoy it without taking any risks . . . . Then came the memorable occasion when I spent the night with somebody and I suddenly realized I hadn't had to consciously think about keeping to what is safe. And that was a real breakthrough, because it meant that I'd become comfortable with safe sex and enjoyed the positive,

imaginative side of it, rather than just being stuck with the negative, difficult side of it all. (p. 142)

Often the therapist opens the discussion of safer sex in the first session and then drops the issue like the proverbial hot potato. The issue of safer sex must be explored frequently and at different stages in the course of therapy. New behaviors are hard to learn, and people at risk for infection often become desensitized to the risk over time. The development of a stable relationship has been shown to diminish perception of risk, even if the partners have not been tested. When partners are known to be negative, they are not likely to practice safer sex in encounters outside the relationship.

The therapist must be willing to talk openly and in detail about sex, recognizing that safer sex for the client must *not* be a matter of obeying rules; rather, it is a sensitive area of personal choice, made in negotiation with the partner. Sexual practices will vary in degree of risk, and each client must assess what level of risk is comfortable for him or her. If the therapist is able to remain nonjudgmental, the conversation around sexuality will remain open and reflective of actual practice. Shame about "slipping" or deciding to perform sexual acts regarded by the therapist as "risky" can drive discourse about sex into the closet.

Knowing what constitutes *absolutely* safe sex is not complicated. Since the virus is transmitted by bodily fluids, most particularly semen, preventing the entrance of semen, vaginal fluids and blood from one person into another is practicing safer sex.

Clients and their partners must be able to identify absolutely safe sexual practices as well as those that entail some degree of risk. For example, dry kissing, mutual masturbation, "on me, not in me" orgasms, body rubbing, massage, and exploration of non-genital erogenous zones, bathing and showering together, are all safe-sex activities. Although deep kissing has not been proven to be a means of viral transmission, it could contain some degree of risk. The use of vibrators or other sexual equipment falls within the area of safe sex only if the equipment is cleaned adequately when exchanged between partners. Anal or vaginal intercourse with a condom, correctly used, falls within the area of safer sex but is not absolutely safe. Lower-risk vaginal or anal intercourse requires both condom use and withdrawal of the penis before ejaculation. Vaginal or anal intercourse without a condom is a high-risk activity even if the insertive partner withdraws before ejaculation because pre-ejaculation fluids contain the virus.

Unprotected oral sex is a subject of controversy. Initially there were few documented cases where oral transmission was the only risk factor. Later studies of infected gay men suggest that there are a number of infected gay men for whom unprotected oral sex was the only risk factor. During oral sex the ingestion of semen and vaginal fluids are hypothesized to be infectious since the mucous membranes of the mouth come into contact with vaginal secretions, menstrual blood, or semen. In the United States, organizations such as Gay Men's Health Crisis recommend the use of condoms during oral sex; in Canada unprotected oral sex is considered to be a safer-sex activity. Most studies show that unprotected oral sex is still common among gay men.

Condoms

The therapist must be able to convey the following rules for safer sex in a simple and clear manner. Men and women who are sexually active should be familiar with condom use. During vaginal and anal intercourse and fellatio, latex condoms, when properly used, have been proven to be effective in preventing the transmission of the HIV virus. Natural membrane condoms should not be used because they contain pores through which the virus can pass. Ribbed or textured condoms, while increasing stimulation, can cause abrasions that increase vulnerability in sensitive membranes to the entrance of HIV infection.

The condom should be put on the erect penis before entering the vagina, anus, or mouth. This is important because pre-ejaculation fluids contain virus. The tip of the penis should be placed against the inside of the condom and the condom rolled down to the base. A small space should be left at the condom's tip as an airspace to keep the condom from bursting upon ejaculation. Some condoms are sold precoated with 5% non-oxynol 9, a spermicide. If not, a drop of KY jelly, which contains non-oxynol 9, can be placed in the tip of the condom for additional protection and lubrication. However, care should be taken to restrict the amount of lubrication inside the condom to decrease the chances of the condom's slipping off during intercourse.

Water-based lubricants containing non-oxynol 9 should be used on the outside of the condom. Oil based lubricants such as Vaseline can damage latex and should never be used. Nor should the insertive partner's saliva ever be used. During withdrawal, the rim of the condom should be held tightly against the penis so that the condom cannot slip off. While condoms do not break easily when used properly, there is always some risk. The likelihood of condom breakage in penile-anal intercourse is upwards of 20 percent; for that reason persons engaging in anal intercourse may wish to use two condoms or to withdraw before ejaculation. If withdrawal follows ejaculation, it should occur before the penis becomes detumescent. Since condoms may deteriorate with age, the user should note the expiration date and make sure that condoms are stored away from heat and sunlight. *Condoms should never be reused.*

Sexualizing condom use as a part of foreplay can diminish the shameful aspects that remind the couple of infection. Bateson and Goldsby (1988) pointed out that condoms have been used as sex toys for years in Japan; they stress that culturally conditioned attiudes toward condom use may be culturally reconditioned. In *Women and AIDS* (1988), Diane Richardson points out that condoms can make sex more exciting. Condoms can help men who climax too quickly delay ejaculation and thus give their partner more pleasure. For men who have trouble sustaining an erection, a tightly fitting condom may make erections harder and orgasms more intense. Lubricated condoms may also make sex easier for women who suffer from vaginal dryness (Richardson, 1988).

Hepworth and Shernoff (1989) have suggested that encouraging men to purchase a variety of latex condoms and to experiment with putting them on and masturbating when alone is an excellent way to increase comfort with condom use. Further practical suggestions include breaking a condom while masturbating, either alone or with a partner, to learn how much stress condoms can take and what they feel like when torn.

Sponge and Diaphragm

Condoms are the best protection from the virus currently available. However, the need to rely on men's willingness to use condoms can present insurmountable problems for women. Some research is focusing on the development of effective prophylaxis against HIV infection that can be used by women. A condom for women, "Reality," is now being tested; it seems to be safe and has been well accepted by the sexual partners of the women who volunteered for the clinical studies (Leeper, 1990). The sponge and diaphragm used with spermicide are only partial solutions for women whose partners refuse safer sex. Leaving the relationship—an option which may not be economically and emotionally viable—would be the only sure solution.

Oral and Manual Protection

Although there have been few documented cases of HIV transmission through oral sex, some risk is always present: The virus contained in vaginal fluid or semen could enter the body through small abrasions in the mouth. As a result, safer sex would require the use of condoms during oral sex with a man; dental dams can be used in oral sex with women or in rimming (oral-anal contact). Dental dams, which are squares of thin latex, can be purchased at medical supply stores. The dam must be rinsed first to remove any substances and then dried. The dam should cover the entire vulva or anus and should be held at both sides. One must be careful not to turn the dam inside out during oral sex, since this would defeat the purpose of using it. *Dental dams should not be reused.*

During manual stimulation of the anus or vagina, or fisting, use of surgical gloves will provide absolute protection of the hands from virus introduced thorugh small cuts. Fisting (the insertion of the entire hand into the rectum and balling it up into a fist) has its dangers because it may cause tears in the walls of the rectum, which make it vulnerable to infection. As with condoms and dental dams, surgical gloves should never be reused.

Since a small amount of virus is present in urine, people who engage in "water sports" should avoid getting urine in the eyes or in any open sores.

Those involved in "S and M" (sado-masochistic sexual practices) must prevent the introduction of blood from one partner into the other.

Kissing

The spread of virus from saliva is rare, perhaps because of a protein which has been found to inhibit HIV's ability to enter a cell. This protein may provide a natural barrier to infection through exchange of saliva (Altman, 1995b). These findings confirm that deep kissing is an extremely low-risk sexual activity. However, some couples will not be able to get past their fear of infection, and such reluctance should be understood and accepted. Logic and scientific studies are not antidotes to primitive fears.

Painful Associations

While using safer sex has obviously positive aspects for preserving a relationship, there are also painful associations. Work must initially focus on helping clients mourn the loss of their customary sexual practices (Palacios-Jimenez & Shernoff, 1986). Exploration of negative feelings associated with HIV infection and sexuality must precede instruction in safer-sex techniques. Unless these feelings are addressed, they may interfere with the learning and utilization of safer-sex practices.

Condom use has the positive meaning of loving protectiveness, but it also signifies a diminution of freedom that characterizes normal sexual activity. Condom use may remind the couple of the presence of the virus and the possibility of illness and death. Inhibited sexual desire may be a defense against the fear that sex, no matter how safe, will result in contamination.

One client spoke about his inability to separate the positive aspects of sexuality from his knowledge that it has resulted in what is tantamount to a death sentence. Another man spoke of religious experience as having replaced sexuality now that he is faced with death. While he has a lover whom he cares about greatly, he feels no desire. Another couple who once had a passionate sexual relationship was shattered by successive diagnoses of AIDS and the belief that the more promiscuous partner had caused the other's infection. Unresolved issues of internalized homophobia in the more closeted partner resulted in a sexual stalemate, as sex became equated with immorality and punishment.

Women such as Sondra may experience safer sex as a painful reminder that they can never have children without fearing for the fetus and themselves; in denial, they choose unprotected sex to sustain their dreams of normal pregnancies. Uninfected women and women who have not been tested have also reported that they feel protective of their infected partners and do not wish to remind them (or themselves) of illness by insisting on condom use. Women's gendered learnings to put the needs and feelings of others above their own are deeply engrained and not subject to simple instruction about safer-sex practices.

"Survivor guilt" can also dissuade a non-infected partners from using safer sex. I worked with a well-educated gay couple in their twenties who were not using safer sex. They are deeply in love with each other, with all the passion of the very young. Peter has tested positive and is showing the first signs of the disease: night fevers, diarrhea, weight loss that begins to show the outline of bone beneath the skin. Michael believes it is he who should die; he was the promiscuous, drug-using partner, while Peter remained faithful and good.

They have been together seven years now and neither feels he could survive the loss of the other. For Michael, asking Peter to use a condom would only remind both of them of the disease at the moment when the sweetness of lovemaking makes them most vulnerable to feelings of loss.

"I am so frightened for him," Michael says, his young eyes filling with tears. Their dream is to die together – a contemporary version of Romeo and Juliet . . . an AIDS suicide pact.

PLEASURABLE ASPECTS

Following the exploration of negative feelings, the therapist should discuss the positive and pleasurable aspects of safer sex. Negotiating safer sex can be seen as a way for couples to deepen their relationships and experience new definitions of themselves as men and women. In a heterosexual couple the man has to learn to be more aware of his partner's needs and more willing to negotiate; the woman, to become more assertive. Many women, whose partners have been receptive to their wishes for safer sex, report that the ability to negotitate sexuality and be open to their own needs and erotic preferences is liberating.

In the wake of the epidemic, and perhaps also because there is more social support available for gay committed relationships, some gay men have sought to change their sense of sexual identity, from a person who defines himself by numerous sexual conquests to one who negotiates and sustains committed relationships. Because a degree of reciprocity and trust must be established before safer sex can be negotiated, the imperative of safer sex may lead people to a more intimate understanding of each other before they engage in intercourse.

Bateson and Goldsby (1988) make an elegant argument for revising the cultural premises that define sexual experience, an argument which could serve as the underlying philosophy of safer-sex education:

> The relatively late cultural elaboration of sexuality has had a number of costs. First you cannot purposefully regulate or reshape an area of behavior you are determined to ignore. Neither can you enhance or enrich it . . . . You cannot introduce choice, caution and discrimination into behavior you believe you cannot control. Gluttony emphasizes impulse, while gourmet eating emphasizes moderation and selection, for subtle flavors are lost in excess; if moderation ceased to be associated with repression, a sexual aesthetic might emerge based on subtlety and careful timing, for sometimes waiting increases pleasure. Sex for the gourmet rather than the gourmand. (p. 106)

We have found two books particularly useful in helping the clinician develop a gourmet's attitude towards safer-sex practices: Luis Palacios-Jimenez and Michael Shernoff's *Eroticizing Safer Sex* and Diane Richardson's *Women and AIDS*. Both books describe in detail erotic practices which are safe and pleasurable.

While the successful negotiation of a protective sexual relationship may be extremely positive in the end, in the beginning most people find the negotiation of each new sexual encounter to be awkward and painful. Typically, sexuality has not been an arena of honest communication and respectful negotiation between partners, but rather one where passion and impulse rule. For the sero-positive person each new sexual encounter can be difficult, as desire must be held in check until safer sex can be proposed and the subsequent questions comfortably answered. Ultimately, disclosure of sero-positivity and the need for condom use may threaten the loss of a critical relationship at a time when the person is most dependent on the relationship. "What if he leaves me and I die alone?" client after client asks.

ISSUES OF SAFER SEX FOR THERAPISTS: DEALING WITH THE URGENCY

Safer-sex conversations touch sensitive nerves in therapists as well as clients. Therapists will have strong feelings about the urgency of safer sex—feelings that may make it difficult to work through patiently the turbulent emotions that are activated. The deconstruction of the sexual feelings that lead to unsafe sex often go to the heart of erotic desire—a territory crowded by complex early relationships that are played out in adult erotic games. If therapists do not address the erotic meanings of sexual behavior, all good intentions for responsible sexual behavior can be swept aside by the onslaught of compulsive desire.

Frequently, clients test therapists. People who carry a sero-positive status have often experienced discrimination *prior* to diagnosis, as members of stigmatized groups or as partners of people who are stigmatized. A gay client who senses a therapist's discomfort with homosexuality may leave therapy if the therapist does not make his feelings an open subject for discussion. Or a client may interpret a therapist's negative feelings about a specific behavior as a more generalized antipathy to homosexuality. A non-hierarchical stance, open dialogue, and the willingness of the therapist to make therapy a collaborative, *human* encounter are crucial elements in the healing relationship.

The following case example, in which I function as supervisor, deals with the bogeyman for therapists who work with sero-positive, ARC, and AIDS patients: the client who seems to be irresponsibly spreading infection, despite a knowledge of safer sex. These clients often arouse a paralyzing anxiety in therapists. The case illustrates the danger of allowing anxiety, fear, and dislike for what one is powerless to control to dominate the relationship; in addition, it suggests strategies for dealing with therapist anxiety and client resistance.

CASE EXAMPLE

Solomon had sought treatment for support in dealing with his recent sero-positive test result. In the first session Solomon reported that he often went cruising and had unsafe sex with young men he picked up. He did not feel that he was putting them at great risk because they were only performing fellatio on him—a relatively safe practice, though not to be recommended. As Solomon discussed the issue with the therapist, he showed no remorse or desire to change his sexual practices. While the team seemed upset by Solomon's apparent indifference to the consequences of his actions, as supervisor I believed that Solomon's having brought the subject to therapy was a sign of his decent intention, which should be respected.

When I returned after two weeks' absence, Solomon had missed the last session and the therapist worried that he might stop coming to therapy altogether. I was concerned about what seemed to be a growing dislike on the part of the therapist and the team for Solomon, who was, admittedly, a rather challenging, angry man in his late twenties. Nonetheless, the therapist was a remarkably sensitive woman, who valued her ability to establish close relationships with clients. In this case, however, she felt repeatedly challenged by Solomon to dislike him; he seemed to sense her feelings and strove to escalate the discomfort.

In his second session, he had described his cruising in even greater detail: He would go to the park and meet young men, boys even, who would perform fellatio on him; then he would warn them in a fatherly fashion to not do "it" with anyone else. The therapist asked him if he felt any remorse. He seemed surprised by the question and answered, "Not particularly. Why should I?" She then asked him why he felt compelled to tell her these things if he had no feelings of guilt. He said he supposed he *should* feel guilty, but just didn't—and that was all. The team tried to help him heighten his anxiety about the health risk to the young men who had sex with him by asking him to explore his own feelings of anger about his infection. He merely became more stubborn and resistant, and missed his next appointment.

I asked the therapist what she understood about his compulsion to confess his cruising to her, the stated absence of remorse, his seeming challenge to her to reject him. Together we outlined a psychodynamic hypothesis, which linked past to present.

Solomon was an older child whose mother had borne twins when he was five years old. The twins had dominated family life, consuming her attention and affection. After the twins' birth, he lost access to his mother, who seemed to favor the twins. Whenever Solomon expressed his anger towards the twins, his mother protected them and was punitive toward him. Over time he learned to accept his peripheral position in the family, but inside he became a sullen rebel. We looked at his behavior with the younger men as being a mixture of the anger he felt toward his twin brothers, his need to dominate them, and protectiveness, which was the behavior prescribed by his mother. Solomon's open challenge to the therapist was a repetition of this earlier pattern, which held the hope that she would not abandon him and the conflicting belief that she would.

This hypothesis shifted the therapist's feelings about Solomon. While his behavior could not be condoned since it put others at risk, we agreed that we could accept his repetitive descriptions of the sexual encounters as a legitimate call for help in handling a bewildering sexual obsession. While he was not aware of actual feelings of remorse, his need to reiterate his sexual encounters to a therapist—who is an agent of both change and social control—could be viewed as reflecting an underlying decency. This gave us a radically different narrative from the previous one of hostility and sexual irresponsibility. Once a more positive view of Solomon had been established, the problem could be deconstructed by linking it to the past and the tension between the two narratives explored.

The first step was for the therapist to telephone Solomon and openly discuss her ambivalence about his behavior: her angry and protective feelings for the young men he was having sex with, as well as her respect for him as a person who was seeking help with a difficult subject. Solomon told her that after the last session, sensing the therapist's and team's hostility, he had sought treatment elsewhere. Nevertheless, the therapist felt that the conversation was helpful to her in clearing the air, and that Solomon was more open to her then than during any of the sessions. They parted with good feelings.

As we reflected on our failure to help Solomon in therapy, we learned several valuable lessons about ourselves. Solomon's behavior had raised difficult moral issues that are central to work with infected persons in this epidemic. What is our role when we know that high-risk behaviors are taking place? When is taking a moral stand helpful to the client? When do we need to take the time to fully understand the meaning of the client's erotic experience, even in the urgency raised by unsafe behaviors? How do countertransference issues affect the therapy?

In retrospect, the therapist's telephone conversation created the open dialogue which should have taken place in the therapy. The feelings aroused by AIDS are often frightening to the therapist, who is then faced with the choice between revealing intensely negative feelings and losing rapport, on the one hand, and trying to hide feelings in the interest of maintaining neutrality and creating an accepting attitude, on the other. Compounding the tension in this particular case was the client's suspicion that a heterosexual woman would secretly despise him. This expectation was projected onto the therapist, whose behavior then began to mirror his beliefs.

As we examined our vulnerability to Solomon's behavior, we realized that we recently had lost many friends and clients to AIDS, and we felt angry and protective of people who might become infected. Solomon, as a kind of Typhoid Mary, had become the bogeyman of the epidemic, magnetizing our feelings of grief and our anger at our own impotence. A superior, even scornful moral stance had become our defense against that impotence. The implicit hierarchy of therapy had permitted this distancing. The development of a different dialogue with the client, in which the therapist was able to describe openly both her positive and negative feelings, would have created a more human encounter—one that would have allowed client and therapist to construct a double narrative reflecting the complexity of Solomon's experience, thus making it comprehensible and potentially open to change.

CHAPTER 10
Living With AIDS:
The Symptomatic Phase

T HE TERM *AIDS* is often misconstrued to mean a single disease rather than the syndrome of infections and diseases that comprise the symptomatic phase of HIV infection. The course of HIV disease is unpredictable in that it can be affected by many factors: the virulence of the virus itself, emotional stress, healthy or unhealthy life style, the natural vigorousness of an individual immune system, exposure to pathogens or reexposure to different viral strains, response to antiviral medication or to medications for opportunistic infections. The idiosyncratic nature of the illness has repercussions on all levels: medical, psychosocial, familial, relationship, and of course, personal.

THE MEDICAL OVERVIEW

HIV is a retrovirus that enters certain types of white blood cells (most particularly CD4 cells and macrophage-type cells of the immune system) as RNA, replicates into DNA, and is then incorporated into the cell's genetic code. These infected cells manufacture at least 110 million virus particles a day. Following HIV infection, the immune system engages in a furious battle to clear out free virus and to search out and destroy newly infected cells before a completed virus is released. Between 100 million and one billion free virus particles are produced and cleared daily, a turnover of about 30 percent of the total found in each infected individual. To replace CD4 cells lost in battle, the immune system must produce approximately 2 billion new cells each day. For an indeterminate period of time the immune system holds its own but gradually, for most people, the HIV begins to pull ahead, replicating faster than CD4 cells can reproduce (Austin, 1995). Medications such as AZT, ddI, ddC, and the newer protease inhibitors may be used to assist in preventing viral replication and allowing the immune system to rebuild its amount of available CD4 cells, but eventually the virus outwits the medication and creates resistant strains (Austin, 1995; Ho, 1995; Kolata, 1995a, 1995b; Shaw, 1995). "Cocktails" of 2 or more medications (e.g., AZT with 3Td) have been used to mount a multi-pronged attack; it appears that when the virus becomes resistant to one drug, it loses its resistance to the other (Cohen, 1995). Unfortunately, the virus has a major advantage: It rapidly stores a reserve army of virus in the lymph system and bone marrow which cannot be eradicated by current medications.

Repeated immune screenings during the course of infection ascertain how the immune system is faring vis-à-vis the number of CD4 lymphocytes available to fight HIV. Evidence that a person is at risk for acquiring opportunistic infections may be derived from a fall in the number of CD4 lymphocytes, and from physical symptoms such as swollen lymph nodes, persistent fatigue, and night sweats. As HIV destroys an increasing number of CD4-helper cells, the body becomes susceptible to a number of microbes to which an intact immune system would not ordinarily be vulnerable. These microbes cause what are termed opportunistic infections. The most common is pneumocystis carinii pneumonia (PCP), which is caused by a parasite and which often starts with a fever of unknown origin and may be present for months with increasing fever, shortness of breath, and cough. PCP was a primary cause of AIDS death, but with more physicians aware that if the T-cell count falls below 250, prophylaxis against PCP (Dapsone, Bactrim, or aerosolized Pentamidine) is necessary, mortality from PCP has declined.

Kaposi's sarcoma (KS) (a rare form of skin cancer) can invade the mouth and internal organs but is most known for its purplish lesions which, like the wasting caused by Mycobacterium avium complex (MAC), symbolize in the public imagination the horrors of AIDS' disfiguration. Chemotherapy and radiation have been mildly effective in clearing up lesions but not in arresting the course of the illness once it has spread internally. Alpha interferon, too, has been useful in slowing down the disease course but not in arresting the cancer itself. KS is diagnosed almost exclusively in homosexual and bisexual men, and can be sexually transmitted independent of HIV infection. The rate of KS has decreased dramatically since the widespread use of safer sex has reduced the incidence of venereal disease among gay men. Other AIDS-related cancers include B-cell lymphoma, which may attack the brain and are often fatal, as is cervical cancer in women.

TB is a serious and increasingly common disease of HIV-infected people, which causes chronic cough, weight loss, fatigue, fever, and blood in the sputum. TB in AIDS patients can also manifest itself as extrapulmonary TB (pericarditis, osteomyelitis, brain abscesses, TB of the wrist, ankles, intestines, and testes). HIV patients sometimes have a particularly dangerous strain of TB, multiple drug resistant TB, which does not respond to standard drugs. A major issue for patients with active TB is the significant infection rate of close contacts. In New York City, for example, the contact infection rate for TB/AIDS was 21 percent (Landau-Stanton, 1993). A second critical issue is the absolute necessity for patients to complete their course of treatment (nine months of multiple standard drugs) so that the mycobacterium does not become resistant to antibiotic intervention.

Fungal infections are common during the symptomatic stage of AIDS, including candida vaginitis in women and oral, bronchial, and esophagal candidiasis. Cytomegalovirus (CMV), a disseminated opportunistic infection, attacks approximately 90 percent of AIDS patients at some point in their disease (Bartlett & Finkbeiner, 1993). CMV is caused by a herpes virus and can cause infections in many different organs. It can cause symptoms as mild as fevers or as serious as blindness (CMV retinitis) or it can attack pulmonary, gastrointestinal, and central nervous systems. It requires early intervention and is hard to treat and impossible to cure (Bartlett & Finkbeiner).

In the final stages of HIV infection, patients are susceptible to MAC, an extremely serious opportunistic infection that disseminates throughout the body and occurs late in the course of HIV infection; aggressive treatment with antibiotics is required. MAC can attack bone marrow (causing a lowered blood count), the lungs (causing pneumonia), or the liver (causing hepatitus). It can also attack the gastrointestinal tract, causing the wasting, chronic fevers, severe diarrhea, and the familiar skeletal image of the AIDS "victim."

HIV infection opens the person to various assaults on the brain itself which require careful discrimination from nonorganic psychiatric conditions. HIV can infect the brain directly, broaching the blood-brain protective barrier, invading the macrophages of the brain, and causing organic damage to the brain itself. At an early stage of acute infection HIV may cause an encephalitis, and in the chronic phase it may cause the cognitive, motor, and behavioral disturbances which have been called AIDS dementia complex (ADC). These symptoms include memory loss, mood changes (apathy or agitation), decreased concentration, as well as speech and motor symptoms (Landau-Stanton, 1993). AIDS dementia is progressive and may affect as many as 60 percent of AIDS patients. AZT has been shown to have some effectiveness in treating ADC (McEwen & Schmeck, 1994). Other neurological infections are possible, including toxoplasma encephalitis (caused by a parasite found in meat and cat feces), which causes seizures and neurological impairment but can be treated with antibiotics; cytomegalovirus, which attacks the central nervous as well as the gastrointestinal systems; and cryptococcal meningitis, which may be prevented by the use of antifungal drugs. B-cell lymphoma of the brain, once a rare disease, is frequently seen in AIDS patients. Changes in mental functioning due to HIV are among the most distressing symptoms for both the patient and his care system.

Opportunistic infections are responsible for most AIDS deaths. The large number of possible illnesses, each with its own shape, treatment protocol, and particular dangers to different systems of the body, makes the course of a person's illness unpredictable and AIDS treatment a protean task. While most researchers have concentrated on the development of antiviral medications or vaccines, there is increasing pressure from AIDS activists to focus research on effective prophylaxis against the opportunistic infections that actually kill patients. Keeping abreast of research advances in both areas of vaccine and prophylaxis is an ongoing process for therapists working with AIDS patients and their families.

Modes of Onset

The work of family researchers John Rolland and David Reiss has been useful to us in conceptualizing psychosocial issues which arise for patients and families during the active phase of HIV infection (Reiss & Kaplan DeNour, 1989; Rolland, 1984). They have described the various modes of onset that certain illnesses may take and the impact of these onset modes on the patient-family-medical system.

The modes of onset of AIDS are as various as the illnesses that are attached to the syndrome. One mode of onset is a moderately discomforting condition characterized by one or more of the following symptoms: excess fatigue, overall feeling of weakness, loss of appetite, night sweats, swollen lymph nodes, occasional mild fevers, and bronchial disturbances. This phase of HIV infection may follow an episodic course during which moderately symptomatic periods alternate with periods of good health. Or, it may result in a slow, progressive physical deterioration following the first signs of disease, culminating in the occurrence of an opportunistic infection such as pneumocystis pneumonia. The early symptoms of HIV are often difficult to distinguish from the symptoms of everyday illnesses and from the psychosomatic symptoms triggered by the fear and stress of knowing one is infected. Close monitoring of the person's immune functioning can give information as to whether the virus is active and likely to result in vulnerability to opportunistic infections.

A second onset mode, described as "a crescendo of symptoms" (Reiss & Kaplan-DeNour, 1989), is characteristic of a phase when the infected person begins to show increased physical symptoms, but has not yet been inflicted with the major opportunistic infections that are the harbingers of the disease syndrome called AIDS. This cluster of symptoms includes diarrhea, thrush infections, high fevers, repeated fungal infections, loss of appetite, memory loss indicating central nervous system involvement, loss of coordination, progressive generalized lymphadenopathy (disease of the lymph nodes), various neurological symptoms, and early phase wasting syndrome. During this stage the possibility that one of the opportunistic infections marking full-blown AIDS will occur is always present.

The third mode of onset is termed "incidental" (Reiss & Kaplan-DeNour, 1989). During a routine medical exam the patient, who has suffered no discomfort or illness, is found to have cancer, most probably a Kaposi's sarcoma lesion. Kaposi's sarcoma carries an AIDS diagnosis but can be a slow moving disease with many patients reporting having no more than one or two lesions for several years.

The fourth mode of onset, called "the medical thunderbolt", (Reiss & Kaplan-DeNour, 1989), creates a medical emergency, is often life-threatening, and requires immediate hospitalization. Here AIDS is diagnosed in a person who has been in good or relatively good health and who may or may not know that he or she is HIV-positive. Pneumocystis carinii pneumonia (PCP) has classically been a life-threatening illness although prophylaxis and improved hospital treatment have reduced its fatality.

Between times of acute illness the person may have long periods of relatively good health. While fatigue, weight loss, and diarrhea accompany the less acute phases when the patient is not hospitalized, these symptoms may not be severe enough to prevent the patient from engaging in normal activities. After leading a relatively normal life with AIDS, progressive immune deficiency may lead to increasing debilitation, ending in death; or death may come suddenly, when the patient seems to be in relatively good health.

PSYCHOSOCIAL TASKS

The appearance of symptoms associated with HIV infection creates a crisis for both the patient and his/her intimate network. During this period there are a number of key tasks for the ill person and family. These include the needs:

1. to unite for short-term crisis reorganization;
2. to learn to adapt to life with HIV-related symptoms;
3. to manage the medical system and establish relationships with the health-care team;
4. to make decisions about disclosure;
5. to begin the process of planning for the future possibility of incapacitating illness or death.

In addition, there are critical tasks of a more general, sometimes existential nature (Rolland, 1987a,b,c; Tiblier, Walker, & Rolland 1989), which may involve both patient and family. These tasks include:

6. creating a meaning for life with illness that maximizes a preservation of a sense of mastery and competency;
7. grieving for the loss of the pre-illness family identity;
8. developing support networks for the provision of care and to reduce isolation.

Short-Term Crisis Reorganization

Each of the various modes of onset will have implications for how the family manages the disease (Reiss & Kaplan-DeNour, 1989). If illness onset takes the form of a crescendo of symptoms, the person will have more time to make decisions about care and disclosure, and the family will have more time to work through the initial emotions and conflicts. A slow or "incidental" onset allows the person the autonomy and ability to continue managing his life and to organize caretaking within his social network. Often, disclosure and involvement of the family of origin remain unnecessary until later in the disease process.

A "medical thunderbolt" diagnosis often forces the simultaneous revelation of sexual orientation and a potentially fatal disease to an unprepared family in the midst of medical crisis. The emotional roller coaster of feelings that follows such revelations is out of synchrony with the tasks before the family: organizing to provide the patient with emotional and practical support. This acute period finds confused and frightened family members suddenly thrust into the strange, high-tech world of the hospital. Health-care providers need to be exquisitely sensitive to the intense vulnerability of the family and to the enormous impact, both positive and negative, that they can have at this crisis point before the family and patient have absorbed the meaning of illness and adapted to its demands.

The provision of care in an acute medical crisis requires the family to demonstrate high levels of unity and coordinated action (Tiblier, Walker, & Rolland, 1989). However, the family may find itself divided by the inability of some members to deal with the stigma of the disease or with the perceived challenge to family values implicit in the revelation of drug use or homosexuality. Further conflicts arise when family members encounter the lover or gay family. For a partner working through emotions elicited by the discovery of secret drug use or of sexual betrayal, or the shock that an infected partner has knowingly engaged in unprotected sex, time is essential—yet there is very little time in an illness typified by a short life span, where decisions about care have to be made immediately. If, for example, a bisexual or drug user's diagnosis constitutes the first open acknowledgment of deviant behavior, his wife may not wish to continue the marriage, perhaps insisting that his family of origin assume the responsibility for his care or that he live alone. The fury of one wife at her husband's secret bisexual life was such that she told him openly that she wished him dead. Although she reluctantly agreed to take him home at the end of his hospital stay, she ultimately persuaded him to return home to his family to die. That a potentially terminal disease should bring revelations that can shatter relationships even as the patient faces death is an unprecedented tragedy in modern medical history.

Adapting to Life With HIV-Related Symptoms

The chronic phase of AIDS, whether long or short, is the time between the initial diagnosis and readjustment period and the terminal phase.

This chronic phase, as noted, can follow different courses: the relapsing/episodic course characterized by the alternation of stable periods with periods of medical crises or exacerbations; or the constant, progressive course of deterioration (Rolland, 1987a,b,c; Tiblier, Walker, & Rolland, 1989). Most often, given new medications and treatments of opportunistic infections, the relapsing/episodic course predominates with a progressively deteriorating end phase, which can take many years.

It is important to remember that the person with AIDS will spend only about 20 percent of his disease course in the hospital. Caregiving requires family flexibility that permits movement back and forth between two forms of organization: one focused primarily on caregiving and one that allows the ill person to resume some of the normal functioning necessary to psychological well-being. The wide psychological discrepancy between periods of quiescence and those of crisis/exacerbation can be particularly taxing and can affect family structure.

During the acute period the family must organize to manage medical care while the patient plays an essentially passive role. In the chronic phase between hospitalizations, the patient, feeling relatively normal, may wish to return to work, resume his or her place in the family, and play an active role in the management of his illness. In this period the family must support him in his dealings with the outside world. For example, he may wish to resume work but have periods of fatigue or anxiety when he has trouble functioning in a stressful job. He may take more and more sick days without wishing to disclose the nature of his ailment. If his employers become suspicious, his job may be in jeopardy— and with it, the medical insurance and financial stability he and his family need, as well as the sense of personal identity that work provides. Although statutes give some protection against dismissal from employment because of HIV infection, the person may be fired because he is no longer able to execute his job.

After a life-threatening crisis the person may question the meaning of work and turn to his family for advice in working out the balance between seeking less stressful, more rewarding work and maintaining job-related medical insurance. While COBRA allows individuals to carry their own insurance for 18 months, the problem of obtaining decent medical coverage for an illness that they have a long chronic period accruing high medical costs places clients in untenable positions.

For some patients, however, an AIDS diagnosis is the beginning of a progressively downhill road, much like that of a terminal cancer. The constant/progressive course of AIDS is one where the family faces a continually symptomatic member whose disability progresses in a step-wise or gradual manner. Because of hospital overcrowding, or because the family prefers home care, the patient may be cared for at home. The family must adapt to progressive deterioration over time, which may include CNS involvement and the mental deterioration of AIDS dementia. Periods of relief from the demands of AIDS tend to be minimal. Continual adaptation and role change are implicit. Increasing strain on family caretakers is caused by both the risks of exhaustion and the continual addition of new caretaking tasks. Family adaptability is at a premium. Within the progressive course of AIDS there will be periods of time when the biological course stabilizes and the family is able to settle on a modus operandi over the short term. During a period of medical constancy the potential for family exhaustion exists, even without the strain of new role demands seen in a progressive phase of AIDS.

While home-care periods are acutely stressful, particularly when the patient is mentally impaired and has lost control of bodily functioning, many families have found such an experience to be immensely rewarding. The work of "buddies," crisis intervention workers, and other volunteers, as well as the generosity of friends, has demonstrated to many families that love can alleviate even the most intense physical and psychological suffering.

Medical issues are always paramount during the chronic phase. The daily routine changes as medication becomes a major part of life. The beeper reminding the person to take his dose of AZT also reminds him of continuing illness. The client has to adjust to episodic or chronic pain and debilitation. Acute infections (such as pneumocystis pneumonia or toxoplasmosis) may leave the patient disabled and weak. Recovery can take as long as two or three months; even then, patients often continue to feel tired, have episodic diarrhea, and lose weight. AIDS patients report that their bodies feel significantly different after diagnosis and the first round of acute illness. For some period of time, or perhaps "forever," they can no longer carry out daily tasks with customary ease. The ill person must learn to take charge of his illness and manage the pain that may have become a constant companion. Resuming control of one's life by engaging in meaningful work or in activities sponsored by AIDS organizations can make physical pain bearable. For many gay men political activism has provided a way of channeling the depression and anger generated by chronic pain and debilitation into work that creates a better future for others.

The ill person must learn to identify the early signs of opportunistic infection. One would think that the unpredictability of HIV symptoms would make people hypochondriacal—glued to the medical system, anxiously awaiting the latest red-cell or T-cell count, misreading every symptom. In our experience, however, people with AIDS learn to be sensitive to meaningful signals from their bodies, diagnosing real danger signs before physicians have objective criteria.

The family, too, must learn to be sensitive to physical or cognitive changes that could signal such illnesses as toxoplasmosis and AIDS dementia. Having recognized these signals, however, family members may find it difficult to help the patient determine when medical intervention is needed. For example, one patient decided to tell his mother about his homosexuality and his AIDS diagnosis. While his "coming out" was traumatic, it was also relieving, and the patient's mother surprised him by her acceptance. The day after his disclosure the patient experienced difficulty breathing. Family members assumed he was experiencing anxiety about his mother's response to his disclosure, because the patient had a reputation for producing hysterical symptoms. In fact, he was experiencing early signs of pneumocystis pneumonia, for which he was later hospitalized. Did the stress following disclosure render the patient more susceptible to infection? In what ways can professionals help patients and their families to reduce stress around such events? These are important questions for AIDS clinicians.

HIV disease is treated with myriad experimental protocols. People who manage the disease with some success usually are well informed regarding new protocols and understand the pros and cons. This kind of knowledge is readily available through gay community organizations and publications, but much less available to impoverished people living in inner-city communities. Therapists in these locations find themselves in the role of liaison between patient, family, and physician, as they help patient and family research new treatment options, locate medication, and join clinical trials. Often, therapists are confronted with suspicion (sometimes justified) about drugs that have been prescribed for family members. These suspicions need to be fully explored with clients and information made as accessible as possible to enable them to gain control over medical decision-making.

When the person with AIDS is not in acute medical crisis, it is important that both patient and family become less focused on illness and pay attention normal developmental needs. Because AIDS is viewed by most people as a fatal illness, the chronic phase can seem like a time of waiting, with both patient and family "living in limbo." To depotentiate this paralyzing attitude, we construct AIDS as a chronic illness of indeterminate length. This emphasis helps the client live as normally as possible and all family members to maintain maximal autonomy in the face of a pull to focus only on mutual dependency and caretaking.

Pediatric AIDS often brings a sequence of severe medical crises in the chronic phase, so that the the needs of other well siblings are neglected or must be met by family members other than parents. In periods of respite it is important that parents re-establish relationships with these children and focus on their needs and emotions in reponse to their sibling's illness (Reiss, Gonzalez, & Kramer, 1986). This task may be greatly complicated by the fact that, in many cases, the caretaking parent is also affected by illness and needs respite to regain his or her strength.

Managing the Medical System

A major task for AIDS patients is learning to deal with the hospital environment (Reiss & Kaplan-DeNour, 1989; Rolland, 1984, 1987a,b,c; Tiblier, Walker, & Rolland, 1989). Hospitalization for the first infection may be a highly unpleasant experience; also, for most AIDS patients, it is their first experience of perceiving themselves as being contaminated. As they watch hospital workers, doctors, and nurses perform routine procedures, they see them using gloves and masks and taking extreme precautions. They realize they are no longer in the world of normal people but have now become fearsome objects to others—sources of contamination and death. Despite the efforts of ombudsmen from organizations such as Gay Men's Health Crisis to improve hospital care, patients sense the fear of hospital workers, some of whom may place food trays just inside the door instead of bringing them to the patient's bed. Family members arriving for the first time see the warning poster of infectious illness attached to the door; they, too, have the shocking experience of seeing their family member ostracized and stigmatized as a dangerous citizen. This initial experience of hospitalization can be a framing event for the family: The brutal psychosocial reality of AIDS can restructure a family to band together in protective outrage or to isolate the person with AIDS.

Hospitals serving as AIDS centers are understaffed, flooded with patients, and unable to give extra services. These conditions make it difficult for AIDS patients and health-care teams to establish the caring medical team/patient relationship so necessary for treating such a complex disease. Even the best AIDS doctors often do not have time to discuss symptoms directly with their patients, but turn over routine discussions to assistants. Some patients feel intensely dependent on their primary-care physician because the disease is so complex, dangerous, and unpredictable. The physician's unavailability causes many of these patients to feel abandoned and even more frightened.

In the gay community the problem of physician unavailability has had the positive effect of creating medical information self-help groups, which encourage patients to become their own experts. Some groups even import controversial new drugs and establish protocols. Such empowerment is healthy for patients, in that it increases their sense of control and willingness to fight their illness. Unfortunately, since many of these information channels have been created by and are located in the gay community, they are not readily accessible to the minority communities who constitute the newest high-risk group and who are frequently homophobic.

Issues of Disclosure and Acceptance

In the asymptomatic phase of HIV disease, infection is invisible and the decision to disclose is a personal choice. Many asymptomatic HIV-infected people choose to tell only sexual partners and their most intimate friends. In the disease stage, however, visible physical symptoms threaten secrecy and force patients to wrestle with the pros and cons of disclosure to a wider network.

As the disease progresses, ill patients may be forced to disclose to family members because of caretaking needs or because they feel unable to conceal illness from the sharp eyes of relatives. If they do not choose to disclose the illness to their family, they are left with the loneliness of maintaining secrecy as they face death. The decision to seek counseling is often around these painful issues of disclosure (Chapter 8).

The need to disclose may come at a time when the client, who is also working out his own meanings for his illness, is particularly sensitive to the opinion of others. If he is not known to be in a high-risk group—as, for example, the closeted bisexual or the occasional or recreational drug user—he may wish to keep the most probable cause of infection secret from everyone, including the therapist. In circumstances where the stated source of infection seems unlikely, the therapist has to judge whether developing a relationship with the client would be jeopardized by challenging the explanation. Perhaps the client first needs to deal with his shame about his own homosexuality or a concealed drug-use problem.

It is also important for therapists to sort out their own countertransference biases about transmission: for example, perceiving one client as a "victim of circumstance" (the blood-transfusion recipient or the unknowing spouse of a bisexual person or drug user), while another is stigmatized as "having brought it on himself." Since these biases are conditioned by the prevalent social constructions of HIV disease, and belong to both clients and therapists, the therapist must continually question his reason for needing information.

What the client chooses to reveal is a private matter, which may be of only secondary relevance to treatment. The vulnerability of the client following initial diagnosis and the belief, often shared by his partner and family, that a socially acceptable explanation will, for now, protect important relationships better than the "truth" seems to take precedence over pursuit of the "truth."

If the client decides to disclose the nature of his illness to family members, he must brace himself for the questions that follow about sexual identity or drug use or the suspicion that "transfusion" is merely a cover for other activities. The therapist must be open to the client's pacing as he handles these questions. Using the genogram, the therapist can help the patient identify family members who are most likely to help the person with disclosure and begin the process of breaking down family secrecy and alienation. Gay men often find that sisters are less threatened by a sibling's being gay than brothers. Also, because the care of elderly parents is often left to daughters, sisters may have the advantage of being close both to the parents and to the gay sibling.

When AIDS revelation is also an admission of homosexuality, some families are overtly hostile and rejecting, confirming the patient's worst fears. Or the family may be torn by conflicting feelings, most commonly splitting on gender lines, with mother and female siblings supporting and protecting the AIDS patient and father and male siblings angry and contemptuous of his sexual orientation. Other families merely need time to adjust to a disclosure of a gay sexual orientation. While the initial reaction to a disclosure of homosexuality may be homophobic disgust, later the family may work towards acceptance and understanding.

Many families experience relief mixed with pain when the person finally reveals what they have guessed but have not dared ask. The person's revelation allows them to fully embrace the patient, to affirm their love and share their mutual grief.

CASE EXAMPLE *

For many people a major task of this phase of illness is arriving at a positive view of their sexual orientation. This process often is particularly difficult for bisexual men, who feel they belong to neither the straight nor the gay community. Several years ago, Vaslav received many blood transfusions following a series of operations. When the HIV crisis occurred, he decided to be tested and learned he was positive. He sought therapy with his wife, Annette, because he found himself afraid to have any sexual contact with her and because ARC symptoms left him depressed and fatigued. A musician, he no longer felt able to work and spent long hours at home brooding. Annette worked to support them. Vaslav refused chemical intervention for his depression, believing that experiencing his depression would help him confront his deepest beliefs about illness and death.

After a few sessions Vaslav acknowledged that, prior to marrying Annette, he had had a number of same-sex relationships, which he had discussed with her and which she had accepted. He wondered if he had been infected back then and if HIV infection was a punishment for his past life. The therapist speculated that his persistent depression was a self-punishment for guilt that he experienced because of his bisexuality.

The issue of bisexuality disappeared from the therapy until quite suddenly, some months later, he said angrily, "Last week, my first wife told my oldest son that she had had a very hard time in her marriage with me because I slept with men." He felt betrayed, believing that this revelation had hurt his relationship with his son. He tried to have a conversation with his son to talk about sexual orientation. "Your mother and I were both damaged people," he told him, "One can't help one's sexual orientation. It is probably a result of damage that was done . . . . At some point this might happen to you. You might be helpless to do much about it." His son answered coldly that he cold not even imagine being attracted to a man.

Vaslav viewed his bisexuality as a result of psychological damage. The therapist believed that it would be helpful for him to create a positive story about his sexuality. She asked Vaslav if he thought that his depres-

---

* The author was the therapist.

sion about HIV infection, as well as his terror of having sex with his wife, might be linked to negative feelings about his bisexual experience. Did he have any explanation for his bisexuality? The therapist wanted to hear the meanings Vaslav gave to his sexuality. Vaslav spoke of growing up in Russia, in a violent, crazy family. He felt his sexual attraction to men was an outcome of his conflictual relationship with his father, a philanderer who had sex with both women and young boys. His father had abandoned his mother after physically abusing her, despite Vaslav's attempts to protect her. Vaslav believed that his father had also sexually abused him. His most bitter memory was of his father humiliating him sexually when he took him to see a doctor because, he said, his son's testicles were not descending. After that his father had often mocked him for being too girlish, a sissy boy, a half-man. Vaslav said, weeping, that despite all this, he still loved his father.

Vaslav internalized his father's view that he was not man enough to be fully heterosexual. "I couldn't escape from the sense that, had I been stronger, I would have been able to be more moral."

The therapist countered this negative story by asking Vaslav to describe positive aspects of his sexual experience with men. What was the particular pleasure it gave him? What was its uniqueness? Vaslav described himself as enjoying being a recipient partner and liking the passivity of the relationship when a man took care of him. There was no commitment, only intense erotic experiences. By contrast, when he was with a woman he was always the caretaker. "I always feel very powerful with women but I never feel that I am taken care of, so I like the passivity that I feel with men." He acknowledged that, while most people had bisexual periods in adolescence, sex with men had been crucial to him and had remained so into adulthood.

Therapist: It must have had a deep meaning for you, if it could override the social injunctions against bisexual experience and your own injunctions against what you thought of as "immorality." If you could find a more positive and independent view of bisexuality than your father's, how would it change your sense of yourself? Do you have any idea as to what it was in him that caused him to have such a negative view of you?

As we did the genogram, Vaslav said that he thought his father, who had been brutalized by his own father, had erotic feelings towards young boys, which he then repressed and projected onto Vaslav. In his father's eyes, it was Vaslav who was a sissy, less than masculine, a girl seducing men. Vaslav's father had always lied about his sexual relationships and, in fact, had never been honest with his son.

Therapist: Vaslav, oddly enough, your ex-wife inadvertently gave you the opportunity to be an honest father to your children, a different father from your own. She could have told them about your sexuality after your death, when you were not around to explain the meaning of your experience. If you were not to see bisexuality as the mark of a failed man, if you were to construct your own independent description of your bisexual experiences, how would you describe them?

Vaslav: Well, it was like a treasure. It was something absolutely beautiful. Very, very intense and very important to me. And I took it.

Vaslav began to separate his positive description of bisexuality from his father's negative view of him, which he came to see as a possible result of his father's discomfort with his own bisexual feelings. Vaslav understood that part of the intensity of his erotic attraction to men was his longing for a closer relationship with his father, to be loved and cared for by him. The pleasure he experienced in being cared for by a man was profound and healing.

Therapist: Whenever you adopt a negative view of your own experience, then you are looking at yourself through your father's eyes. You have a choice about whether you wish to do that or whether you want to claim your own experience. If you are able to reclaim your unique experience with men, making it your own, not your father's or anyone else's, then you will be able to convey this feeling about yourself to your children in all its complexity and richness.

I asked Annette what her experience had been listening to Vaslav discuss sexual experiences with men. She said she felt excluded, in that Vaslav allowed men to care for him sexually in a way which he forbade her. Vaslav said that he was uncomfortable allowing women to care for him. He shared his father's belief that a man must always be in control because women were powerful and all engulfing.

Annette wondered whether Vaslav gave up his relations with men out of fear or as a choice. If it was out of fear, she would worry that somewhere he might have another sexual life without her. "I don't want him sleeping with anyone else. I love him; I want him to be all mine." Vaslav laughed. The tension in the session dissipated, and the couple held hands as Annette tearfully spoke of her love for her husband and her fear that she would lose him. At the end of the session Vaslav said that he wanted to call each of his four children and have a discussion with them about his bisexuality. He felt that he was ready to experiment with allowing Annette to be more sexually assertive. The couple resumed having sex, although not as frequently as before infection, and they went away for their first vacation since diagnosis, which was a magical experience for both of them.

Beginning the Process of Future Planning

Once the person has been diagnosed with one of the opportunistic infections that comprise the AIDS syndrome, it is time to begin planning for the eventuality that another bout of serious illness will cause mental and physical incapacitation or death. Since AIDS is spreading rapidly into communities where it affects families with young children, critical tasks include helping infected parents and single mothers identify and develop support systems that can take charge of the children during times when illness incapacitates the parent and to help the family prepare for the parent's death. A family resource genogram is useful in helping mothers identify family members who could raise their children.

For example, Beatrice, an African-American single mother with AIDS, initially felt that her 21-year-old daughter, Nikki, could raise Beatrice's four-year-old daughter, Ruth, when she died. After some consideration she realized that raising Ruth would keep Nikki from finishing college, thus perhaps keeping her trapped in a cycle of poverty. She decided that cousins in Virginia whom she had known as a child could provide a network of "siblings" for Ruth. With the support of relatives who knew her situation, Beatrice moved to Virginia and reestablished close ties to her cousins, who agreed to raise Ruth if she were to die. Beatrice felt relief that her child was in a better environment than she could have provided in New York.

For gay men future planning is important because gay life partnerships are not accorded the same status as marriage. A life partner may find himself in a battle with a hostile family of origin over who has the right to make medical decisions for his incapacitated lover, or after his lover's death become embroiled in legal battles with the family over entitlement to property that was jointly owned or a shared apartment.

The therapist and the client may be hesitant to raise such issues because making a will or planning for the future care of children seems to inject a note of pessimism at a time when family and client are trying to marshall hope. Family members may not be able to think about family reorganization because it is hard to deal with the finality of the person's death while there is life and may seem presumptuous to plan for the assumption of new responsibilities before the family member actually dies. However, the idiosyncratic course of AIDS makes such planning prudent. Furthermore, clients who have been able to work out arrangements when they are healthy feel a sense of peacefulness and relief about having set things in order, in preparation for an unexpected exacerbation of the illness. Addressing the taboo fears of death in a practical way actually increases the client's sense of control and mastery.

In the following case it can be seen that, while future planning is delicate, skirting the possibility of death and loss, it can be done with humor and joy that do not diminish hope.

CASE EXAMPLE *

Loretta, a single mother with three children, had suddenly been diagnosed with AIDS. She came to therapy because her 16-year-old daughter, Cara, was cutting school, staying out late at night, and defying her mother's rules. Cara, the oldest of the children, was the only one who knew that her mother had AIDS. In the first session it became clear that Cara was overwhelmed by her belief that if her mother died, she would have to raise her younger siblings. Once Loretta was able to reassure Cara that, if should she die, Loretta's sister Susan had agreed to assume primary responsibility, Cara's symptoms subsided.

Working with the genogram, the therapist learned that Loretta's greatest fear was that she would abandon her children as she and her siblings had been abandoned by their mother, a drug user who had disappeared when Loretta was five. Future planning, which would reassure Loretta both that she had been a good mother and that her children would be cared for in the way that she wished, was the central task of therapy.

The therapist invited Loretta's sister Susan to join her in the therapy. In the beginning of the session the sisters discussed the way in which

* The therapist was Nellie Villegas.

each saw Loretta's illness. Loretta feared that each time Susan saw her she imagined her dying. She felt despondent because she did feel that she had little time and her health was poor. She was bitter that she would not live to see her children grow up and she worried that Susan was not up to the job of raising them. Susan firmly stated that she did not see Loretta as dying soon; rather, she saw Loretta as having a chronic illness of indeterminant length. She felt that some of Loretta's health problems existed because she failed to seek adequate medical care. Susan's tough optimism was infectious. Once Loretta could begin to construct her illness as chronic, she could lay the groundwork for a possible time when Susan might have to care for her children.

In the following dialogue, the therapist asks the sisters to address their different styles of mothering, so that Loretta can feel that her vision of how her daughters should be raised has been conveyed to her sister. The tone of the session is intentionally playful and light as the sisters weave back and forth from present to future.

Therapist: Susan, how do you see the difference between the way you mother your children and the way that Loretta mothers hers?

Susan: Loretta is more quick-tempered than I am. I'll try to reason with them until reasoning doesn't work anymore.

Loretta: But you're also more of a pushover than me.

Susan: Yeah, plus that's true. [*They laugh.*]

Loretta: They get over on her all of the time.

Therapist: Is that a concern for you . . . that your children will get their way with Susan in the future, when you're not there?

Loretta: I'm afraid because they'll tell her anything and she might fall for it, 'cause she's sweet and kind and loving, and she loves her nieces and she never wants to think anything wrong about them, and they'll just take advantage of it. You know. And my daughter, Alise, she is a hell of a liar. She is. And she could tell you a lie with a straight face. And she'll have you so convinced. She will have you totally convinced and you know it.

Susan: My oldest daughter is a big liar, too. So Alise can't be any more of a liar than . . .

Loretta: Yeah, but you are still doing the babysitting for April and everything—April's still getting over on you.

Therapist: So you are both similar in that you both give them a lot of attention and you're very available to them. But Susan, you tend to be a bit more lenient with them? Whereas Loretta, you tend to get firmer with them and set limits and . . . ?

Loretta: I get to the point when I say the heck with it, I say, "You're punished, that's it," and then start snapping at them, you know, I can't see . . .

Therapist: Susan does well up to that point, but you think maybe she could be firmer? How do you think it could be different?

Loretta: With my kids, she would have to be very, very firm. Because I know how they are. You know, I know how they are and they would try to manipulate her, oh God.

Therapist: Do you think Susan is capable of withstanding that?

Loretta: I don't know.

Both sisters laugh and the session moves on to untangle issues from their growing up that have shaped their relationship and that have become reactivated by this crisis. Loretta discusses her jealousy that Susan, the oldest daughter in the family, had the privileged position of filling their mother's place; it is a jealousy that is mixed with a compassion for the burdens her sister had to bear. These feelings re-emerge when she thinks that her sister may have the privilege and the burden of raising her own girls. As the sisters complete the process of future planning, they begin to focus on the everyday issues of living with an illness and raising two families of adolescents.

Creating a Meaning for Life with Illness

In earlier chapters, we have spoken about societal meanings given to AIDS and of the need for the person with HIV disease to create a narrative about both pre-illness life and life with illness that has positive meanings. Even when a person has disclosed illness to family members, symptoms may bring terror that outsiders will begin to suspect and that suspicion or knowledge will bring shame on the family. If the ill person attaches this stigma to earlier behaviors that gave the family pain, such as drug use or a relationship with a person whom the family disliked, the ill person may prefer to die quickly and essentially alone as a way of sparing the family further shame and hurt. One ex-drug user barely responded to affectionate approaches made by family members; rather, she seemed locked in a deep depression. When asked if it was painful to experience her family's love and support, she said that, because she did not deserve it, she could neither allow herself to wish to get better or to feel happy. When the therapist then asked her to use the session to comfort her grieving sister, she was able and willing to do so. After this the therapist was able to construct a meaning for illness as a time when the ill person has the important task of helping family members deal with their sorrow.

In creating a positive meaning for illness, it is important to counter the popular belief that AIDS results in certain death with a belief that AIDS is a chronic illness during the course of which personally important goals can be realized. As AIDS and ARC symptoms appear, the invisible virus becomes real—the enemy inhabiting the infected person's body and now, active, seemingly eating away inexorably at his life. Doctors may have reassured the patient and his family that people can survive indefinitely with ARC, but most people, experiencing ARC as the harbinger of AIDS, see death just around the corner.

Since AIDS is perceived by most people as a fatal illness, life may be colored by anticipatory grief and pervasive hopelessness. While the majority of diagnosed persons have indeed died, if HIV disease is perceived as uniformly fatal, the patient may be less willing to take realistic measures to preserve his life, and his life with illness may be marked by depression and hopelessness. Since research (Borysenko, 1989) shows that patients do better when they are optimistic about illness, feel control over decision-making about illness, and have a fighting spirit, it is important to help the patient understand that there are a number of long-term survivors from whom hope may be drawn and that these people survived AIDS at a time when far less was known about the management of the opportunistic infections that account for AIDS fatality than is known today. Such optimism, however, should not be confused with a Pollyannaish cheerfulness which may not allow the patient and the family latitude to express feelings of sadness, fear, and even despair.

It is tempting to believe that the right attitude can cure a powerful medical illness. As a result, many people with HIV infection seek illness meaning and nonmedical techniques for recovery in the growing illness self-help literature. The Simontons (Simonton, Simonton, & Creighton, 1978), Louise Hay (1990), and others give the event of biological illness psychological meaning by stating that illness vulnerability is related to negative psychological states. For example, vulnerability to cancer and AIDS is seen as due to repressed anger and to emotional resignation and a failure to hope (Sontag, 1979, 1989). For some writers AIDS vulnerability is due to what is seen as the damaging psychological aspects of gay sexuality and gay lifestyle (Monte, 1990).

Disease course clearly can be influenced by psychosocial factors, events, and even patient attitude, and the Simontons have described useful techniques for stress reduction, for improving quality of life, and for creating an optimistic and courageous attitude towards illness. But some skepticism should be maintained about the underlying premise of all these books: that serious illness should be equated with the failure to achieve a positive, healthy psychological state and death with the failure to maintain it. In the case of books that attribute AIDS to the psychological effects of gay sexual mores, underlying homophobia and prejudice endow AIDS with moral meaning cloaked in psychological language.

Sontag (1979, 1989) has mounted an eloquent argument against the application of such beliefs to illness, showing historically how poor understanding of the mechanism of illness, the absence of remedy, and certain cultural fears created metaphors and mythologies (often punitive to the patient) that became attached to specific illnesses, most particularly, tuberculosis, cancer, and AIDS. While the Simontons and others assure us that they understand the danger that a person who embraces their beliefs may feel a sense of failure if he becomes ill, nonetheless everywhere implicit in their work is the idea that illness recurrences contain messages about psychological failures.

> Patients may have unconsciously surrendered to the emotional conflicts they face . . . . Patients have not yet found ways of giving themselves permission to meet their emotional needs except through illness . . . . Patients may be trying to make too many changes in their lives too fast—in itself a physical stress . . . . Patients may have made important changes but have slacked off and become complacent . . . . Patients may not be taking care of themselves emotionally; their behavior may be self destructive. (Simonton et al., 1978, pp. 231–232)

The above, quoted from *Getting Well Again,* is apparently only a partial listing of the messages that illness bears bout one's psychological peccadilloes. If one embraces this philosophy, it is hard not to feel that one is always doing something wrong and therefore in constant danger of receiving the illness message. In this landscape where mind rules body, death is surely the patient's fault, a failure of the *esprit de corps* the ill person is supposed to achieve, a cowardly succumbing to a tension generated by a stressful event. But the Simontons, who have an elegant ability to reframe, do give the patient a graceful way out, so to speak. The dying patient need not feel that his death is an abject failure to clean up his psychological act. Mind controlling body to the end, he can choose to reframe death as his "redecision" (Simonton et al., 1978).

Where the self-help literature is useful is in its underlining of the importance of quality of life for people with chronic illness and in describing techniques for relaxation and visualization, which give hope and a sense of control and for pain management. But perhaps most critical to the patient's ability to live a satisfying life with AIDS and to set realistic goals for himself is understanding that, with current medical intervention, *AIDS is a chronic illness with an indefinite time frame.*

In the following case, therapists John Patten and Carol O'Connor utilize a client's behavior to help him conceptualize AIDS as a chronic, rather than an imminently fatal, condition. When he is able to do so, rather than living in "frozen time," he begins to be able to make future plans.

CASE EXAMPLE

Michaelangelo and Fiametta were a young couple with a four-year-old child. Michaelangelo was a paramedic who believed he had contracted AIDS during the course of his work, perhaps from the blood of an injured addict who had struggled with him as he tried to take her to the hospital. His attempts at documenting the source of his infection had been scoffed at by his superiors, who clearly had a more blaming scenario to explain his infection. Michaelangelo and Fiametta thought of themselves as devoted family people. He was her hero; she loved to hear the stories of the sometimes heroic efforts he made on behalf of others. Her admiration was all the greater because she had been in an abusive and troubled first marriage to a drug user.

Fiametta was deeply loyal to her husband's version of the infection. The possibilities that he might have been infected in another way or that she could have been the source of infection were never considered. Their child seemed healthy but had also never been tested. Fiametta had been test but never picked up her test results. The couple kept the illness a secret from their families.

When they sought therapy, Michaelangelo had just had a terrifying case of pneumocystis, which led to his being diagnosed with AIDS. He was depressed, thought that he would die soon, and felt helpless to get any kind of acknowledgment of the source of the infection from his employer. At this point he had been placed on permanent leave from his job.

The initial task of therapy was to increase his hopefulness about illness, first by introducing medical information and advocating for proper medical care, which he had not received prior to coming to therapy. John Patten negotiated with the medical systems until he located the appropriate physicians for Michaelangelo. This attention to his most basic needs enabled Michaelangelo to begin to fight his disease. The next step involved changing his gloomy perspective on the fatality of his illness.

In the following dialogue the therapists have a discussion in front of the couple in which they introduce the idea that, despite illness, Michaelangelo and Fiametta might be able to change their perception of the illness and move out of the limbo of waiting for death. Then they might be able to see themselves as setting goals and realizing them. By tying Michaelangelo's style of dealing with illness to a critical aspect of his pre-illness identity—his perception of himself as a fighter—the therapists construct a linguistic frame that encourages him to see the illness as chronic.

John: What do you think would happen if he didn't base his thinking on the idea that he was going to die? If he based it on something else, like he had a chronic illness and that he was going to be around for a while? How would he be different?

Carol: You mean, if he didn't believe he was going to die?

John: Just supposing, hypothetically, that Michaelangelo was able to see his illness as being a chronic illness rather than a fatal one where he's about to die any month. If you were able to change his perception of the illness so that he was able to see it more as a chronic illness, all right?

Fiametta: Well, that's how I see it now. I don't see it as fatal, I don't see him as dying, you know, within a certain amount of time. Because look at him—he's gained weight, he's healthy.

John: But that's your perception of him, not the way he sees himself . . .

Carol: No. He looks good to me, too. But I know what you mean—how would he be if he thought he had a chronic illness and not a fatal illness?

John: Right.

Fiametta: I think he probably would open up a business and would, you know, get into something—yeah, he'd go on.

John: It's quite valid that he does.

Carol: But John, the dilemma might be that, if he lets go of the big challenge that a "fatal" disease suggests, he may not stay as on top of everything as he does.

John: That he might not be as in control . . .

Carol: As in charge of it—you know, he's a fighter. As long as he looks
     at it as fatal, it keeps him geared up to fight. But he fights it as
     though it's chronic.
John: Even though he believes . . .
Carol: That it's terminal.
John: But if he believed that it were truly terminal, he would just . . .
     lay down and die. There's a part of him—
Carol: I don't think changing that idea would be that big a switch,
     because I think that much of what keeps him that determined is
     that he fights this as though he can win.
Fiametta: Right.
Carol: And you can't win a terminal illness. But you can beat a chronic
     illness, by the quality of the life you lead.
John: Okay. But maybe he needs to keep that—I'm sorry, we're talking
     about you, is that all right?
Michaelangelo: It's making a lot of sense.

The interview changed the couple's belief about illness, and this
switch allowed them to define themselves as people who were fighting a
chronic illness. Little else, except the sensitive, supportive presence of
the therapists as witnesses to their struggle, was as important to Michaelangelo and Fiametta as this change of definition.

Grieving the Loss of Pre-Illness Family Identity

Family identity following an AIDS diagnosis will never be the same, and
the family must grieve this profound loss. The grieving process, which is
a normal developmental task after diagnosis, may be, in fact, a grieving
for the family itself. But for many families in crisis, time to grieve is a
luxury. Children of ill parents must be cared for and raised and the sick
must be tended. In an increasing number of families seen at Ackerman
and elsewhere, as many as five adult siblings are infected, ill, or have
died of AIDS. Overburdened well siblings and parents dealing with extreme loss are attempting to form new families for orphaned children.
The therapy session may be the only protected time the family members
have in which to express their grief.

Families with AIDS must find a way of maintaining a sense of continuity with past history. This may be especially hard since the power of
the illness, the medical necessities, community isolation, and the media
lock the family in a painful present, with a future that does not bear

contemplation. Remembrance of past experience may increase the anguish of present reality, bringing to the surface feelings of guilt, failure, and betrayal. The illness may create personality changes in the ill person, making him seem very different from the way the family experienced him before illness. One wife described her ill husband, who had infected her and a baby, as violent and abusive during his illness—"not a lot of fun to be around." When reminded by the therapist that she had at other times described him as a gentle and loving father, she summed it up by saying, "Yeah. When he was violent that was not the *him* him; that was the *sickness* him." Since she adamantly refused to disclose to her children the nature of her husband's illness, his transformation into a furious, violent person created a discontinuity that was hard to bridge when they were grieving his death.

Many families must go through extended periods of self-examination and self-laceration before they can accept the illness and forgive themselves for not having protected their family member from the lifestyle that exposed him to it. Reviewing the past can be an agonizing, although necessary, experience for the parents of a gay man, a drug user, or a hemophiliac. The therapist's task is to help the family mourn for its failures and losses as well as to construct a more positive narrative about the ill person, his relationships with the family, and the family members' life together. While parents may never be able to fully accept the fact that a child is gay or has a problem with drug use, they can be reminded that these behaviors make up only a part of the person's identity. Within a more positive frame, the parents may be willing either to examine the nature of their prejudices or to put aside issues of gayness and to focus on those qualities that they love and admire in their child. In the case of a drug user, a psychoeducational approach, which validates the family's distress, constructs addiction as a disease, and gives the family techniques for handling its relapsing course—all in the context of validating the parents' attachment to the positive aspects of their child—enables family members to better adapt to the needs of the drug user.

Developing Support Networks

A major task for the family in the symptomatic phase is to develop appropriate support. The therapist can encourage disclosure to key family members and help the family organize to provide care. With gay young adults, two families may be involved: the family of origin and a family of adoption or friendship network that plays a quasi family role.

Therapy can be useful in negotiations between these systems, which otherwise may conflict over the establishment of lines of authority if the person is incapacitated by illness. Such a situation can be seen in the case study of Mitchell in Chapter 13. In a planning session the therapist should include key figures from each of the caregiving networks, which may include lovers, buddies, crisis intervention volunteers, home atten-dants, friends, and family.

Given the isolation of AIDS, particularly for inner-city families, for the wives of bisexual men, and for parents of gays, the establishment of various forms of support groups is essential. Preserving confidentiality is often difficult. For example, convenience for hard-pressed families would dictate that the group be easily accessible; however, if the group meets in the community where the family lives, members may worry that atten-dance is tantamount to announcement of their secret.

Couple groups are helpful, particularly for addressing issues of safer sex. Multiple family groups provide social networks for families who are often isolated, as well as socialization for children. Women with HIV infection are often isolated from other women who would normally make up their support system. Because their work is often in the home, as they care for children, or because the demands of childcare preclude a social life after work, they are often socially isolated at a time when they are carrying responsibilities for raising children and worries about illness. Women's groups seem critically important as a source of support and nurturance.

Involvement in an AIDS activist organization also affords socializa-tion and opportunities to discuss concerns. Some people find this infor-mal structure preferable to a more formal group. Activism counters help-lessness and provides informal care networks.

Volunteers attached to AIDS organizations should be used to provide caretaking and companionship and, in families where children are ill, respite care.

CHAPTER 11
The Illness Family:
Therapeutic Intervention

THE COMBINATION OF illness, actual or potential loss of family members, and the powerful stigma of AIDS creates an AIDS family, with new coalitions, structures, secrects, and boundaries. The family members may become divided in their interpretation of the meaning of an illness event or over the best course of treatment. For example, neurological complications can be hard to distinguish from psychological states. Families can become divided, with one side fiercely defending the psychological explanation, the other the physical. In one case of a gay man with undiagnosed AIDS dementia, the parents attributed his depression and apathy to his relation with his lover whom they detested. His lover believed that the behavior indicated some organic change. Early neurological tests were inconclusive, but later tests at the lover's insistence confirmed an organic process.

Gay couples are under additional pressure at times of crisis because they do not have the social recognition of marriage, which would insure that parents and relatives would acknowledge and facilitate the primacy of their attachment, nor do they have the economic security of mutual insurance plans. Financial stress may make it difficult for the well partner to take time off from work to provide caretaking. Furthermore, parents often live far from their gay children, making conflicts of loyalty inevitable. For a gay couple, the decision of one partner to return home may be devastating, since it involves giving up critical aspects of adult identity, as well as betraying the primacy of the relationship. If a gay adult child does not return home, parents may have to disrupt normal life, being ready to travel to a distant city at short notice to nurse a child through bouts of infection. Such dislocations may stress their own marriage, particularly if, as is often the case, there is controversy between the parents over the child's sexual orientation.

As we will see in Part IV on inner-city families, the marriages of drug users are often volatile and may exist under the shadow of powerful unresolved attachments to the family of origin. The crisis of diagnosis may stir up in the drug user a primitive longing to return to his parents, together with the guilt that he very likely has infected his spouse and possibly his children. These feelings and his spouse's anger may create a crisis in an already precarious marriage. Solutions for the drug user include precipitating a crisis that will cause his partner to throw him out, deciding to return to the family of origin, or increasing drug use until it leads to life on the streets. Some recently diagnosed drug users seek substance abuse treatment, but treatment slots are hard to come by and treatment programs are only recently beginning to provide beds for drug-using persons with AIDS.

In other families the crisis of a prolonged acute illness may lead to reorganization and ultimately to reconciliation and family unity. When her brother was diagnosed, one sister realized that her closeness to him had made staying in a loveless marriage for the sake of her children bearable. Shortly after her brother's diagnosis, she fell in love with another man and found the courage to divorce her husband and to remarry, despite fierce family opposition. "I knew," she said, "that if my brother died, I would have lost the only person I had allowed myself to trust and confide in. It was an unbearable thought." As she turned away from him and toward her new husband, her brother felt that, at the time of his greatest need, he was losing his closest confidante. This realization, in turn, precipitated his leaving a difficult and unsupportive relationship with a lover. As the longstanding coalition of brother and sister against the rest of the family weakened, the mother, who had always felt herself to be in an outside position in the family, was able to meet with her son in a therapy session and discuss her feelings about his being gay. The other son was able to put aside conservative beliefs to support his brother.

BOUNDARIES

HIV illness changes family boundaries. Secrecy may create a coalition between the parental couple when one of the parents or a child has AIDS, separating them from their extended family. Or the couple may admit one or more family members to the inner circle of those who know.

As decisions to disclose take place, internal family structure shifts, with sympathetic family members becoming involved in the caretaking process and others refusing. Since an increasing number of poor, single-parent women are contracting HIV disease, caretaking for children in the face of the mother's illness or the illness of one or more children forces the nuclear family to open its boundaries to include members of the extended family or kin system who are willing to help. As David Reiss (1987) has noted in his studies of family response to end-stage renal disease, often poor families have a flexibility of organization that permits them to adapt to illness needs better than more highly organized middle-class families. Furthermore, despite the stigma of AIDS, African-American and Latino families have a tradition of providing kin support, even if providing such support entails an elaborate masquerade of "not knowing" the nature of the illness. Nevertheless, the incorporation of other family members may bring its own difficulties, since there are often residual angers, feuds, and jealousies among competing subsystems.

Boundaries between the family and the immediate community may become more and more rigid as the family has to guard its secret. Inner-city families learn to keep their own counsel for fear of being stigmatized in the schools, work places, or even within the extended family system.

While the boundaries between community and family are becoming more rigid, those between the family and medical system are likely to become more permeable, so that numerous health-care workers, including buddies, home health attendants, and medical and social work personnel, can be absorbed. If the person with AIDS is also the family executive and is becoming increasingly incapacitated, she may turn to an involved health-care worker to help her make decisions. If the health-care worker does not explore whether other family resources exist and comes to play a major role in the woman's life, the worker may find herself in a coalition with the client against the family members who must ultimately take over. This coalition is likely to be a replacement for a coalition that has been disrupted by illness. For example, frequently a difficult relationship with a spouse is consolidated by mutual anger at one or both families of origin. When illness divides the couple and forces one partner to return home to the family of origin, the health-care worker may be triangled into the place vacated by the spouse and find that she is expected to carry the flag of opposition against the family.

In some cases, as various family members step in to assume the executive functions left vacant by the ill person, rivalries occur between health-care workers and family members or between different factions in the family. In one family, the introduction of an educated male GMHC worker disrupted the fragile balance of a marriage where the wife with ARC was better educated than the non-infected husband. In other cases, the health-care worker may be absorbed into the family and should be included in family sessions. The relationship between health-care worker and family is often loving and intense; in at least one male couple, following the death of the partner, the health-care worker and the surviving partner became lovers.

ISOLATION AND SUICIDE

Because the secret of AIDS may rigidify PWA/family boundaries or family/community boundaries, disrupting normal social and familial discourse and support, isolation poses psychological risk for the AIDS family during a time when support systems are critical. The AIDS patient may become depressed and think about suicide. Suicide is a complex dilemma for the clinician: On the one hand, he is professionally bound to take steps to prevent it; on the other hand, when a patient is severely impaired, he may personally agree with the patient's wish to take control of his dying (Glazer & Strauss, 1965). While religious beliefs make suicide untenable for some clinicians and clients, others see it as an act of surrender to processes of nature with which medical intervention has interfered.

Suicidal ideation may be a response to familial and social isolation, to guilt at having infected family members, to the perceived hopelessness of the disease, to the actual debilitation of illness, or to the loss of a critical relationship. If suicide is a response to social isolation, the most important task for a therapist is to reestablish active contact with the person's support network, which might be his or her family of origin, the family of choice, or the family of helpers created by the illness. If this network is firmly in place, it may provide an alternative to psychiatric hospitalization. If a person has infected one or more family members, guilt may be overwhelming and he may actively engage in suicidal behaviors, as in the following case.

CASE EXAMPLE*

Sid, who was an IV drug user, learned that he had infected his wife, Doreen, and their baby. Even though Sid had married and become a

*The therapist was Ruth Mohr.

hardworking family man, he continued to use intravenous heroin on weekends. Because he was good to his family in so many ways, his wife overlooked his drug use. Sid's diagnosis and the loss of the baby to HIV infection and cancer were devastating. Sid resumed full-time drug use, using every last ounce of strength to get to his dealer and obtain drugs. His wife managed to get him to come to one session, in which he explained to the therapist and his wife the depth of his fear and despair.

Therapist: Most of the time you fight because you don't take care of yourself.

Sid: Yeah, mainly. And the drugs.

Therapist: And the piece with the drugs is that maybe you are harming yourself, you are putting yourself into . . .

Sid: Well, from what they tell me, every time I do it, it is taking something, uh, you know, it's probably advancing the AIDS and weakening my body.

Therapist: Is that what you want to do?

Sid: [*Sigh*] I think about it. I honest to God think about it. Before, on the way, I asked myself, "Why?" And I keep asking myself, "Do I want to die, do I want to get it over with?" And to be honest, I don't know the answer to that question. I know what I'm doing is wrong and bad for me. I'm not a child, I know the difference between right and wrong. I know that she knows what I'm doing when I'm gone a lot of the time. I know what I have to face when I go home, and I know she knows. Even if she didn't, she's going to say I did drugs anyway, but it just doesn't matter. I just get so down. And really, I don't know. They tell me I have anywhere from now to two years. I don't know if I can deal with this for two years. You know, every morning, you know, every cough, you can get—scares me. Right now I feel like I have a cold coming on. It's scaring the hell out of me because I don't know if it's just a normal little virus reaction or another attack. So, you know, it's a lot of stress. It shouldn't be an excuse, but it is. And whether I use it as a crutch, or whatever, it's happening. I've never been that strong.

Therapist: [*Emphasizing the suicidal aspects of his decision*] A crutch or a dagger, right?

Sid continued to use drugs, telling his wife that he hoped each injection would be an overdose. He hid all AIDS medication. After his death, Doreen found unopened bottles of AZT. He isolated himself from his family and refused to see his children in the hospital — so great was his shame about what he had done and the physical disfigurement of illness.

A patient may believe that illness is fatal and has irrevocably destroyed his ability to control his life. For example, one patient came to therapy to ask the therapist to help him plan his suicide. What soon became clear was that by planning to take charge of his death he resumed control of his life, a control that had been eroded by illness. Because he came from a religious family, he needed the therapist's sanction to feel justified in doing what he needed to do.

CASE EXAMPLE*

For Rustin, being in control of his life had been a guiding premise, which had actually grown out of a revolt against his mother, who believed that humans have no control because everything has been ordained and fated by a rather punitive but all-seeing God. Clearly acknowledging that he was gay, thereby violating his mother's faith, was Rustin's first step in taking charge of his own destiny.

Rustin's wish to end his life was exacerbated by social isolation due to a precipitous move, generated by his upset about his illness, away from the city where he had lived and had friends. The therapist helped him see that euthanasia was a legitimate wish for control, but that he could also take charge of life with illness. He would know when he was so ill that ending his life would be an appropriate act in accord with his deepest beliefs.

Once Rustin felt both in charge and, because of therapy, less isolated, he allowed the suicide deadline to pass and he went on to take charge of his life in ways that gave it new meaning. He made numerous friends through involvement in AIDS activism; he used his experience to counsel others with AIDS and to bring new depth to his work as an artist. However, when physical debilitation became very real, he again considered euthanasia (see Chapter 14). For Rustin suicide was a way of dying with dignity and forestalling extreme medical interventions, which he had learned from experience are almost impossible to prevent, despite living wills.

*The therapist was Ruth Mohr.

Isolation that is exacerbated by the loss (or perceived loss) of a critical relationship in the context of illness can also lead to suicidal fantasies.

CASE EXAMPLE*

George came to a session after a crisis with his lover, during which his lover threatened to leave. He told us that the reason he looked so haggard was that he was in the midst of committing the perfect suicide. He had decided to go off all medications and neglect his health; he knew that, shortly, nature would take its course. We knew that George's style was to be independent and to rebel against anyone's attempt to control him. Consequently, we intervened by telling George that, while we respected his decision, we hoped that we had his permission to continue to see him until nature took its course. George considered us to be part of his family, and our offering to stay with him until he died deflected the challenge implicit in the suicide threat, acknowledged his control and autonomy (which were being threatened by his lover's decision to leave), and broke the pattern of isolation that had pushed him to this dramatic cry for help. Shortly after this session George spent a weekend with his mother, which further increased his sense of connection. The crisis was followed by a realization that, despite his illness and his lover's distancing, his life still had meaning. George began to address issues of his own identity separate from his relationship. Equally important, he joined the PWA Coalition, which provided him with a new family.

As time progressed, George became more and more empowered to manage his life and his illness. However, when his lover died of AIDS, no amount of therapeutic intervention could give him the will to live. Because he was gay, there was no legitimization of his long relationship with his lover, who for complex family reasons had not left a will. As a result, George lost not only his apartment but also many of the possessions that they had bought together, which went to his lover's family. While the parents had been polite to him during their son's life, they secretly held George accountable for their son's infection and had no wish to continue their relationship with him after his death. In short, George's world had vanished with his lover's burial. Reconstructing a world would have been an overwhelming task for a seriously ill

---

*John Patten and Gillian Walker were the therapists.

person. From George's perspective, joining his partner in death seemed the most desirable option. While he did not choose to commit suicide, he neglected his health and soon died.

ILLNESS DEMANDS: ROLE
REDEFINITION IN COUPLES

Illness threatens the delicate balance of any relationship, since the roles that we take with our partners are often fundamental to our sense of identity. We resist the emotional disorder spawned by physical disorder. AIDS requires shifts in the structure of a couple's relationship and changes in role definition. For example, if the AIDS patient was the dominant partner in the relationship, to admit his new dependancy on his partner might threaten a fundamental belief about himself, "I am worthwhile because I am a caretaking person." His loss of control in the relationship, compounded by loss of control due to the ravages of illness, may lead to increased anxiety and stress. On the other hand, if he does not give up control and allow his partner to care for him, he may become exhausted and perhaps vulnerable to further infection.

The paradox is obvious. As one sensitive care partner expressed it: "If I take over more, he will lose the stubborn way he controls everything, and that stubbornness is what he uses to fight his illness. Things might go better for us, but I would worry for him." He refused to come to couples counseling because he feared for his partner (and himself) if they were to change their interpersonal "dance."

If the partner with AIDS has been subordinate in the relationship, he might fight what he experiences as the dominant partner's attempts to assume total control, by resisting his attempts to get him needed medical help. This statement might seem contradictory, but, in fact, complementary relationship systems are stabilized by both the dominant and subordinate partners' having areas where the roles are reversed or equalized. If the dominant partner controls too many areas of the couple's life, the relationship will become unstable. The subordinate partner may threaten to leave the relationship, either literally or by retreating into a depression or other symptomatic state.

In his classic work, *Naven*, Gregory Bateson hypothesized that if the disparity between the powerful and the subordinate becomes too great among the subgroups which comprise a social system or if there are no brakes on a symmetrical escalation between subgroups, the system must either find a rebalancing arrangement or it will go into a "runaway" that will lead to its dissolution. In his study of the New Guinea tribe, the Iatmul, Bateson noticed that when a transitional event involving a male child created a power imbalance between conflicting kin groups (father's relatives, mother's relatives) which became too great, a rebalancing ritual called a "Naven" took place. During the Naven, men and women from the different kin groups dressed in opposite-sex clothes and performed ritual actions that comically reversed the traditional power arrangements. Father's sisters, whose position as women was normally subordinate, dressed in men's clothes and beat the men; mother's brothers, who as men had a dominant position, dressed in women's clothes and acted as wives to the child. The Naven, together with cybernetic theory, provided Bateson with a model for examining rebalancing processes that ensure the stability of natural systems in the face of processes or transitional events which might lead to destabilizing change.

A dramatic and tragic example of a complementary relationship pushed beyond its normal balance by illness was seen in the first session with a gay couple. Terry, the PWA, had always played the role of an entrancing child, very similar to the "Petit Prince" of Saint-Exupery's fairy tale, while his lover, Jack, had enacted the role of the kindly older caretaker. When Terry developed a serious thrush infection, he ignored his lover's urging that he seek immediate medical attention. A childlike non-chalance masked his underlying need to regain some control, of which illness had robbed him. The more Jack warned, the more Terry found ways to avoid the medical care he needed. As the interactional pattern became clear during the initial session, the therapist was able to help Jack drop his parental tone and admit to his fear and grief that he was losing Terry to illness. When Terry realized that Jack needed him to soothe his fears by seeing a doctor, he had regained enough power in the relationship to be willing to help Jack by seeking medical care. It was, however, too late.

The example just described taught us to examine couples' relationships from the perspective of complementarity or symmetry in both their pre-illness and post-illness identity. In that way we can evaluate whether a couple is flexible enough to adapt to the caretaking needs of illness and to adjust to the chronic phase. At least temporarily, the dominant partner may have to permit caretaking; the subordinate partner may have to take charge. In a predominantly symmetrical couple, the ill person may have to tolerate an uncomfortable passivity in the acute phase and fight his way back to a more symmetrical relationship in the chronic phase.

These changes can be painful or exhilarating. Problematic shifts are often the presenting problem for therapy. People who experience the exhilaration of changes – that is, partners who can use role shifts to learn about new aspects of their lover – are not likely to seek help. If, for example, the partner who has taken a subordinate or dependent role in the relationship begins to take charge, he may discover aspects of himself that he has overlooked. And if the "in charge" partner, who often has indirectly satisfied others' unacceptable dependency needs, can overcome beliefs that he is not entitled to care or that admitting dependency needs would be wrong or humiliating, he may find the experience of being cared for to be deeply satisfying. However, if the pattern is rigid and deeply entrenched, there may be no way that the therapist can help the couple change to meet illness needs or preserve the relationship.

The person with AIDS may derive secondary gains from the diagnosis. He may be shrewd at manipulating family beliefs and guilt about his situation in order to gain power over other family members or to maintain control when he is faced with increasing disability. Often the illness itself shapes to fit the person's emotional or relationship needs. But if one wishes to lead as normal a life as possible despite the disease, one may have to relinquish some of the secondary gains that illness status may grant.

CASE EXAMPLE*

Jay and Frank are partners who both have AIDS; while Jay is showing symptoms, Frank has been able to maintain perfect health. The roles that they play in the relationship influence the course of their illness. For Jay, the acute phase of AIDS brought about a change in the relationship that he had always desired. Frank, who had always been distant, became much more available and assumed a caretaking role. As Jay finds himself feeling better, instead of, as he had expected, dying, he has a dilemma: If he wishes to become more hopeful and survive and thrive with AIDS, he must relinquish the attention he is receiving as a sick person, attention that he has always wanted from Frank. The clinician helps Jay understand that illness is not an acceptable price to pay for nurturance. She introduces other ways that Frank can nurture Jay and helps the couple to reestablish less extreme and more flexible boundaries of closeness and distance, within which AIDS plays a part but does not rule.

*The therapist was Lauran Kaplan.

The following case describes a couples therapy that addressed the problems inherent in a rigid relationship structure. It also illustrates a pattern of deepening disclosure, which often occurs in the therapy of people with HIV infection. While the case was a "failure" in that the couple left therapy precipitously, like many failures it taught the AIDS team many things—in fact, more than perhaps any other case about the myriad issues for couples where a person has AIDS.

CASE EXAMPLE*

Stewart and Rick have been together for two years. They had had a passionate sexual relationship prior to Stewart's diagnosis with PCP. Rick has never been tested but is in a clinical study that monitors the immune systems of gay men. Stewart is much older than Rick. He is a human services administrator, whose identity depends on seeing himself as a caretaker, teacher, and protector of others. Rick, by contrast, is a singer who, until diagnosis, had played the role of the refractory son who must be cared for and advised by his older lover. While Rick looks to Stewart for caregiving, he also rebels when Stewart attempts to reorganize his life and preserves a feisty independence. Illness challenges this arrangement, as Stewart clearly needs help from Rick but rebuffs his attempts at caregiving. The cycle escalates because, as Stewart feels more impaired, he defends himself against role loss by trying ever harder to parent Rick. The couple fights more and more, and Stewart's shame about illness and his feeling that he is contaminated and dangerous to the partner he loves impede his ability to have sex.

In the intial assessment the therapist (1) defines a presenting problem; (2) ascertains the medical and psychological consequences of AIDS for the relationship and its rules as they exist before and after the onset of illness; (3) explores the existence of support systems; and (4) does a genogram, which allows her to understand isomorphic patterns in the family of origin that inform the relationship and to assess what role the family of origin is likely to play in the illness.

The couple defines the presenting problem as Stewart's inability to have sex. This problem is behavioral and seems relatively easy to solve because the men have had a passionate and satisfying sexual relationship prior to diagnosis. Indeed, for many people, exploring each partner's feelings about illness in relation to changing sexual practices and as-

*The therapist was Carol O'Connor.

signing some safe sensate focus exercises are enough to begin to reestablish a climate for sex (Palacios-Jimenez & Shernoff, 1986).

In the first session we learn that, although Rick had always been scrupulously careful to use safer sex with other lovers, when he met Stewart, he decided not to do so. The reasons lie in the underlying contract of their relationship: Stewart will protect and father Rick. Stewart opens the first session by confessing his inability to perform sexually.

Stewart: It's not a problem for Rick, but it's a tremendous problem for me. I don't feel good about myself. I feel contaminated. I feel dangerous. I just cannot get close to him because I am so fearful for him. It's something we need to resolve and talk about. My temperament ranges from being very loving to extremely hostile . . . very volatile. I try to hold it down. But there are little things that just send me into great explosions . . . the little things don't justify the explosions that occur. I think it has been very hard on him. He bears up under it pretty well. But I'm concerned about his mental welfare.

As the session continues, it becomes clear that illness has changed the balance between the partners. Stewart feels out of control, an unusual experience for him. His sense of himself as a loving protector is threatened by his extreme irritability. But in the session the only concerns he voices are about the effects of his illness on Rick's well-being. Stewart's absolute insistence on being the good father, the protector, the caregiver, to the exclusion of permitting satisfaction of his own emotional needs, is a way of proving to himself that he is a good person despite his sexual orientation. Despite the fact that Stewart is openly gay in his own community, with his family it is still a shameful secret. He is determined never to tell anyone in his family that he is sick or that he is gay.

Stewart: I have not dealt with telling my family at all. I come from a generation where you were living in a closet, and it's very difficult for me. My mother is 81, she is a very small town, provincial lady. I don't think she even understands what homosexuality is . . . . I showed her a picture when I was there the last time. And I said, "This is my friend, Rick." I thought it was a good, informal "fun" picture, and I thought she should be aware of his existence. I have had a lot of lovers over the years. My parents, my family, have known some of them. But they have not known the relationship.

Homophobic family attitudes are internalized and exacerbated by illness, and may be reflected in Stewart's inability to have sex with Rick. Rick, by contrast, is comfortable having sex with Stewart.

Therapist: Rick, do you share Stewart's worries about you?

Rick: Well, of course, you can't help but be concerned about your own health, especially since we've been intimate. Somehow, I'm very fatalistic about this. I don't know what to think. It seems to me as though I'm going to come down with it sometime.

The therapist asks Stewart how he handles AIDS. Does it preoccupy him or can he lead a relatively normal life with illness?

Stewart: My approach to fighting the illness is a little bit bizarre. I am not so sure that it's bad because it works: I don't allow myself to think about it.

Therapist: How does that work for you?

Stewart: It works very well. Apparently, I have had no illnesses. I keep myself going, and really going like a dynamo until recently. Rick put his foot down.

Stewart's need to be in charge results in difficulty admitting to what extent illness impairs his functioning. It also makes it hard for him to adapt to the emotional and physical changes in himself and in the relationship. Shame also limits his support network.

Rick: One of the problems that we've had is that Stewart would rather avoid thinking about it. But at the same time, he's spending more and more time inside. He's only told a few friends. The few friends that he's told have more or less disappeared. I'm sorry to bring that up, but it's true.

Stewart: [Defensively] I think that happens always.

Rick: [Placating Stewart] It's inevitable on some counts.

Stewart: My friends are not terribly sturdy friends. I have not spent my life developing and nourishing friendships. I've been very busy working. I've been a workaholic my whole life. I'm sorry to interrupt. I have a tendency to do that.

The therapist, realizing that Stewart is ashamed of his inability to keep relationships, offers him a way to save face.

Therapist: Is the workaholism the reason you're successful in your career?

Stewart: Yes.

Rick: I don't think that Stewart can do it as much on his own as he wants to. And what I finally did two weeks ago was say to him, "I can't do it alone. I need help. I can't be the only one in the house. There have got to be other people around." I decided I was going to buy him a punching bag and some gloves. I've been going to the gym and just knocking myself out. There's a lot of release there. I think that Stewart would just like to beat AIDS up and go at it. He's used to having an office to sit in and a phone to scream in; if someone does something wrong, you can get results. But AIDS isn't a tangible thing. And I can see it tearing him up. It's not his fault.

Stewart: I was trying to say that the anger wells up before I realize that it is there. The tears come the same way. I mean, I can cry like that [*snaps fingers*].

Therapist: But those are very natural feelings.

Stewart: I guess. But not when the anger is directed in a direction that you don't want it to be. And then when it's out, you want to cut your tongue out. You have this terrible feeling of...this awful bad feeling, because you've done something that you hate yourself for.

Therapist: It's Rick's perception that he is the only support you have.

Stewart: Yes, I think that's largely true.

Rick: Maybe, but I think the choice was yours, not to tell people, to stay out of circulation. I think you can only cut yourself off from the world for so long before you explode. Because there's no vent for it. I'm there, I'm not leaving, I'm there. But I want to stay healthy, and I don't think that living in a constant or variable state of hysteria is any better for him.

Stewart: You see, that's all a matter of degree. My state of hysteria has always been there. And I've got to tell you that my priorities have changed dramatically. If I find myself in a situation at work where the stress becomes agonizing and that's when they need me to be there, now I get up and I go home. I've been told that stress is one of the most dangerous things that I can get involved with, so I try to avoid the stress. Stress builds up almost, I think, like a boil. If I can't get relief, then I walk away from those stressful situations. I think it comes out when I'm at home.

Therapist: Does it come out when you're alone or does Rick need to be there to witness it?

Stewart: It comes out when I'm alone. I beat the walls, I cry. I do a lot that he's not aware of. And that I don't think it's necessary for him to be aware of. But it comes out a lot when he is there. I don't want to do that to him.

Therapist: If you were to give him some advice, like how to help him through this, what would you tell him?

Stewart: I don't know. I don't know that I can do it myself, let alone help him.

Therapist: So maybe that's one of the things that we can work on.

Stewart: Yeah. I think our caring about each other and our love for each other have grown since this has happened. I think it has brought us a great deal closer in some ways. But there are tremendous voids. The sexual void is one thing that... I mean, it started out being a sexual relationship. That is now totally removed. And I have been a sexual being my whole life.

Stewart goes on to speak about his fears that he will infect Rick. At the same time he is jealous and thinks that Rick is promiscuous, which Rick vehemently denies. In the exploration two things emerge. First, this is both Stewart and Rick's first committed relationship, in the sense that they have chosen to live together most of the time. This proximity exacerbates struggles over dominance that might have been resolved had they been able to come and go. Secondly, it becomes clear that Stewart projects his own behavior in past relationships, when sexuality waned, onto Rick, and therefore expects Rick to be unfaithful, as he was. Stewart's new feelings of incompetence in an area that was his chief way of expressing and receiving affection have made his fears all the more intense. Stewart's obsessive jealousy may also be a way of reaffirming his attachment to Rick at a time when his guilt that he may have infected Rick is propelling him to end the relationship. In the area of sexuality and in other areas, partly because of illness and partly because of Rick's personality, Stewart for the first time does not feel in charge. The therapist explores the relationship contract.

Therapist: So you've always been in charge in your relationships.

Stewart: I was always providing.

Therapist: Did you provide for Rick?

Stewart: No, he's very independent. Very independent. The very first time we dated, we went out to dinner and I tried to pick up the check. And he got highly insulted . . . I'm very proud that he's independent. Sometimes I think that that is one of his strongest attributes. But I think that at the same time there is a lot of stubbornness that shuts him away from opportunity. Because he insists on being independent. I mean, the independence sometimes becomes the issue.

Therapist: If he were less independent, would you feel more secure?

Stewart: Of course.

Therapist: What's the other side of the thing? There's always a flip to it.

Stewart: Well, I've been used a lot in my life and I think that his independence protects me from that.

Therapist: In some ways, that may be a relief to you. In other ways, that may confuse you.

As the therapist does genograms on both partners, the origins of the patterns that they play out in their relationship become clear. Stewart was a responsible oldest child, close to his divorced mother, the caretaker of his younger siblings. Rick was the youngest of three children, the only son, from a conservative, middle-class, upwardly mobile family. To his family's dismay, Rick chose a career in the arts. His father was successful and authoritarian. No one would have dared to argue with him. Like Stewart, Rick has not officially come out to his family, but some family members know his sexual orientation. Rick's lifelong battle with his father is reenacted with Stewart, as though this relationship offers Rick a chance to symbolically work things out with his father by being able to argue and define himself with a powerful older man. Stewart's illness has confused this working out.

At the end of the first session, the therapist contracted to work on restoring the sexual relationship and on helping the couple recalibrate their relationship so that Stewart could feel more comfortable with being less dominant. By the third session the couple is beginning to renew their sexual intimacy. As in many therapies there is a rapid relief of symptoms in the early sessions. In work with people with AIDS, this change may precede the revelation of painful underlying issues that AIDS has brought to the surface.

Stewart: We've had safe sex intercourse . . . something that I hadn't been able to tolerate. Using a condom—I think a condom is an impossible way to have sex.

Rick: I just said, "This is the way."

Stewart: So finally, just out of sheer necessity, I'm facing up to that now. I'm able to manipulate that now, so to speak. It's not great, but it certainly is a lot better than the way it was before, which was nothing. The last couple of times we've had very loving, very good sex. And I'm the one with a handicap – the fact that I feel unclean – so therefore I have to be wrapped in gauze from head to foot. There's a great deal of difference between someone who is trying to protect himself and someone who is trying to protect someone else from himself. The dirty part comes from me because I'm the poison in the situation. And I'm dangerous.

The therapist links the reemergence of sexuality to a shift in the relationship towards more symmetry, but she does it in Stewart's language, implying that he is teaching Rick to take responsibility for his choices.

Therapist: You're giving Rick an opportunity to share in responsibility and he's choosing to be with you sexually, and that gives him a chance to share. And you are equalizing your relationship a little bit. And in a way, it's taking you out of that father/caretaker/overseer/in charge/protective role. It's a nice new quality developing in your relationship.
Stewart: It hadn't occurred to me. But maybe it's true.

Illness requires the ability to adapt to its demands without losing integrity and identity. The therapist asked Rick to help Stewart identify moments when he allowed himself to depend on Rick. She was looking for what Michael White would call "unique outcomes" (White, 1988). She points out that behaviors that are different from the rigidly complementary positioning of the partners also exist but go unnoticed. In this session each person struggles to remember moments when there was a difference, which might become a blueprint for each to play different roles. They describe a recent moment when Rick ordered for Stewart at a restaurant.

Rick: After the waiter left he looked at me and said, "No one has ever done that to me before." And I said, "Done what?" and he said, "Ordered for me." I said, "The waiter was talking to me, so I told him to bring you a cider." He just couldn't get over the fact that I had the upper hand.
Stewart: Well, what did I say?

Rick: You said it felt kind of good. . . . There is going to be a time when
    Stewart is going to have to lean on me and give me responsibility. I
    wish he'd learn to do it.

Therapist: You think he will give it to you?

Rick: I will have to seize it with tongs if I don't want to get burned! I
    would rather not have to fight for it.

Therapist: There seem to be several things that you've done recently
    that have been different, but not because Stewart is getting sicker or
    weaker. You're negotiating the relationship in a different way.

The improvement in the relationship leads to what seems like a
regression. This storm after the calm frequently occurs at a midpoint in
work where a partner has AIDS, after there has been substantial
improvement in the presenting problem. This storm may take the form
of a confession of behaviors that led to infection or guilt about the past.
It often constitutes a testing of the relationship and a seeking of either
forgiveness or punishment. On the one hand, Stewart feels safe enough
to raise deeper, more troubling issues; on the other, as he plays a less
dominant role, he is becoming more in touch with his own vulnerability.
In the next session both Stewart and Rick report an increase of fighting
and emotional volatility on Stewart's part.

Rick: Yesterday was like a roller coaster all day. Within an hour of being
    awake there was a fight going on. Half an hour after that it was all
    patched up. But two hours after that it was on again.

Stewart: I cry so easily. I don't know how to turn it off. And it just seems
    like it's right under the surface, so the least little thing sets it off. I
    don't feel very proud of myself. I don't feel very good about it. I feel
    like Dorothy in the whirlwind and I'm being sucked down and I
    don't know how to stop it.

Rick: So I'm getting more and more afraid to open my mouth because I
    just don't want to be misunderstood, and I don't want to trigger
    something. We're spending more and more time with him watching
    TV and me sitting in the corner reading a book.

Therapist: What do you suppose he's thinking about?

Rick: Do you have any ideas? 'Cause I could use some help.

Stewart: It's not the sex that's the problem—the sex or the lack of it.
    That's not the thing that is festering in me. Well, I'm back to that
    topic again. If you don't feel good about yourself, you don't want

sex. Well, I don't want sex. It terrifies me. I've said that before. Rick knows that. But occasionally the intimacy is there and you feel like you want to break through and then I . . . it's like I'm playing this awful game. I feel like I have a mask on. I don't feel very real about it. My concerns are for him. I don't know how to operate. I'm very jealous. I haven't said that, but I am terribly jealous.

Rick: I don't think you need to verbalize it.

Stewart: Well, I guess you know it after yesterday's . . . Something happened yesterday that . . . I banged out of the house and it was because of my inability to perform, which then multiplied into something else, which triggered my jealousy. It was how he responded.

Rick: Who was I with last night? You. Who was I with the night before?

Stewart: I don't know.

Therapist: Do you go out?

Rick: No I don't, because I'm still with him.

Stewart: I still think he does.

Therapist: Stewart, if the roles were reversed . . .

Stewart: I might be doing the same thing . . . worse.

Therapist: Doing what?

Stewart: I don't know . . . stirring the pot! I don't know. I think probably I see in him the sexuality that used to be in me and I don't trust it.

Therapist: If the tables were turned, can you imagine yourself being faithful to someone who was diagnosed with the disease?

Stewart: I've lost a lover to this. I was faithful to him.

Therapist: You've never said that before.

Stewart: I've lost more than one ex-lover, but I was living with a guy who died.

Therapist: When?

Stewart: Three years ago, four years ago. Mike.

Rick: Mike who?

Stewart: Mike Walling.

Therapist: So this is news to you, too?

Rick: I've never heard that name before.

Stewart: Yeah, you have . . . . I don't think it's ever really penetrated. I don't discuss it much. I went through two and half years of therapy because of this.

Therapist: Was this a person you loved?

Stewart: Very much.

Therapist: So you know what's happening, you can imagine what's happening. How did you help him? How did you help yourself?

Stewart: The two and a half years of patchwork was because I felt I wasn't there as I should have been. I was faithful to him, but I was not there as much as he needed me. I'll never get over the fact that I wasn't . . . . So I know, I know how it is when this thing happens, and I know that even love and good intentions and all those things don't always come out the way you mean them to.

Therapist: Is this news to you, Rick?

Rick: [*Frozen, just barely containing his anger*] I don't feel very good about it, because whenever I hear news or something I didn't know about, I just wonder.

Stewart: His picture is on the bookshelf if you wanted to ask. I brought it up a couple of times. He painted the painting over the bed.

Therapist: So what could you beat yourself about? How weren't you there for him?

Stewart: He died alone.

Therapist: By that you mean he was physically alone, you left him, he was in the hospital?

Stewart: He was in the hospital in Philadelphia.

Therapist: You had stopped visiting him?

Stewart: I had visited . . . it meant taking the train and the bus and it was very hard because I didn't have a car. And I rationalized. I rationalized . . .

In this painful session Stewart addresses two of the most painful issues of his life—the fact that he abandoned a lover who had AIDS, and the fact that he has never told Rick that his former lover died of AIDS. The betrayal of Rick is more symbolic than real. Although Stewart clearly thinks of himself as a criminal for not having warned Rick that he was probably infected, Rick might have been infected through other lovers. Nevertheless, Stewart holds himself responsible for not using safer sex, because of the role he sees himself taking in the relationship. When Rick challenges Stewart about the concealment of his former lover's death, Stewart is angrily defensive. His emotionality over the past few weeks is probably due to the self-laceration that precedes confession.

This confessional session was critical to the couple. In some couples such sessions are followed by separation, at least for a period of time, while the partner absorbs the information and processes his or her feelings. Often after a period of separation there is a reconciliation. But separation may precipitate a terminal phase of illness, perhaps because in an AIDS version of suicide the person neglects necessary medical care or simply because the stress of losing the relationship triggers an illness process. It was hard to know what Rick would do. His anger was just under the surface, but he was seething. How could he express it in the context of his deep love for Stewart when Stewart was already so vulnerable because of his illness? Furthermore, the complementary structure of the couple's relationship had never provided a forum for Rick to express critical or negative feelings.

Two difficult sessions followed. The therapist commended Stewart on his courage in discussing with Rick the complex issue of his last lover's death. At the same time she tried to get Rick to voice his anger. At last Rick was able to acknowledge that at times he was so angry he felt like destroying the world. The father whom he had trusted to repair his relationship with his own father may have destroyed him.

In the weeks following his confession Stewart actively considered suicide. While Rick could not tell Stewart fully just how angry he was, Stewart sensed his anger and could not stand the truth it carried about himself. He who had always seen himself as a caring and loving person had put the man he loved at risk. The imagery of danger and contamination, which was part of his early self description, had a still more powerful meaning in the context of revelation. Suicide would be the ultimate self-punishment — a fitting, lonely death, which would in some way expiate the abandonment of his earlier lover.

But gradually Stewart and Rick were able to work their way through these feelings. Stewart's revelation had offered a powerful challenge to the structure of the relationship. The crisis initially offered an opportunity for a more symmetrical relationship to emerge. However, illness and the fear of loss so stressed the thin skin of a fragile equilibrium that both partners were terrified that pressing for change would jeopardize the balance.

The couple gradually moved back towards its familiar balance, with Stewart as father and teacher, Rick as sometimes rebellious son. Symbolic of return to a complementary relationship was Stewart's planning of a vacation for the couple. There were some changes, however. Illness had intervened, making it impossible for Stewart to continue to manage his demanding job, forcing him to rely on Rick. Rick had at last begun to be more successful in his career.

In the final session, which took place after several calm and seemingly productive sessions, Stewart was highly agitated, seemed furious at Rick, and tried to hit him in the session. He asked to end therapy, saying that it was too painful. Two weeks later, Rick called to explain that the therapist had not had the crucial piece of information that fueled Stewart's outburst. The morning before that last session he and Stewart had found out that Rick's T-cell count, which had been normal, had fallen dramatically, indicating that he was infected.

In retrospect, the therapist was so stunned by the vehemence of Stewart's anger that she failed to grasp that this anger must be related to a repetitive pattern in their relationship. Historically Stewart's anger at Rick was most often a reaction formation occasioned by his underlying guilt that he had harmed him. While Stewart could manage his own illness, he could not manage his guilt about Rick. And because he could never openly acknowledge how much he depended on Rick and cared about preserving their relationship, he was not able to be honest about the real danger he presented.

Despite this crisis, the ending of therapy, and the turbulence in their relationship, Rick would not leave Stewart. While Stewart gave Rick conflicting messages, with Stewart the teacher saying, "If you don't stay with me until I die you'll feel as I felt," and then Stewart the person saying, "But I deserve to be abandoned," Rick saw fidelity as a sign that he was a good person.

Two years later the couple ended their relationship when Stewart became increasingly ill and insisted on leaving for another city where, like his lover Mike, he would die alone.

PART III
Journey's End: Beginnings

CHAPTER 12
In the Shadow of Death

T WO EXTENSIVE CASES will form the basis for discussion of the last phase of AIDS illness, when death is near. How the family and the ill person handle this time will resonate throughout the period of bereavement following death (Parkes, 1982; Parkes & Weiss, 1983) and will have important implications for the family's recovery and reorganization. Transcripts and case descriptions will be used throughout Chapters 12 and 13 to illustrate the attitudes of clients towards death, issues of terminal illness, and clinical interviewing techniques demonstrating how the family therapist conducts conjoint therapy with spouses, friends, and family members who are at different stages of awareness and acceptance of death (Kübler-Ross, 1970).

MOVING FROM DENIAL TOWARD AN
ACCEPTANCE OF DEATH

I will begin with notes taken after watching the interview with Michaelangelo and Fiametta, introduced in Chapter 10—an interview that dramatically illustrates the way in which denial of death as a natural process truly beyond technological control can create a situation of isolation and terror for the dying person and his family. The work with Fiametta and Michaelangelo, and later with Jacob and his family, flow from our belief that the most fundamental task for the dying person and his family is to establish those connections that give the final separation meaning. A second and related task is for the therapist to find a way of respecting what Lifton (1983) has called "the patient's middle knowledge of death" (p. 17), a stage hovering between complete acceptance and repudiation of the imminence of death — a stage in which conversations about death and loss may alternate with conversations about the ongoing life of the family.

CASE EXAMPLE

Michaelangelo has asked for a session with Fiametta after a three-month absence from therapy. He has had AIDS for three years now and was managing his illness well, but for the last three months he has been very ill with rapidly spreading internal Kaposi's sarcoma, CMV infections, and wasting diarrhea. He can no longer tolerate AZT. Doctors are experimenting with ddI, but without apparent benefit. Michaelangelo is still a darkly attractive man with melancholy eyes and a general sadness; Fiametta is pretty, slight, nervous. She buttons and unbuttons her coat.

"It's coming unravelled," she says, pulling at the tweed. As noted in Chapter 10, her husband has been her hero; this is the longed-for marriage to a good man after a marriage to an abusive drug user. Michaelangelo has always claimed that he got AIDS in the course of duty as a paramedic. The question of the nature of viral transmission hangs in the air: Although there are records confirming that Michaelangelo did treat a prostitute who later was diagnosed with AIDS, all attempts to get his supervisors to recognize that this experience was the cause of his illness have been fruitless. The therapists, John Patten and Carol O'Connor, have decided not to question Michaelangelo's explanation; the couple has made it clear that only by accepting this explanation can the therapists remain in the couple's trusted inner circle, in a coalition with the couple against unbelieving outsiders who treat Michaelangelo unfairly. The couple's battle against the outside world seems to be central to maintaining the marriage and to bolstering Michaelangelo's ability to fight the illness.

In the beginning of treatment, Michaelangelo was depressed and had no will to live. He felt surrounded by accusers who, not believing his story, seemed unwilling to help. The gentle compassion of John and Carol, combined with John's willingness to act as an advocate to support Michaelangelo in his battle with his superiors for work-related benefits, seemed to be critical in helping him turn the corner. Since Michaelangelo could not work without jeopardizing his civil suit against his employers, John helped him become an expert on his illness. In ways, Michaelangelo became the expert for our entire project, researching new treatments and reporting back to us. In this active role Fiametta could continue to see him as a hero and Michaelangelo could continue to feel in charge. For as long as he was physically able, Michaelangelo functioned as boss of his family. The couple even allowed themselves to dream of starting their own business.

But AIDS is a cruel destroyer of dreams. During the months away from therapy, as Michaelangelo's condition worsened, his battle against illness became the only subject of discussion between the couple. It was as though, just as disease was eating away the body, so the obsession about illness and finding a technological cure was eating away at Michaelangelo's soul and at the soul of the relationship with his wife, until there was nothing but a shell constructed of the obsession.

I observe the session. John is working alone, clearly distressed about the change in Michaelangelo, for which he has had no preparation. The session is unbalanced by Carol's absence. John has always represented the doctor who can manage the medical systems and lend the couple a power that counters their feelings of humiliation and hopelessness in the face of discriminatory situations. Carol is the good mother who gives comfort and raises emotional issues. I think John feels very much alone with what appears to be Michaelangelo's impending death.

Michaelangelo is in pain from Kaposi's sarcoma, for which he takes medication that fogs his thinking. He has chronic diarrhea and has trouble walking. Most of the time he is at home lying in bed, thinking. He feels very alone. He and his wife don't talk. "What is there to talk about?" he says, "I'm not alive this way." Each time he tries to speak about his despair, his wife becomes angry.

"He is full of self-pity. He should be fighting this thing."

"I'm losing weight," he interjects.

She corrects him, "You lost weight when you were sick—from 160 pounds to 140 pounds. But you gained back ten pounds. Then when you had diarrhea last week, you lost three pounds—but only three pounds."

Each time Michaelangelo tentatively raises the subject of his deteriorating health, Fiametta invites John to collude with her in offering her husband hope of medical intervention. But the conversation is paradoxical. Even as she offers hope, Fiametta uses phrases such as "at this stage of the game," implying that the concluding point is near. But if Michaelangelo moves to discuss his feelings of fear, pain, and exhaustion from the long battle against disease, she immediately shifts back to asking about further medical interventions. It is as if Michaelangelo must forever be the warrior knight who fights unrelentingly for the princess against overwhelming odds. When he seems crushed by the opposition, she presses him for further efforts. Watching this dejected man, I feel he wants to implore: "*I'm not a knight. I'm scared and I'm going to die. I want to sit and rest and not fight anymore and just be held and allowed to die.*"

Fiametta continues: "Sometimes he wakes in the night. He feels he cannot move his legs. He's frightened and he says, 'Take me to the doctor.' I am tired of running to doctors all day. That's all I do. I tell him, 'Wait until morning. If you are still ill, I'll take you to the doctor.' In the morning he does not remember what has happened. You see, it was all in his mind."

For most of the session Michaelangelo cooperates with the script, attacking his doctors for their incompetence. "All I do is fight this disease, but the doctors don't help. I went for another test for the diarrhea. The test won't be back until next week. 'What am I going to do, Doctor?' I ask. 'Try Kaopectate,' he says. I didn't need to go to a doctor to have him tell me that!"

Fiametta joins in with some enthusiasm. "He's right. I could have told him that. Couldn't they give him something else?"

Michaelangelo adds: "The doctor said I have to wait for the tests to get back. A week. They don't help. I don't think they care."

Fiametta interrupts. "It's because you are on so many medications. They don't want to add more. But what does it matter at this stage of the game?"

The session has an odd, disconnected rhythm. Michaelangelo starts to talk about his aloneness — the aloneness of one who has already half left us, the living.

Fiametta talks about doctors and medicine with the collusion of the therapist. Michaelangelo abruptly changes the topic. "Your sons don't care. They never ask me how I'm feeling. They avoid me."

"They do your chores," Fiametta counters. "They shovel the snow from the walk, take out the garbage — boy things." In an aside to the therapist she adds, "They are only boys, 19 and 21. What do they need to know about all this?"

Her husband responds despondently, "I am alone all the time, just lying there. The little one — she's only three — has more understanding than they do. She says, 'You're sick, Daddy.' She puts her little blanket, her security blanket, over my feet and says, 'This will make you better.'" He starts to cry.

Fiametta changes the subject. "He's had trouble with his eyes. He went to the doctor for his eyes." Michaelangelo stops crying and joins her with some bitterness. "They saw a lesion in my eye and they did a test. They think it's an old lesion from CMV. I have to wait for the ophthalmalogist, though. Fiametta asks, "Isn't CMV a bacteria? Can't they give him something for it if he has it?" They talk for a few minutes about medical issues.

Michaelangelo says again, "I feel so alone. I think about nothing except this illness." The wife adds, "That's all he thinks about. He's giving up! He doesn't take any interest in anything." Looking for an opening to raise emotional issues, the therapist asks if they talk to each other. Both shake their heads. "There's no conversation, nothing," Michaelangelo answers. "I have nothing to talk about. I can't do anything I used to. What's there to talk about, except this illness?"

"I asked him about our daughter," Fiametta says. "Maybe she should be in school next September. He wouldn't answer."

"I had nothing to say. What's the point? I might not be around in September. My opinion is of no importance."

Missing once again her husband's invitation to notice the imminence of his death, Fiametta responds angrily, "Of course you have something to say! She's *your* daughter."

At the end of the session, John offers to speak to Michaelangelo's doctor in order to understand the medical situation better. Michaelangelo seems fearful. "Do you mean you think there is something he isn't telling me? Of course, if there was, I wouldn't want to know." Fiametta moves to protect him.

"Don't worry, Michaelangelo. If the doctor knew anything, he would have told me."

The frozen quality of the session raises a number of issues that must be considered in working with the last phase of illness. It is clear from Michaelangelo's description of his increasingly debilitating symptoms and his decreasing responsiveness to medication that death is near. On the one hand, he says that he is afraid to know his fate; on the other hand, he gives a number of openings to discuss his feelings of despair, isolation, and his fear of dying. The therapist has to balance Michaelangelo's need for comfort in the face of growing isolation against Michaelangelo's fear of disclosing what he knows and having his fears of dying confirmed. Furthermore, for family, patient, treating physicians, and even therapists, dealing with oncoming death has become awkward and fearful.

The process of facing the fact that a beloved person is dying is made more difficult by the development of a belief that one can "survive and thrive" with AIDS. This belief countered the overwhelming negativism of the media and was enormously important to patients and their loved ones. Developing such a belief was critical to Michaelangelo and Fiametta's initial ability to live with an AIDS diagnosis. But, as discussed earlier, beliefs that illness can be held at bay by maintaining a positive attitude can lead to a denial that the patient is actually dying, compounded by a negative perception of death as a personal failure. The failure is attributed to the patient's assuming a "negative" attitude toward illness or to "giving up" his belief in the omnipotence of medical technology (or even alternative cures). To escape guilt about failure, the patient has to lie to himself about what he knows to be true. Michaelangelo feels horribly frightened and alone, ashamed of his impending death, but equally afraid of acknowledging to others what he secretly knows.

Once fear of illness and death have made the medical profession the substitute for community, once society has come to rely on the medical technology to cure any disease, then in times of mortal illness the lie becomes essential: It makes the work of the medical profession easier and it minimizes the experience of failure that death represents. Glazer and Strauss (1965) have called this lie "the drama of mutual pretense" in which both medical personnel and patient know that the patient is dying, but no one verbalizes this knowledge and the doctor continues to offer an endless procession of treatments. Ironically, while studies show that between 69 and 90 percent of physicians want their fatally ill patients kept in ignorance, between 77 and 89 percent of patients want to know the truth (Hendin, 1973). If the patient is in the hospital and kept in ignorance, the "sentimental order of the ward" (Glazer & Strauss, 1967) is preserved from disruptive emotion. The maintenance of this pretense, however, requires extraordinary vigilance; since each interaction threatens to reveal the truth that must be concealed, fewer and fewer interactions with the dying person take place. Furthermore, all conversations are superficial, lest topics that might reveal the secret be stumbled upon. At a time when many patients need spiritual comfort and a safe environment for reviewing their lives and relationships, mutual pretense makes this impossible. From the partner's perspective, "mutual pretense" can damage the intimacy and honesty of a relationship at a time when the need for these qualities is greatest. However, a family may be correctly reluctant to break down the defenses of denial if they believe the ill person truly does not want to know.

The therapist can offer the ill person openings to speak of death with statements and questions such as:

- "Tell me about your illness."
- "How sick do you believe you are?"
- "What have the doctors told you and what ideas do you have about what they have told you?"
- "What do you know or believe about your situation?"
- "What does your partner (wife, lover, mother, father) believe?"
- "What do they believe you know?"

In the case described above, Michaelangelo cannot prepare for his death because he is not allowed to reveal that he knows he is dying. He has nothing to say because any conversation may veer toward dangerous ground. Discussing his daughter, for example, leads to uncomfortable references to a future when he will not be present. He and his wife have the choice of inventing a fictitious future in which neither really believes or letting the barrier of silence fall between them, cutting them off from one another's comfort. They choose silence.

Michaelangelo is angry at himself, Fiametta, and the world, although he only allows himself to vent his anger at the doctors "who don't care" but who are not present. One feels his rage at the living, but he is too dependent, ashamed, and guilty to speak. Meanwhile, Michaelangelo's doctors maintain the pretense that he will overcome each infection. For physicians the payment for concealment is increased patient coopera-tion, decreased patient emotionality, and, perhaps, not having to deal with their own feelings of impotence. Privately, one doctor asked John Patten, "Doesn't he realize his situation is hopeless?" The doctor, how-ever, will not discuss the hopelessness of the situation with his patient, whom he has decided does not want to know.

Denying the visibility of approaching death robs the patient of the dignity and personal integrity involved in taking charge of or possessing one's own process of death. As the gay community has had to confront the overwhelming needs of its ill and dying members, a discourse about community, illness, and death has begun to challenge contemporary ways of dealing with death. Just as many people with AIDS have challenged beliefs about the omnipotence of medicine and analyzed the connection between medicine and power operations of the government, so are they teaching us to treat death, once again, as a sacred event. Gay families, buddies, and lovers make it possible for the person to die at home; if he must be hospitalized, they make sure the patient is seldom left alone. The emphasis is on helping the person face and shape his illness and death as well as his life by performing such tasks as writing a living will, discussing his impending death with others, choosing whether he wants to die at home or in the hospital, deciding whether to allow extraordinary life-sustaining measures or be helped to die, and designing his own memorial service. The process is healing for all involved.

For "surviving and thriving with AIDS" to have its fullest meaning, death must be experienced not as a medical or psychological failure, but as part of the natural context and flow of human existence. And it must be located safely within the context of family or community. Though desperately /ill, one young man, Jay, decided to take a last trip to the Smoky Mountains to a place he had loved from his Tennessee child-hood. Family and friends gathered from all parts of the country to be with him on this, his last trip. They camped together, shared memories, and said goodbye. A month after Jay's death his lover, Frank, said: "We always talked about our flags. We always tried to keep up his flag. 'I can fight this illness. I can beat this.' And after the trip to Tennessee, which was magnificent, I think he knew his fight was over and he stopped being afraid of it. He talked a little about being afraid no longer and being glad he had made the trip. I think, for him, it was a cap of finality. I think he was at peace. He took the time to say thank you – an amazing thing to do when you are lying there not feeling too comfortable."

CASE EXAMPLE

Jay was able to make peace with his death and to share his experience of living and the process of dying with friends. Michaelangelo, though also dying, is at a very different place. While some patients deny their illness to the end, we felt from the last interview that Michaelangelo was giving us a number of openings to discuss the issue of his dying. Before the next session two weeks later, John Patten, Carol O'Connor, and the team discussed various concerns. As therapists we had to acknowledge that our own vulnerability to loss often interfered with our ability to enter the client's world or to follow the openings that the client offered us to talk about death. We realized that Michaelangelo's fear of talking about what he really knew created a loneliness that was almost unbearable. It seemed necessary to open some communication between the couple to enable Fiametta to comfort Michaelangelo during his dying as well as to prepare for his death. Beginning this process was important for Fiametta; once Michaelangelo had died, it would be comforting to her to feel that they had together prepared for her future without him.

We knew that this might be our last session with the couple and we wanted to be sensitive to the family's openings and closings, allowing the family to modulate the discussion and signal when it had gone too far. Both therapists felt that one task of the therapy was to restore something of the old marital balance. They knew that both Fiametta and Michaelangelo did best when he was able to take charge and provide for his family, if only by his leadership. Michaelangelo's present depression was related to his sense of defeat and his humiliating submission to Fiametta's frightened nagging. The therapists had to find a way of helping *him* help her.

The therapists reasoned that John would have difficulty engaging the couple around emotional issues involved in preparing for death. The couple saw John as having rescued Michaelangelo from the crippling depression that followed his diagnosis by offering respect, hope, and medical advocacy. As a result, there was a danger that if John were too active in the interview, the couple would retreat from the emotional side of the experience by attempting to draw him into the technical issues. John decided to sit back so that Carol could begin to explore this vulnerable, uncharted area.

Michaelangelo opened the session by listing all his symptoms. Carol used this emphasis as an opening to explore his grief and sense of loss. She knew that Michaelangelo must mourn the physical and mental disintegration involved in the terminal stages of his illness and, at the same time, come to a reintegration of personal identity. The theme of loss and reintegration recur throughout the session.

Carol: [*To Michaelangelo*] Do you let yourself cry?

Michaelangelo: No.

Carol: Do you cry together? [*Silence*] Will you know when it's time to cry?

Michaelangelo: The medicine doesn't let me cry. It dries me up. [*The normal process of weeping is impeded by technological intervention.*]

Carol: If you could cry, would you?

Michaelangelo: I don't know anymore. It doesn't do any good. It doesn't help. If it helped, I'd do it every day.

Carol: Crying is a symbol that you are at another place. [*Carol is attempting to punctuate her work with the couple and acknowledge that she is open to hearing about the "other place."*]

Michaelangelo: Yeah, but what do you say? Why me? Help? I've said it already.

Carol: Are you scared?

Michaelangelo: Yeah, I'm scared.

Carol: Do you share that?

Michaelangelo: Sometimes I yell out.

Carol: When you are alone or when there's someone to hear?

Michaelangelo: Both *[pause]*, but sometimes I need a little comforting.
  *[This is one of the few times in the therapy that Michaelangelo has
  allowed himself to acknowledge his loneliness and need. Such an admission is at odds with his traditional sense of himself as the macho-provider.]*

Carol: How do you go about getting that?

Michaelangelo: I don't. Sometimes Fiametta comes over.

Carol: You both are at a new place. You both have handled everything
  for so long and you are now at another place. Maybe you can let
  John and me help you handle this new place.

Michaelangelo: *[Softly and with some relief]* That's why we are here.

Fiametta: I am less alone than Michaelangelo. I have friends to talk to
  and who comfort me, but I don't cry with them. If I cry, it means I
  have accepted it. But I haven't accepted it yet. I've not given up yet.

Carol: And crying would mean you have given up?

Fiametta: Yeah.

Carol: If Michaelangelo has to cry, does that mean he has given up?

Fiametta: We all know Michaelangelo gave up. *[There is some anger in her
  voice. His giving up is a betrayal of his contract with her to be the
  protector.]*

Carol: I didn't know.

Fiametta: He gave up a long time ago. He keeps to himself and doesn't
  communicate. He lays there and looks at the ceiling. Every once in
  a while he'll say something, but we don't talk.

Carol: How does it feel not to talk?

Michaelangelo: Sometimes I'll say something and she'll get sarcastic with
  me.

Fiametta: If we talk, we really have to face this issue and I don't think I'm
  ready for that.

Carol: Do you think Michaelangelo is ready for that?

John: What would be each of your greatest fears if you faced the issue?

Fiametta: I don't know what would be worse.

Michaelangelo: *[Opening the subject]* Your greatest fear is that you are
  going to die. That's it. Sometimes I just lie there, praying that I have
  a heart attack in the middle of the night so that it's over, one way or
  the other. I'm putting her through hell. I am getting put through
  hell, the baby, our friends, my sister, and brother.

Carol: Feeling what's happening and not talking about it makes it more difficult between the two of you.

Fiametta: What can we say?

Michaelangelo: We know where we stand, where we are. We know there's not much time left. We know all that. *[Yet this is the first time he has acknowledged the closeness of his death.]*

Carol: Are there things you want to say to Fiametta about the future— perhaps about a future when you are not here. . . lessons you want to teach, things you want Tina to know?

Michaelangelo: *[Avoiding Carol's invitation to talk]* No. I've showed her everything, I don't want to scare the baby. She doesn't want me to go into the hospital.

Carol: You both know what's happening, but you and Fiametta are going through it separately. Maybe that's the way your family wants to do it. If I were in your place, I would be scared to death to say the things on my mind, but on the other hand, I would be scared of what would happen if I didn't say those things. What if I never said them? *[Silence]* What is it like when you start to talk and get sarcastic with each other?

Fiametta: Maybe I've been fighting more with him lately.

Carol: I think it's been very important for you to have this strong husband. You both have been coping with this disease with the idea that Michaelangelo is a "tough guy." That's how he's helped you through this and that's been the deal between the two of you. But how to be tough now, nobody knows.

Michaelangelo: I don't have any strength left—that's one thing, for sure. I walk around like a zombie.

Carol: Yeah, physical strength, but what about other strengths? Are they gone or not discovered? *[Carol is too quick in attempting to ameliorate Michaelangelo's depression. Having just touched on the feelings of loss, he is not yet ready to move on.]*

Michaelangelo: Everything's gone. My nerves are shot. I'm a completely different person than I used to be. If they found a cure tomorrow, it would take a long time for me to get back to my old self. *[Turning to John and changing the subject from the frightening sense of physical and mental deterioration]* I know some good news, by the way. The proctologist said it's just an inflammation. If it had been colon cancer—I could not take all that.

Carol: *[Taking another tack as she senses Michaelangelo has shifted to the safer ground of medical issues, she indirectly appeals to Michaelangelo's sense of himself as Fiametta's protector.]* Fiametta, is there any way your husband can help you? You look so alone. Maybe he can't help himself, but is there a way he can help you?

Fiametta: He can help me more. I'm not talking about the disease. He can help me just by talking. I've got to instigate everything—the talking, I mean. I just want him to acknowledge that we are there once in a while. Now he just yells at the baby. Once in a while, when he's in a good frame of mind, he'll play with her. But basically he ignores her.

Michaelangelo: *[Defensively]* You say I yell at her? Why do I yell at her?

Fiametta: But if you don't talk to her the rest of the time and you just yell, what is she going to think?

Carol: Why do you yell at her?

Fiametta and Michaelangelo: *[Both answer simultaneously]* Because she's bad! *[Both laugh]*

Carol: *[To Michaelangelo]* Look at the grin on your face!

Michaelangelo: Because she'll jump on the bed!

Carol: To be with her Dad.

Michaelangelo: And she'll bounce a few times and fall off and hurt herself. I told her to stop, but she runs and, I'm telling you . . .

Carol: The epitome of life!

Michaelangelo: I'm telling you!

Fiametta: Yeah, she's got all this energy. *[Carol and the couple discuss Michaelangelo's difficulty in playing with Tina. He admits he can't manage her energy.]*

Carol: Tina's not treating you like a man who is dying.

Fiametta: She knows something's wrong.

John: She pulls the blanket over you sometimes.

Fiametta: I told her the other day, I said, "Daddy doesn't feel good. I think he's broken." So she said, "What do you mean?" I said, "Maybe we should send him back and get another Daddy." She said, "No, I love my Daddy! I don't care if he's broken or not." *[Pause]* I don't want to focus on the future—I mean, there's always hope.

Carol: Well, you are thinking about the future. You are coming for marital therapy. Something's not right.

John: If they are not talking now, there's an amount of tension here.

Carol: And sadness.

Fiametta: Because we are focusing on the future, because we are thinking about it—about death.

Carol: That was tough even to say, wasn't it?

Fiametta: Death. I don't want to believe. I try and try and try to be optimistic.

Carol: Is there a way of maintaining a balance so that you stay with what is real? Is there a place inside you where you can also maintain optimism and hope and take into account what is happening now?

Fiametta: Every time I go to the doctor with him and they give me bad news. When I didn't go, it wasn't so bad. I wasn't involved. Now, I'm involved. It's too much. I don't want to be there. Sometimes I feel I'm going to be next.

Carol: Being afraid for yourself is another part of it.

Fiametta: [Weeping as she speaks] What's going to happen when I'm next? Who is going to take me to the doctor? No one. Then I'm going to be left with the whole problem. Who is going to watch over me? Who is going to take care of me and my daughter?

Carol: That is, *if* you are infected.

Fiametta: I don't have enough courage to find out. I'm going to have this problem for the rest of my life. I'm never going to know. If I had some guts, I'd know what the deal was. But I don't. I don't know how to handle it. I keep it in here. If I never know, I don't have to worry about it, but I worry anyway—I'm worried sick.

Carol: Can I guess something? While you are worrying about that, you are feeling guilty because you are not thinking about Michaelangelo. And when you are thinking about him, it makes you think you also might be infected. So the circle goes around and around and you end up feeling worse and worse.

Fiametta: [Nods as Carol speaks] I feel that I could be a little more supportive—not supportive so much, but more compassionate.

Carol: What keeps that from happening?

Fiametta: I don't know. Maybe I'm just selfish. Maybe I don't want to believe it.

Carol: You're stuck.

Fiametta: I'm in a rut.

Carol: [To Michaelangelo] But you know what she just said. It's not news to you. Does Fiametta talk about that sense of not feeling like a good person and that she should be more compassionate?

Michaelangelo: No.

Carol: What do you think when you hear her saying that she is selfish?

Fiametta: He thinks I'm a bitch.

John: Last time he said she was a saint.

Fiametta: [*Laughing*] A bitch and a saint—I'm like all women!

Carol: If I were in your shoes, Fiametta, I would be caught in that, too. Michaelangelo, sometimes she is a bitch. Probably that's the only way she can survive it.

Michaelangelo: She's got to be strong. She's compassionate sometimes.

Fiametta: [*Dabbing her eyes*] That's why I don't want to cry. Just look at my face.

Carol: [*Laughing*] You could go out in dark glasses!

Fiametta: Oh my God, I forgot them!

Michaelangelo: Sometimes she'll come over to me and squeeze my hand or give me a hug. I'm not looking for more than that. Sometimes I just need it. Maybe she could do it a bit more often. It's funny, she mentioned the attitude of non-caring. Her sons are that way. Oh, the hell with the boys. But there's a touch of that I can see in her sometimes.

Carol: Is it a way that Fiametta is trying to take care of herself, protect herself from the pain?

Michaelangelo: Oh, sure. Most of the stuff I try to understand.

Carol: Tell her, not me.

Michaelangelo: I try to understand her. I know she's scared sometimes.

Carol: Tell her, please.

Michaelangelo: [*Silence*]

Carol: When she is scared, she does what she has to do.

Fiametta: He says I run away from the problems. He told his sisters, "She's always running away." But before I run, I make the dinner, and I take care of the baby. So when I run, I don't have to come back for a while and nobody suffers. I run, but I take care of all my problems. I have to get away. In fact, I told him for my birthday— I just turned 42 today—

Carol: Congratulations.

Fiametta: I look 42 today.

Carol: [*Laughing*] Oooh.

Fiametta: I told him for my birthday I want to go away by myself to a spa or something. His sister would stay with him and Tina.

Michaelangelo: I understand.

Fiametta: He said I have to get away sometimes.

Michaelangelo: I know it's getting too much for her. [*Fiametta's suffering*

is a reproach to Michaelangelo. If she is unhappy, he blames himself.]
Look, I'm the one who caused this problem.
Fiametta: You didn't cause the problem.
Michaelangelo: Sure I did.
Fiametta: It just happened.
Michaelangelo: It happened to me. I could have been more careful. Stupid me. I should have been on top of these things and I wasn't. I should have had gloves on and I didn't.

Michaelangelo's insistence on self-blame and the hesitation with which he speaks makes one wonder again whether he is circling around another explanation for his infection. Or does his hesitation seem to have meaning only in the beholder's suspicious eye? Michaelangelo has always seen his role as the protector of Fiametta. Is the self-blame arousal because he is now failing in that role? Perhaps. The therapists have always decided to accept his version without asking any questions. In doing so, they have certainly won his trust—but have they also closed off discussion and forced him to maintain what may be a fiction? It is impossible to know.

Carol: I have never heard you talk about it.
Fiametta: Never?
Carol: Never in two years. Do you talk about it together?
Fiametta: We don't talk about much.
Carol: I'm getting that picture.
Michaelangelo: There is nothing to talk about with me.
Carol: You only think that you are empty.
Michaelangelo: Oh, I'm empty.
Carol: Just now you weren't empty at all.
Michaelangelo: [*Tearful*] I'm empty, empty.
Carol: Do you think that Fiametta thinks these things? That you should have been "on top of it"? That you should have worn gloves? You *should. . . .* you *should.*
Fiametta: You know, it's funny. In all this time, I haven't blamed him. I haven't blamed him for anything. I don't know if he realizes it, but I don't. It's just the way it happened. Bad luck.
Michaelangelo: I blame myself.
Fiametta: Bad luck.
Michaelangelo: Bad luck, but I blame myself—putting all these people through what I'm putting them through.

Fiametta: There's no way you could have known. You are going through worse.

Michaelangelo: She was looking at the neighbor today and she said, "Why can't that be us?" You know the neighbor, the wife, and the little girl.

Fiametta: Oh, and they're out there with the family portrait and the whole yuppie routine.

Carol: How did you respond to what she said? Did you turn it on yourself? Did you blame yourself?

Michaelangelo: Yeah, probably.

Fiametta: You said, "I wouldn't wish this on anybody."

Michaelangelo: Yeah.

Fiametta: That wasn't blaming himself. He meant, it had to happen, better it should happen to him. He wouldn't wish it on anybody else.

Carol: [*Picking up the change in tone, lightening of affect*] I think we have gotten away from the important things you both were saying to each other. I think it was hard to bear what each was saying.

Fiametta: [*Crying*] I don't remember.

Carol: Scared?

Fiametta: Yeah, I'm scared.

Carol: [*Again using her own feelings to bring the conversation back to the issue of Michaelangelo's impending death*] Can I say that I am scared watching you? I love someone very much and I can imagine—it's only imagining. I can't be where you are now. But it's got to be excruciatingly painful. I would find all kinds of ways to dance away from it or build whatever I believed would keep it from hurting so bad—like getting angry or running away or hiding—and then I would feel like shit.

Michaelangelo: [*Nodding in agreement*] That's how we are. That's the way she is. I am not saying it's wrong, but that's what she does. I can't run because no matter where I am . . .

Carol: Maybe because you can't run, you can help Fiametta through this.

Michaelangelo: [*Eagerly*] How? Tell me how?

Carol: Talk to her. You've been a man who has taken care of your family and I know that the way to take care of your wife now is to *talk*. She may give you a hard time, because it's hard for her, too. But she needs you to persist, to try again and again.

Michaelangelo: I've always wanted to take care of her.

Carol: [*Softly*] I know.

Michaelangelo: I've always loved her. It's just that I've got a lot of guilt. There isn't anything I wouldn't do for her–anything. You see, I guess nothing is important to me–TV, all that stuff is so menial and so stupid. They're not real to me.

Carol: Is Fiametta real?

Michaelangelo: Sure, she's real. She's real and I would do anything I could for her.

Carol: She's telling you that you can do something for her.

Michaelangelo: Talk to her?

Carol: Even sharing that stuff you don't want to let out of your mouth. This is the time to do that.

Michaelangelo: What do I have to say? What do you say? I'm home most of the time and nothing is changing with me.

Carol: What do you think about when you are lying in there? Look at her. [*Fiametta is crying.*]

Michaelangelo: The disease–that takes most of my time.

Carol: She thinks you have given up. [*Carol's meaning here is not clear. She is referring to Michaelangelo's retreat from participating in family life, but he interprets her as meaning that he has given up the fight against illness.*]

Michaelangelo: What she said before: You go to the doctor and it's always bad news. The doctors don't care. There's no doctor-patient relationship.

Carol: They are scared, too, aren't they John?

John: Sure.

Fiametta: Doctors?

Michaelangelo: Yeah, people are scared. No one wants to touch you. Dentists are scared, everybody is scared.

Carol: I'm not so sure that it is only the fear of infection that makes doctors scared. I think it's being impotent. [*The session has moved as far as it can. Michaelangelo has returned to a focus on symptoms and attempts to draw John into a conversation about doctors.*]

John: Michaelangelo feels more comfortable being angry at the medical system.

Carol: I wonder if we have ended one part of the session and begun another.

John, Carol and the team take a break. We decide to clearly delineate the two realities: the reality that the battle against physical illness is over (which Fiametta, in particular, denies); and the reality that they still have a life as a family in these last days of Michaelangelo's life, and that as a family in this different place, there are tasks to perform.

Fiametta: Got a cure for us?

Carol: I think you have your own cure — not the cure for AIDS, but for what's ailing you.

John: It lies in the strength you both have as a couple.

Carol: It's hard to shift focus, Michaelangelo. You are a sick man.

Fiametta: *[Interrupting somewhat anxiously]* I was telling him when you were out of the room that we should take an hour or two each day and talk of something else.

Carol: You have to learn to accept that illness is always there. But you can have two things going on at the same time. The illness can be there, but at other times you can let another story come into play. There is also your life together as a family.

Fiametta: Last night we had a picnic on the bed, eating Chinese food with Tina while watching *Jeopardy*. I asked Michaelangelo, "Were you able to put the disease out of you mind?" and he said, "It's always there on my mind."

Carol: It can always be there; at present it is the most important thing in your life. But, remember, it is going on *in* your life. And you can have two and three things happening at the same time. Michaelangelo, I think that's how you can help Fiametta: by letting her know you are *connected*. But, Fiametta, you cannot expect him to give up entirely the reality that is defining him now. I wish it weren't, but it is. However, remember that *you are more than an illness. You are a husband and father, a person.*

John: You have to give yourself permission to feel more things than the illness.

Michaelangelo: Sometimes I feel like a leper and she's running away from a leper.

John: Sometimes you feel that, but there will be times when you do not feel that.

Michaelangelo: I feel responsible. I feel that it's all my fault. I feel like a leper.

Carol: Michaelangelo, are you painting yourself as a leper, or are other people?

Michaelangelo: I guess other people and myself. Other people treat me like a leper.

Fiametta: What other people? [*She continues reassuring him about how friends and family treat him well, discounting his need to talk about his painful sense of being polluted. The team intervenes. It is clear that Michaelangelo has issues that are painful to both of them. He needs the space to talk about his feelings and Fiametta needs to tolerate this conversation.*]

Carol: Fiametta, hard as it is to hear him talk that way, you are going to have to let him talk about that. Just as I opened the way for you to talk about your fears that you are not a good person, that you are bitchy, he needs the room to talk about those dark things that are important to him. You struggle to keep him strong and fighting, but part of the struggle is to come to grips with what you feel inside. That's a part of the fight, too.

Following this session, the couple reported that they talked a great deal with each other. Michaelangelo became rapidly weaker and died a month later. Both felt that this session was a turning point in that it enabled them to become closer to each other as they accepted the inevitability of Michaelangelo's death.

The transcript of this session with Fiametta and Michaelangelo illustrates the complexity of working with issues of dying when a partner has AIDS. In a society where death becomes invisible and is even considered a somewhat ignominious defeat, dialogue between a couple about impending death is difficult to achieve and sustain. Only a rare kind of grace and wisdom allows a couple to comfort and heal each other during the time when a partner is dying. But with AIDS, discourse about death requires still greater courage because it also raises the specter of the infection of the other person. Each time Fiametta thinks about Michaelangelo's disease, she is reminded of her own jeopardy; each time Michaelangelo thinks about his death or accepts Fiametta's embrace, he feels guilty. Anger is just below the surface and almost anything can trigger it. Loss is mixed with the general rage of grieving and the particular rage of a disease, the dominion of which does not end with the death of the beloved.

The therapeutic task during the last phase of AIDS is to help the patient make plans both for his dying and for the future of the people he loves. Unfortunately, families are often not in synchrony with the patient in terms of their acceptance of death. Studies show that even when the well partners are told the seriousness of the illness, the majority either disbelieve what they have been told or find a way of minimizing or denying the information (Parkes, 1982). As a result, patients wishing to speak about the full range of their feelings about dying are dissuaded by partners who have difficulty in handling the emotions. The therapist's challenge is to open a space that allows this crucial dialogue to take place.

CHAPTER 13

Preparing for Death:
The Last Tasks

WHILE MICHAELANGELO'S CASE demonstrated the communication difficulties confronting a family dealing with death, the following case illustrates how a remarkable young man and his family were able to carry out critical psychosocial tasks common to the final phase of AIDS. For the ill person these include: (1) finding self-acceptance and coming to terms with personal identity; (2) facing impending death and making clear one's wishes for care; (3) healing rifts with family and friends; (4) saying goodbye. For the family the tasks center on (1) acceptance of the patient's identity; (2) acceptance of his wishes for medical care and in relation to his death; and (3) as a prelude to saying goodbye, reviewing everyone's life together.

CASE EXAMPLE

The presenting problem in this case (Kaplan & Patten, 1989) was a mother's painful sense of isolation and her need to come to terms with her son's sexual orientation. Emily sought treatment because she had recently learned that her youngest son, Jacob, age 30, was ill with AIDS. She lives in a conservative community in Florida, where she feels that people would be shocked if she told them about her son. She has been divorced for many years and cannot share her grief with her ex-husband. She has two other sons, one of whom she describes as a "redneck" from Virginia who has never been able to deal with Jacob's homosexuality, and a second to whom she talks occasionally.

"I realized that I never came to terms with Jacob's homosexuality," she confesses. "I feel ashamed. I can't tell anybody. I've never told anybody that he's gay and now I'm stuck with the idea that he's gay and sick and I'm alone."

Isolation is a common theme for parents and lovers of people with AIDS and makes the task of tending the dying and mourning the dead infinitely harder. Support groups for family members are essential.

Laurie Kaplan and John Patten were the therapists. In the first session Laurie asked Emily to identify one friend in whom she could confide. By the third session Emily had begun to develop a support network both in New York, through a group of other mothers whose children had AIDS, and in Florida with selected friends. She now felt it was time to talk to her son. In the first session with Jacob and his mother, Jacob was able to consolidate his positive sense of gay identity by discussing his difficulty with his mother's feelings of shame about his homosexuality. He shared some of the feelings he had experienced when he "came out" to her, including a wish to provoke her to anger so that she would punish him.

Consolidating a sense of personal identity that includes acceptance of sexual orientation is a critical psychosocial task that needed to be accomplished before Jacob died. As one gay client put it, "Because I have finally learned to like and value myself, I can accept my death." Jacob had always felt different from the other males in his family; he was more artistic, more sensitive; he liked to sew and design things and he liked to sing. He felt the family mocked him for being different. When Jacob speaks of the straight world's reaction to him, he often uses a camp, feminized voice, as if by appropriating mockery he protects himself from the pain of others mocking him.

Jacob's hurt about his mother's attitude toward his homosexuality (which was tolerant, if not joyful) covered a much deeper hurt concerning what he perceived to be abandonment by his father. As the youngest son he had been caught in the middle of a bitter divorce and was forced to take his mother's side. After the divorce when Jacob was 13, his father vanished for seven years. Jacob longed for his father's approval, closeness, and acceptance. The difficulties he observed between his parents and his position in the family had made his acceptance of himself as a gay man difficult. He could not allow himself to seek a long-term relationship. While being openly gay, he punished himself by not allowing himself to have gay friends. Even in adult life he played the role of social misfit—a gay man in a straight world—as he had in his family of origin. Self-acceptance, including acceptance of sexual orientation, was a critical issue that needed to be resolved before he died. Because Laurie had seen Jacob's mother for a few sessions before he joined the therapy, Laurie found herself cast by Jacob into the role of his mother's confidante. She became the recipient of Jacob's confused anger against his straight family and no amount of interpretation could dislodge Jacob's projections. When Jacob began to have headaches and increasing pain, Laurie used that as a pretext to have John Patten join the therapy, ostensibly to do some hypnotic work, but more importantly as an ally for Jacob who could work with him on issues of gay identity. John's involvement freed Laurie to help Jacob understand his mother's position.

The therapy could be seen as containing a tension that was isomorphic to the divorcing family. Indeed, Jacob often attempted to set up conflicts between the therapists. In his original family he had felt bound to support his mother but had yearned for his father; in therapy he made an alliance with John and often fought with Laurie. The therapy was reparative in that John and Laurie remained united in their concern for Jacob. They were able to use the tensions in therapy to have conversations about Jacob's conflicts between loyalty to father and mother and between membership in the community of gay men and belonging to a straight family, whom he also loved.

John's entry into the system enabled Jacob to acknowledge his difficulties, his loneliness, his struggle to find himself and to make gay friends. He began to get involved in different kinds of spiritual healing seminars, which provided support groups. Through them he developed friendships with other men. He became very close to a young man named David whose family struggles mirrored Jacob's. While Jacob had been adamant about not bringing his father or other family members to therapy, he advised David to go to the Ackerman Institute with his family. David, stubborn as Jacob, sent his family to Ackerman, but he stayed home. Shortly after his family started therapy, David died. For Jacob, David's death represented an opportunity to begin to feel the depth of a friendship and its loss and to value himself as a member of a community of gay men. In a tragic sense, the ritual of funerals has had a bonding and politicizing effect on many gay men who have experienced the necessity to celebrate being gay in the face of community loss. Jacob, like many others who have experienced the death of a friend to this epidemic, became active politically and developed other gay friendships.

As Jacob began to feel more comfortable with himself and Emily felt supported by other mothers of gay children, her visits to her son became less conflictual. As their relationship deepened Jacob felt it was time to talk to his mother about the way he wanted to die. Earlier, just as Jacob

was passive about being gay, not actively seeking gay friends or relationships, he would have been more passive about his death. Now he felt it
important that he take charge of making his wishes clear. However,
broaching the subject was clearly too painful for both mother and son.
Each time he tried, Emily cut short the conversation by saying, "Look, if
I'm successful, and I take good enough care of you, you'll live, and if I
don't, you'll die." Jacob decided to bring the subject to therapy.

Jacob: [*To mother*] You have options because I'm going to be dealing with
     it. I'm going to sign legal papers and I'm going to assign power of
     attorney and I'm writing a will and I'm taking care of some business.
     So, you can be part of it and help me make decisions or not. Because
     I want to have as much control over my life in the hospital and with
     my possible death as I do in my life. I know you have certain feelings
     about how things might be. I don't know what they are, but I
     definitely have feelings about how I want my life to go and how it
     might end.
Emily: But do you feel that you have to do it now?
Jacob: Definitely. Before this infection turns into that infection and that
     turns into this and then I end up with that and – it would be much
     easier on me and I'll get proof from professionals that I'm sane
     because I don't want anything contested, I don't want anything
     fought. There is a problem with control and that's why I want it
     done. Because I'm afraid you might want things from me out of love
     and concern and continuation – that may not be the best thing. I'm
     afraid of that. So . . .
John: You mean in terms of – talking about things like life support?
Jacob: Respirators – things like that. I want dignity to the whole thing.
     That may not seem fair to you but it's – that's why I think I'm
     working on my spirituality because when it's time to go, I can say
     that I learned a lot and I had a full life. I don't need another two
     weeks. I don't need to live on morphine. So, I think it's very
     important that I know that I have that secure. I think that I'm even
     a little late. And I think it's time to get going on this stuff.
Laurie: It's like in some ways, I sense, Jacob, you're making your own
     separations in your own life. As you are talking about death, you
     are talking about the things that we all do, which is we become
     adults in our own ways and we keep becoming adults, each of us, at
     different times.
Jacob: The bottom line is that I want to go out with as much class as I

lived. I don't know how you'll be in the hospital if I'm real sick, so I want you to work with my nurse, not against him. What he's going to tell the doctor to do and not do is just going to be my wishes, nothing that he's thought up or decided by himself. But I know he understands the hospital and understands the medical treatments and he'll just be cool and calm about it. I think you'll need someone there like that. It kind of takes a lot of pressure off of you. I've been with friends in groups whose mothers come to the hospital, screaming, "Get your spleen taken out, get the surgery done, get this and get that." They say, "I don't think so, I don't know . . ." "You gotta do it, you gotta live, you gotta take this out!" And then just four or five months of morphine after that, when the infections never heal—I've just seen too many things. We see them back in group and say, "Congratulations." They say, "Don't congratulate me, I really made a mistake, this is horrible. I can't walk, I can't eat, I can't sit, I just—it's just prolonging death, making the last few months hell. I just should have left everything intact and just kept my respect." The stuff really gets to you, you know? Because you're really getting someone's opinion of his life—the core. And you can really learn from their mistakes and from their wishes.

Laurie: Yeah.

Jacob: I don't want to be dragged through hell for months and months and months and months because someone can't let go or whatever.

Laurie: Then you know that your mom will have a hard time.

Jacob: Yeah.

Laurie: Like?

Jacob: Like who wouldn't? That's why I'm trying to do this. I mean, I almost want to open up an envelope that says, this is where we're going and this is what time, like a wedding invitation. You know. Because I find with my friends the more I can talk about it, the more we can make jokes about it, laugh at it, the easier it is. I told Irene I want five thousand yellow roses. And Jenny, you know, takes photographs of me. It's my way of saying goodbye.

Although the pain in the room as Jacob talked seemed almost unbearable, the session was ultimately relieving to both Jacob and Emily. Later Emily said that this was perhaps the most wonderful moment of her life, when her son gave her the gift of letting her know that he was in charge and that he was going to help her to prepare for his death, which he felt she could not do alone.

HEALING THE RIFTS WITH FAMILY
AND FRIENDS

Jacob has completed a great deal. He has taken charge of his death and he is at peace with himself as a gay man, but perhaps the most difficult task of all is still ahead, that of reconciliation with his father before he dies. The completion of this task becomes increasingly urgent as his illness worsens. He is weak from almost incessant high fevers. He has a home-care attendant and friends, and his mother travels back and forth from Florida. As he grows weaker he feels safest when he is being cared for by his mother, but tension and fighting increase because they are both scared. The stress shows on Emily, who is losing weight. Jacob calls to ask Laurie and John if they would do a session at home. "I'm really sick. My mother's driving me nuts. We need a session, we're a mess."

John and Laurie hold the session in Jacob's bedroom. Despite a high fever Jacob is quite clear that the cause of the recent tension between himself and his mother is that his father had sent him a crystal to wear around his neck. Overwhelmed by this beautiful and longed-for token of affection from his father, Jacob showed the crystal to his mother and expressed his joy. Emily, quite understandably, exploded with a litany of accusations at her ex-husband, whom she saw as having abandoned his family and then, with a single gesture, winning the love and affirmation that Jacob seldom gave her. Jacob told her that he'd had it and she should leave immediately.

The therapists first reframed Jacob's anger as concern about his mother's heart condition and a way of pushing her to get some rest, even though he was scared to let her leave. They told Emily that it was critical for Jacob to spend time with his father, which he hadn't done since he was 13 years old. Furthermore, Emily needed a break and there was nobody whom Jacob would trust to care for him while she was away as he would his father. Difficult as it was for Emily, since she had not spoken to her ex-husband for 15 years, she called him and requested that he come to spend a week with Jacob. Jacob could never have asked his father directly. He always protected himself from disappointment by making excuses for his father and by mocking his attachment. "My father can't. He doesn't know how to cook an egg. He couldn't possibly survive. There's no way. He's a wimp. We've never spent more than ten minutes together, how could we spend a week together?"

When his father arrived in New York Jacob invited him to therapy. Before the session he described his father as the kind of man who lives and talks "Scottsdale Arizona"—a nervous superficial patter that drives Jacob to withdraw into moody introspection.

Because frequently therapists have only one session in which to reconcile past hurts when family members come to visit a dying child, these sessions are overdetermined, the pressure on both the therapist and the family intense. Furthermore, the parent and adult child arrive feeling sure that the subject of discussion will be sexual orientation or drug use. The adult child wants his parent's acceptance; the parent often feels guilt, failure, and distaste for his child's lifestyle. Both feel that sexual orientation or other behaviors have caused a rift, for which they feel guilt.

The idea that the rift will be resolved by discussion is often a trap, since both are likely to be defensive. Also, focusing on sexual orientation, drug use, or parental abandonment draws attention to the "problem saturated narrative" (White & Epston, 1990) and reinforces the assumption that the "dominant narrative" is the person's identity. Sexual orientation or drug use is only a part of a person's identity. A homophobic society and a gay culture operating in reaction to the political oppression of homophobia have emphasized "sexual orientation" until it has subsumed personal identity. It must be remembered that the politics of homophobia shaped gay identity, a social construction that enables a person with same-sex sexual orientation to claim the protection of minority status and gain the comfort of belonging to a community with its own traditions and culture when, without such recourse, stigma would bring social isolation, shame, and secrecy. Similarly, the socially constructed vicious cycle of poverty and racism creates a context where drug use provides short-term relief. While the tyranny of a drug habit may organize much behavior, other behaviors coexist but are overshadowed by the dominant category "drug user."

For both drug users and gay men, the relationship with the parents is disrupted by the need to maintain a secret life. The parents' lives may be affected by shame and the need to hide from their community what is perceived as "deviance." Secrecy and accompanying shame displace normal interactions. Because Emily was available for therapy over a long period of time, Jacob and his mother had the time to process emotional issues revolving around Jacob's sexual orientation. By contrast, Jacob's father is only available for one session. During this session the therapeutic task is to build relationship narratives as bridges between father and son in less controversial areas of their shared experience. The session opens with Jacob's father rather nervously filling time.

Father: [*Anxiously, a little too fast*] Can I start? I'd just like to say thank you. No more than that. Thank you very much for all you've done for my family.

Jacob: I was just telling him how I can always come here.

Father: You're there. I'm not, you are, and I'm very grateful. Jacob lies a lot, he tells me how good things are. I lie to him, I tell him, usually the father protects the son. This son protects the father. [*The father cries a little and changes the subject.*]

The therapists ask what the father's fears are about meeting and spending a week alone together. Both father and son are awkward, father evasive. Neither wants to speak of the illness, nor of their relationship. Nor does the father want to speak of his relationship with his ex-wife.

Laurie: So coming here today, I was interested in what thoughts you had in your mind, if you had any thoughts.

Father: A little bit of trepidation in a different sort of a way. I don't know what can of worms might be opened. It's not so bad if Jacob and Emily are in touch with you, but when I leave you today, we probably won't be in touch for a long time, so whatever is opened or transpired, it will start and have a very definite ending and that's it. There's no chance for clarification on my part, your part.

This is surely an oblique warning not to explore what Jacob and his father fear stands between them. "The can of worms," once opened, can never be closed. The critical issue is to create a yes-set between father and son.

During the next 15 minutes we engage in an uneasy back and forth as father and son evade the issues. Father continues to worry that the conversation would never be resolved if they opened up any difficult issues. John takes another tack by asking father, "What would improve the relationship?" Again he is evasive. Jacob talks about the formal distance between them but says that the distance is healthy.

Next Laurie asks about the end of the marriage, the bitter battles, father's disappearance from the family; she raises the subject of Jacob's coming out when he was in college. Father becomes increasingly defensive, filling in facts, going off on tangents about business. Jacob interrupts to say, "Why rehash the past when this session is all we have?"

In response the therapists try to bring the subject to the present, but Jacob begins to describe his father as a lecturer, talking too much about inanities and too little about emotional issues. Father insists that he is a salesman who is trying to put a nervous customer at ease. He senses

Jacob's depression and nervousness and tries to entertain him. Jacob now worries about opening a can of worms. He feels strange about being at home alone with his father, embarrassed about being so thin and so introspective. He does not want to drag his father into his depression and despondency. He doesn't want to talk about the illness.

The team decides to create a bond between father and son by asking the father to reflect on his early life with his children and on his own experience as a son.

Father immediately opens up. He talks about his life as a son of a traveling salesman, who was never there and was absent emotionally when he was there.

Father: My mother was my father and my mother. She took care of me always. In my marriage Emily was not demonstrative to me or to the kids. When I wanted to hug and kiss my children, I held myself back. I thought somehow that it would be pitting mother against father and so I didn't. The rule for me was that Mom took care of children.

Laurie: How did you try to make things different for Jacob and his brothers?

Father: I tried to get involved with all things that my dad never got involved with. Boy Scouts—my dad never got involved with Boy Scouts, he never encouraged me to do any of these things. I tried to encourage my sons to be a part of what I assumed was modern-day life with youth.

Laurie: And that worked better with some of your sons than others?

Father: Yes.

This small beginning opens an entirely different exchange between father and son. During the break the father tells his son that whenever Emily was away, he was able to hug and kiss his boys. He says it with relish and pleasure. Jacob looks surprised and appreciative at his father's open discussion of his disappointment that he had not been openly affectionate and his wishes for a closer relationship with his own father. Father admits that he allowed Emily to run his life and to dictate the way in which he treated his children. He is about to begin a discussion of his marriage when Jacob cuts him off. He makes it clear that he does not want to be caught in that triangle again. The intimacy and excitement dissipate and we wonder whether they will find a way to reestablish it in the next week.

The next session followed Jacob's father's return to Florida. The

therapists use Michael White's technique of looking for unique outcomes, the unexpected moment that can be constructed into the beginning of a different story (White & Epston, 1990).

Laurie: Were there surprising moments?

Jacob: Yeah, there were some...but somehow it got onto the subject of
flowers, because there were none in the apartment for weeks and
weeks. He just said, "Did you want some?" and I said, "ummmm,"
and he said, "Tell me yes or no," and I said, "Yes." So he went down
to the corner and he was gone for a really long time – a good hour
and a half. So I don't know where this man has gone or what bum
he's talking to . . .

Laurie: Who he's telling about Scottsdale . . .

Jacob: Yes, that's what I imagined. The florist is saying, "Just go home."
So it was really a long time and I was watching the clock wondering
what to do. It was just down the block and he's not the type to just
go to the store and shop. So he finally comes back with this huge
thing – beautiful, like something from Hawaii – and he says, "Well,
I was coming back and I had this four dollar thing and I said, 'This
is a piece of shit. I can't give this to my son. This looks like four
dollars. Let's get some flowers.'" So he went back and he got violets
and he got some lilies, magenta, he got some chrysanthemums,
some purple and white spotted things, and it was just beautiful, lots
of greens. It was really nice.

Laurie: Must be where your artistic flair has its roots.

John: Or that he was sensitive enough to respond to that.

The story is used to emphasize a web of connections between father
and son. It also refers indirectly to Jacob's experience in his original
family as the sensitive and artistic son, an experience that came to be
associated with being different, later with being gay. The team intervention frames the moment as a metaphor of acceptance between son and
father, father and son. Each therapist emphasizes a different aspect:
John, the father's attempt to symbolize his love and acceptance in his
son's language; Laurie, the son's gift to the father, a lesson about
sensitivity whose learning is symbolized by the gift of flowers.

John: The team members were struck, as we were, with the image of your
father, who didn't know how to get along with his father, standing
there in a flower shop for an hour and half. Probably he's not too
good with flowers.

Jacob: No, he asked the woman for help.

John: And choosing expensive flowers, and trying to decide which one was better, and somehow coming up with that arrangement. In the end he came up with something that was right with your aesthetics, your needs—something that you would find beautiful. That image of your father in that flower store, looking around, and making the decision that this was not a four dollar deal.

Jacob: It's more relaxed. Even knowing that it doesn't have to change and that's it just on this level and you can relax about it.

Laurie: And there's this part of you that has given something to him by being who you are, by your sensitivity. He has a chance to be sensitive with his son, to go pick out lilies. You've given him something that he never had. And you respect the awkward parts of your father, so that when he "talks Scottsdale" you know things are not going to change in that way. You accept that this is who he is. It's very nice to imagine you two during this week.

John went on to hypnotically suggest the possibility of organic growth in their relationship, a gentle hypnotic suggestion that underscored Jacob's "relaxation."

After Jacob's father left, Jacob's physical condition deteriorated. He had difficulty dealing with his loss of independence. In his depression he began to cut himself off from friends. His mood in the session reported below is one of hopeless resignation and apathy. Laurie is not clear where Jacob is in relation to his illness. Does he want to talk about how ill he is? He does not. He acts like someone who is waiting to die. He complains about isolation. Remembering Jacob's usual feistiness, she wonders whether people are withdrawing because they think Jacob is dying and do not know how to behave around him.

Laurie: If I were to yell at you, Jacob, and say, "Get out of bed even though you're sick! Screw it, you look awful, but move! What would you do?"

Jacob: It would help me. It's what I need and what I've always needed in my life. I'm used to being feisty. I don't really want to talk about dying. I'm a pain in the ass. I like people who give me a bit of a push and a nudge and I can fight them and they can tell me I'm a pain. That's what keeps me alive and enables me to live with the pain and struggle with it. I'm prepared to die. Living is harder than dying. This is what I need.

Jacob puts the dilemma of the dying person well. He needs to feel that he is not abandoned by the living; he wants friends to "kick" him back into their company because they love him and don't want to lose him yet. He also needs them to accept the reality that he may die soon, to share their feelings with him, and to be open to hearing his.

The therapists decide to conduct a session with Jacob and his friends so that they may open a discussion of Jacob's difficulty in relating to them. During the discussion, Jacob tells his friends that when they are too soft with him, it only increases his depression.

Friend 1: I asked you how your feet were and you said, "Stop playing nurse." I wanted to say, "Fuck you, what do you mean, 'Stop playing nurse,'" but of course I didn't.

John: With any chronic illness the person who is ill is put in a powerful position by those around him — the walking-on-eggshell effect.

Laurie: But it's lonely at the top.

John: Family and friends become frustrated that they cannot tell him their feelings.

Friend 1: Sort of protective — but out of love. What I've been learning is that I have to be who I am. If I'm not what I want to be, I won't call him as much. I want to be with him because he is my friend. So now I call him up and tell him everything. It's a learning process.

Friend 2: I remember that Terry talked about her feelings about Jacob's dying and he talked to her about his feelings.

Laurie: [*To friends*] What do you think about talking about dying? We all avoid the subject. We all wonder whether or not we should talk about it.

Friend 2: [*Denying the reality of Jacob's impending death*] I don't like to talk about Jacob's dying because it's not the reality. Jacob is living, more than most people . . . . It's arrogant of me to believe he is going to go first. I don't want to set it up that Jacob is going to die. Maybe he's not. If he wants people to talk about it, then he should say, "I want to talk about the practical and emotional aspects." I don't want to put restrictions on it.

Jacob: But it's not fair if you don't share with me your feelings, call me up and say, "I'm feeling this or that. I want to talk." My friends *must* be fearful and want to talk to me about it sometimes. They probably haven't lost another friend. They must be on eggshells part of the time. It must be confusing for them to know what to do for me. One day I'm fine; then zap, I'm like this, zap like that. Confusing. But if they don't come to me with their feelings, it's hard for me to feel I can go to them with mine.

Laurie: [*Summing it up for us all*] We are all in this together, all young, all in these incredible situations where people our own age are dying. None of us really knows what to do. We are finding our way, like pioneers.

The session makes it clear that the issue is not just that the person must talk with his friends about death; rather, a frame must be created in which it is understood that death can be talked about if either the friend or the dying person needs to do so. Jacob makes clear the importance of reciprocity, insisting that his friends come to him and talk about their own feelings, about their relationship to him, about his behavior. At the same time he makes it clear that he wants them to treat him as if he is alive and a full member of their "family."

Jacob: You keep saying to me, "What do you want?" I'm so alone. You're all asking me what I want, how you should be. I need some reciprocity. Am I a pain in the ass? Yell at me. Have a relationship with me. Don't make my illness the thing that you're relating to.

After this session his friends were more comfortable with him. They could let him know, "Well, yeah, I am upset that you're dying. It's very painful for me. I don't know what to do. I do feel powerless." And they could give him the "kick" he needed.

SAYING GOODBYE–LETTING GO

As Jacob's health deteriorated, Emily needed assistance with the help she was getting from the holistic healers to whom both she and Jacob had turned. She began to believe that Jacob's attitude, mediated by his relationship with her, could keep him alive or lead to his death. The possibility of failure became tangled with her feelings that she had failed him growing up, that she had failed somehow to protect him from being gay. As Jacob became neurologically impaired and lost touch with reality, his family of origin and family of choice began to fight. The friends worried that Emily would not allow him to die, and she worried that his friends were going to kill him. The session below, the last before Jacob's death, is about letting go, allowing a beloved son, for whom one has fought so hard, to go in peace.

Emily: He thinks he has lymphoma.

Laurie: Lymphoma, right.

Emily: If he does, then he has to be treated completely differently. The doctor wants him to come in on Wednesday, so he can take his CAT scan and some other tests if this hasn't stopped by then. He said he felt the wound had reached his stomach. So I said, "That means you think he's going to go." And he said, "Well, you know, we can do some drastic things to help him for a little while, but if that's what it is, they won't help for too long." And Jacob is unhappy—he's cranky. And I was just kind of holding his hand going home and I felt the fever in his head, so he said to me, "What are you, a home-care nurse or a mother?" So I said, "I'm a mother." And he said, "Mothers don't do that." I said, "Yes, they do. If they care, they do."

Laurie: You and Jacob both said that you saw it as a kind of mission. And you said to me before that you would be successful if you were to keep Jacob well.

Emily: Alive? Keep Jacob alive? Right.

Laurie: And if Jacob were to die, you would see yourself as a failure.

Emily: [*Pause*] I don't know that I would see myself so much as a failure. I think I would just be heartbroken. I don't know whether that connotes failure; maybe it does to a certain degree. I know that every mother goes through this. Our women's group has more mothers who come whose children have died than are alive.

Laurie: Um-hum.

Emily: And I see what they go through. And it's . . . . [*shakes her head.*]

Laurie: I know that the most important thing for you right now, despite how exhausted you are, is to be helpful to your son. And I guess what's most important is to sort out how to do that.

Emily: [*Sigh*] I don't know whether it was that last weekend we sort of lost a lot of what we had as far as togetherness was concerned, or whether it's because he's feeling so ill now and so irritated with what's going on, but it's a little hard to reach him.

Laurie: I think part of the struggle is that Jacob knows that it would kill you to see him die. At the same time, he wants you there helping him. So sometimes, I think, he pushes you away to push you away from the pain of the situation.

Emily: Do you remember that session we had this past summer where he wanted me to know that the end was near for him? I think that Jacob was preparing me. I don't think we ever talked about it, because I was always saying, "We're gonna do this so you'll get well;

we're gonna do that so you'll get well. Work hard and you'll get well. I'll help you." That was always the contention on my part. It was never "Time will pass and you're gonna get worse," but "Time will pass and we'll try to make you better." And I guess he wanted me to know that as time passed, it would probably be more difficult for him to get better. He was preparing me for this. And I don't know that he did that for any of his friends. I think that was the most wonderful hour that I've ever spent.

At the end, when Emily suspected Jacob's death was imminent, she brought him to the emergency room. But when asked if they should put him on a respirator, she made what was probably the most difficult decision of her life, answering, "No, that's not what my son wants. I'm going to let him die." And she took him home. After his death, when other mothers in her group challenged her decision, Emily wondered if she did the right thing. As she grieved for her son, she would watch the tape of the session in which Jacob had prepared her for his death. Hearing once again his wry but clear voice outlining his wishes, she knew that she had done what Jacob had wanted.

Jacob's funeral was healing to the therapists, too, for it was as he had wished, in a gay synagogue with the 100 yellow roses, the photographs, and all the people in Jacob's life who were important to him. Jacob's brothers spoke about how their brother's courage had changed their views about gayness. Jacob's legacy was that he had brought an extraordinary sense of community to people from different worlds as they shared the experience of his living his death. He had used therapy in a terminal period of illness as a process of self-integration, which also had enormous impact on the lives of those who survived him.

CHAPTER 14
Providing Care: The Family and the Medical System

T HE TERMINAL PHASE of AIDS may be acute or protracted; in either case it is critical to the bereavement phase which follows that the family members, both as a unit and as individuals, feel they have done "everything possible" within reason to help the person who is dying. A family's sense of competency about this task is integral to successful navigation of the subsequent bereavement and reorganization phases. What constitutes sufficient involvement will vary greatly among families and among different cultural/ethnic groups. One family may be satisfied that they had provided compassionate care; another only with heroic efforts to save the dying person.

Often decisions about care for the dying are guided not by the best interests of the ill person or even by his wishes, but by unresolved relationship issues including guilt because the dying person was addicted to drugs or beliefs that family relationships were responsible for sexual orientation. In its anger the family may abandon the patient or dedicate itself to saving the patient when all reasonable avenues of cure are exhausted. Unresolved losses or failed rescue attempts from a previous generation, rigid beliefs about control, or an inability to define limits or develop a balance between self-sacrifice and self-care can intensify family members' refusal to accept the finality of the patient's last hours.

A family's driven efforts at saving the PWA can result in the dying person's feeling guilt that he/she is letting the family down. One patient begged hospital staff to get the family therapist to help the family accept her acceptance of death. The family was unable to do so and continued to insist that she would recover. Even as she was dying, family members were busying themselves trying to get a new medication from Israel. The patient was forced to remain in her accustomed role, being the parents' protector and reassuring them, at a time when she needed reassurance and comfort about her own dying.

As children are now harboring infection for many years before becoming symptomatic, issues around the dying older child will become more and more prevalent. As we consider issues of how family and patient interact around dying, the reader is referred to an eloquent book by Myra Bluebond-Langner, *The Private Worlds of Dying Children*, which describes the clarity and detail with which dying children understand their medical situation. Langner notes that children pick up cues from staff and family that let them know that, in order for social roles not to be utterly disrupted by terminal illness, they must enter into a mutual pretense, never acknowledging what everybody knows. In actuality this pretense forces a hierarchical inversion, as the dying child calibrates his interactions with the parents and staff in accordance with what he perceives to be the needs of his significant adults. In this way he enables the parents and staff to perform their social roles of parenting and caretaking.

Langner reports the following dialogue with a dying child who, though he and his mother had never spoken of his dying (rather the opposite), knew that he must help his mother with the ultimate separation of death.

Langner: Jeffrey, why do always yell at your mother?
Jeffrey: Then she won't miss me when I'm gone.

Later she asks the mother for her explanation of Jeffrey's yelling at her. Mother answers: "Jeffrey yells at me because he knows I can't take it. He yells so I can have an excuse for leaving" (Bluebond-Langner, 1978, p. 232).

Such mutual pretense permits family members to act as normally as possible under the circumstances and to make normal developmental demands of the ill child. Staff members feel more comfortable when they can deny the reality of impending death, at least to the child, and go about their roles of "preserving life." In the case of children, open awareness does not lead to increased interaction between adults and their ill children; in fact, Bluebond-Langner presents some evidence that the opposite occurs.

The demands of care for dying family members may mean that emotional and practical needs of other family members are neglected. Children and adolescents may deny their own needs for nurturance out of loyalty to a parent who seems overburdened by the demands of caregiving for a partner, child, or other relative. The parent, impossibly overloaded, may indirectly express a wish for this kind of loyalty by expressing his/her admiration for their children's ability to "take care of themselves." Expressions of need by a son or daughter may not only imply disloyalty, but also become fused with any eventual unresolved guilt felt by the parent-caretaker who has been unable to heal the dying patient. Such situations can have far-reaching, long-term implications for the entire family.

During the terminal phase, effective decision-making requires that family members work together as a team and that they establish a good relationship with the medical system. If there are preexisting rivalries in the family or conflicting loyalties, as, for example, between a gay man's family of origin and family of choice, the family may not be able to act as a team. Splits should be addressed in network sessions that include all the concerned parties.

For example, staff at one hospital were unable to discharge a patient because family members kept vacillating between choosing to place him in a chronic care facility and choosing to take him home, in which case home-care attendants would need to be trained to provide for his quite extensive medical needs. In a case conference we found that family members were in fact deeply split. The young man had been living with his mother, who had been so stressed by his illness that she became ill herself. Although she could not care for him, she wanted him home, as did her sister. The idea of sending him to die in a chronic care facility was abhorrent to mother and daughter. From a Spanish culture, they believed that a person should die at home with his family around him. However, there was a longstanding feud between the sister's husband and his ill brother-in-law. The husband was jealous of his wife's relationship with her brother, whom he regarded as a no-good junkie, and he opted for a chronic care facility. As long as the family was able to stall the hospital, the wife did not have to choose between her husband and her brother. Finally, she decided to risk her marriage and move in with her brother and her mother so he could be cared for at home. Temporarily at least, her decision cost this woman her marriage, as her angry husband left her, taking the children. Had family and couples work been done, the family might have been able to resolve the impasse in a less destructive way and the hospital staff would have been spared many hours of work around the sister's vacillation.

Deciding whether to maintain a patient at home or to let him die in a hospital or chronic terminal care facility is difficult for families. Hospice care, when available, may afford a solution, allowing palliative medical intervention when the person is too ill for home care or when the family cannot manage 24-hour coverage; when the disease process abates, the patient can return home. Hospice care, in fact, has been shown to be preferable to hospital care for the dying patient and his family in terms of managing the bereavement period. Parkes and Weiss (1983) reported that survivors whose family members were at home or in hospice felt less anger and guilt than did relatives of patients who had died in hospital. Hospitalization during a person's dying may mean better medical management and spare the family dealing with the ravages of bodily disintegration, the unhygienic aspects of death; however, the price paid is often increased isolation for the patient and a loss of control for both patient and family of medical decisions and of access to each other (Aries, 1982; Glazer & Strauss, 1965, 1968). While all studies show that it is critical for the bereavement phase for the family to be involved as much as possible with the dying person, the efficient running of the hospital ward may require the curtailment of family visits to avoid emotional disruption. This limitation of access may hinder the family in sharing grieving with the dying patient and prevent the dying person from sharing his wishes for his family or lover before his death.

At home the family and patient can to some extent control how the patient is to die and let the patient choose whom he wants to have near him, for how long. The family and the patient have more freedom to decide to let the patient die and to refuse heroic measures. While for children the experience of living with a parent who is incoherent and ravaged by illness may be immensely disturbing, it also demystifies death and allows them to experience gradual separation and anticipatory grief. Nevertheless, the often lingering death of a person with AIDS is stressful to families, especially if small children require care. Balancing the needs of the patient and other family members may ultimately mean relinquishing the natural human longing not to let a beloved family member die.

For example, a poor African-American family moved a neurologically impaired patient home. While doctors pushed for a new medication that would prolong life but would have to be administered in the hospital, family members were able to ascertain that it would not reverse the neurological damage. They felt that a continuation of this young mother's lingering illness was neither in her best interest nor in the best interests of her children, to whom she had been a devoted mother. The children could not be placed with relatives as long as she was alive and the strain of her long illness was beginning to cause them to have problems. They were bewildered by their mother's erratic behaviors, which resulted from the neurological damage. And yet the family felt guilty about turning down a treatment that offered to prolong life. With the encouragement of the therapist, they invited their pastor to pray with them at the mother's bedside for the strength to resist the doctors and to let her go in peace, if that were God's will. A week later she died at home.

Rolland (1984, 1987a,b,c) has written about how the attitudes and behaviors of the medical team can either facilitate or hinder family decision-making concerning where the patient will die and whether, if the patient is in the hospital, heroic efforts should take place. A medical team that insists on taking heroic measures to delay death may convey confusing messages. How does a family know how to interpret continued lifesaving efforts by the health-care team? Is there still real hope, which should be read by families as a message to redouble their faith in and support of medical improvement? Do the physicians feel bound to a technological imperative that requires them to exhaust *all* possibilities at their disposal, regardless of the odds of success? Often physicians feel committed to a heroic course for ethical reasons (a "leave no stone unturned" philosophy) or because of fears concerning legal liability. Is the medical team having its own difficulties letting go emotionally? This situation can be caused by staff's own emotional attachments to a patient or their history with similar expectations.

Health-care professionals and institutions can collude in a pervasive societal wish to deny death as a natural process truly beyond technological control (Becker, 1973). Strong relationships with certain patients can be fueled by identification with losses, often unresolved, in health-care professionals' own lives, and endless treatment can represent the medical team's inability to separate from the dying person. Professionals need to closely examine their own motives for treatments geared towards cure rather than palliation, particularly when a patient may be entering a terminal phase. The family's beliefs about control and right to participate in medical decision-making must be taken into account, as well as its beliefs about palliation vs. cure.

Decisions about palliation vs. attempts at cure are made more complicated by the very medical nature of AIDS, which sounds a number of "false alarms," with the patient appearing to be dying of an opportunistic infection and than rallying and going on to live for weeks, months, or years. As family members keep vigil, they may go through anticipatory mourning and come to accept the loss of the dying person, only to have him recover, leaving them somewhat bewildered as to how to handle their feelings and proceed with their lives.

This terminal phase can go on for months or even a year. A painful or lingering death can place intolerable strain on family members, who often feel guilty and wish the ordeal were over. During this time the doctors may be trying a series of medical protocols to save the life of a patient who may have already suffered major physical and neurological impairment. Often, in the attempt to save the patient, little thought is given to the needs of a larger system. Yet the children, burdened by worries they cannot assimilate, may become symptomatic.

In one family where the child was diagnosed as school phobic, the mother, who had AIDS, had not been designated as ill enough to have a home-care attendant, but was ill at home alone during school hours when her boyfriend was at work. It was clear that the boy stayed home to be with his mother. In order to cover his real mission, he told his mother he was afraid that children at school knew about her illness and as a result he was ashamed to go.

The social worker in the hospital accepted the boy's explanation. A family therapy interview that explored the larger system established that the mother was without friends or other family members to support her and that a more plausible explanation for the boy's school phobia was his refusal to leave his mother alone. He was responding sensitively to her fear that she would die alone.

PLANNING FOR THE FUTURE

During the terminal phase, the family therapist must encourage the family and dying person to plan for the future. Clearly, the time to begin this process is when the patient is still active and can express his wishes. If the patient has been the sole caretaker of her children, the therapist must help her determine custody so that legal disputes can be avoided. It is healing for the dying person to actively discuss parenting with the person who will be designated as the custodial parent, as Loretta did in Chapter 10. Sometimes, however, when the therapist wishes to raise these issues, patients are in denial and want to believe that they will recover and resume taking responsibilities for their families. Many therapists are so caught up in meeting immediate family needs that they do not think about long-range family planning, or they may busy themselves with practical details as a way of joining patient and family denial that death has become imminent.

For all these reasons decisions may take place de facto or at a time when the parent is too ill to think coherently or consider all the options. As a result, after the death of one parent, the family may be thrust into family court to deal with litigation over where the children should live and who the custodial parent should be. Or a decision may be made that reflects some current family feud and does not seriously consider the best interests of the children.

For example, an African-American drug-using mother had formed a close relationship with a white social worker. After her death it was learned that she had designated him as guardian for her children. The social worker was a good man and in many ways the mother was right in feeling that he could better realize her dreams for her boys in terms of education and financial opportunity than her own rather chaotic and poor family. But her oldest son, aged 16, was deeply connected to his blood family, even though he liked the social worker, whom he had known for many years and lived with for a while during a period of his mother's addiction. He worried about his relatives as he had his mother. He was also struggling with issues of identity as a young black man. Removing him from this kin group looked like the best decision, but it did not take into account deep loyalties of race and family. Eventually, he rebelled, quit the school chosen by the guardian, and returned to live in a difficult but familiar network, where he was welcomed.

LOOKING DEATH IN THE EYE

Glazer and Strauss (1965) write of the many ways in which medical professionals may make it possible for the terminally ill person to end his life, whether by giving an overdose of painkillers or by prescribing a medication that, if taken in sufficient quantity, will cause death. Because medical technology often prolongs life beyond the time when it has quality or means, doctors respecting their patients' right to control their lives and deaths have provided the means to end their terminal suffering. The ancient tradition of honoring a person's right to auto-euthanasia has become common practice in the AIDS epidemic. Clients speak of feeling at peace because they have the means to take their lives if physical and mental deterioration threatens to rob them of dignity and meaning. For many, the knowledge that they can, if they choose, make such a decision restores a sense of control that is calming. Planning for their death allows them to face it, give it meaning, and make peace with it.

CASE EXAMPLE

Rustin, whom we met in Chapter 11, had had a long and trusting relationship with the therapist, Ruth Mohr, which had begun when he had initially sought treatment with the goal of establishing criteria for ending his life. At that time Rustin was recovering from his first opportunistic infection. The loss of control, which occurred because illness forced several simultaneous upheavals in his life, was overwhelming. The sensitive work that the therapist was able to do around issues of control and meaning in a life with chronic illness allowed him to develop a new life, one of AIDS activism and giving comfort to others, as well as continuing a career in the arts that he had thought was over. During the next two years he developed a wide network of friends and made several trips home to his family, even though he chose not to reveal his diagnosis. He became an eloquent spokesman for people with AIDS; tonight he was a spokesman for their right to die.

Now Rustin was ill, with increasing neurological complications. The pain in his legs was intense. Medications made him unable to think and work. He knew that it was merely a question of time before he became unable to function on his own. He tried to work, spoke at important conferences on behalf of PWAs for as long as he was able, but at last he came to a session, this time to say goodbye. What was remarkable was his stillness; certainly pain made movement difficult, but the stillness was more than just physical. He no longer felt he was one of us. For the last few weeks he had been considering auto-euthanasia. He had decided to die. How or by what means, or even when, he would not say. His decision about his death was not ours but his alone. He wanted to die alone, partly because he did not want to have anyone else held responsible, partly because he did not want to be bound to the living by ropes of tears and loss.

He said, "I'm not in a position to take care of people. I can only take care of myself. It is as if I am in a whole different space. I've been through it so many times with other people that I am real clear that this is the best thing and ultimately easiest on everybody, certainly on me. In a way there is no sense of loss on the other side. It's not that I won't miss people.

I don't know how to explain it. It's such a sense of peace. What I miss now is that I am alive and not able to do the things I want to do. Living like this is a much larger sense of loss to me. It's just different. When I made the decision, it was the most peaceful moment I had experienced in the last year. That's why, for me, I know I am near that point and that this is for the best. I've done good work and left behind all I can. And that's all I can do. I am beyond the point of being able to do any more work. I can hardly even think. There are better times when the pain is not so bad. I can think a little more clearly then. But those are fleeting moments. I'm just very ready to let go. I guess it's a space you can't really understand until you are there."

Rustin's voice breaks for a moment as he speaks for a second about the sadness that life is over, but he goes on to explain the finality of his decision. There is extraordinary peace and dignity about him. The young friend who has come with him weeps silently, tears of mourning. He is gentle with her but lets her know that her tears are hard for him, because he is no longer really here but concentrated on the sacred act of his passing. I think of Ivan Illich's meditation on folkloric death practices:

> People learned to be ready when death came, to have the steps learned for the last dance. Remedies against a painful agony multiplied, but most of them were still to be performed under the conscious direction of the dying, who play a new role and played it consciously. Children could help a mother or father to die, but only if they did not hold them back by crying. A person was supposed to indicate when he wanted to be lowered from his bed onto the earth which would soon engulf him. But bystanders knew they were to keep the doors open to make it easy for death to come, to avoid noise so as not to frighten death away, and finally to turn their eyes respectfully away from the dying man in order to leave him alone with this most personal event. (Illich, 1976, p. 185)

Rustin went on, "There's some sadness that it's here, but given the choices, this is better for me. This is not depression or an attitude problem. This is cold reality and there is nothing that can be done about it, and the possibility that it will get worse from here is practically 100 percent."

In his generosity Rustin has tended to many people through their dying. He has seen people clinging to life, exhausting every medical alternative, spending their last days on respirators, and he has also been with people who have taken death into their own hands. He makes no judgments, but he is clear about what he wants for himself. He wants to die with a full sense of his own identity. He does not wish to become merely an AIDS victim managed by technicians.

Rustin's acceptance of his own dying, his sense of completeness of the passage of his life and of his work, brings to mind a quote from the writings of the Renaissance physician Paracelsus:

> Nature knows the boundaries of her course. According to her own appointed term, she confers upon each of her creatures its proper life span, so that its energies are consumed during the time that elapses between the moment of birth and its predestined end . . . . A man's death is nothing but the end of his daily work, an expiration of air, the consummation of his innate balsamic self-curing power, the extinction of the rational light of nature and a great separation of the three: body, soul and spirit. Death is a return to the womb. (Paracelsus, 1969)

CHAPTER 15
Bereavement and Reorganization

EVEN IF THERE IS no logical reason to hope, the existence of the relationship during the terminal phase of illness is comforting. A seductive hope that one can trick loss always hovers on the sidelines, making anticipatory grief utterly different from the grief that follows the finality of death. Death shatters security; death forces significant changes in the economic and social status of the bereaved; death is accompanied by absence, loneliness, and longing. In the case of AIDS, death is further shrouded by stigma. Many of those who lose people they love to AIDS choose not to reveal the cause of death and thus must carry a secret that prohibits the sharing of grief with friends and family.

From a family systems perspective death brings a critical period of disorganization, as it forces the family to reconstruct itself without the lost person. A family with a fluid emotional structure will reorganize, utilizing the experience of death and bereavement as a dramatic opportunity for growth and change. Families with more rigid structures, more limited possibilities for emotional expression, may cling to old patterns and substitute other family members for the dead person.

While bereavement issues differ for the various subpopulations affected by AIDS, what is common to most of the bereaved is that, as in war, their loved ones died young, out of phase with their expected life cycle. Children die before parents; parents die leaving young children; young lovers, unprepared for the death of someone of their own generation, lose a partner and a lover. Normal grief processes become entangled with the dilemmas of the disease itself.

If the bereaved are parents or siblings, death from AIDS may bequeath a legacy of guilt and the stigma of failure to rescue the person from the behavior or situation that caused infection and death. If AIDS is revealed in the community to be the cause of the person's death, the family may be subject to social ostracism at a time when family members most need friendship and support. If the survivors are children or sexual partners of the deceased, the revelation of the secret brings the dreaded suspicion that they also may be carrying the disease. A wife of a drug user or a bisexual is left to deal not only with normal grieving, but also with the ambivalent feelings caused by the partner's legacy of infecting her, and through her, their child. A male lover may be fearful of his own infection, feel nagging guilt over the possibility that he infected the partner who has died, or blame himself for a failure in the relationship that put the lover at risk (Monette, 1990). Families may be grieving for more than one family member lost to the disease. Each subsequent death threatens the survival of the family itself.

Under normal circumstances, bereavement suppresses immune functioning and leads to an increase of morbidity and even mortality among the bereaved; to a person who is immuno-compromised or already ill with AIDS, the death of a partner constitutes a serious threat to health. In many cases we have seen partners who were HIV-positive but asymptomatic show rapid deterioration after their partner's death. Infected children and parents often die in close proximity to each other. As a result, it is critical to encourage bereaved partners and family members with AIDS to enter support groups and counseling.

It is important to note here that the dissolution of a significant relationship within the context of HIV disease also may constitute a loss that threatens health. The vulnerability of a person with HIV infection to the stress occasioned by such loss magnifies the seriousness of such events. Techniques used to resolve bereavement can also be applied to the mourning of a lost relationship.

AIDS creates a shattered world that demands extraordinary measures of compassion, thoughtfulness, and support for its healing. The task of bereavement is to accomplish separation from the deceased as well as a sense of deep connection (Lifton, 1983). Using the classic work of Parkes and Weiss (Parkes, 1972; Parkes & Weiss, 1983) to provide a theoretical framework for the bereavement process, this chapter explores aspects of bereavement and reorganization that are made more difficult by AIDS. A clinical case example illustrates interventive techniques with families.

DETERMINANTS OF GRIEF

Parkes and Weiss (Parkes, 1972; Parkes & Weiss, 1983) provide a useful clinical outline of factors that determine whether the bereavement process will be resolved, prolonged, or become chronic. Their studies have identified six critical variables influencing the mourning process: (1) the mode of death and the way in which partner or family members related to it; (2) synchronicity of death with the expected life cycle; (3) the presence of multiple stressors; (4) socioeconomic changes resulting from death; (5) support available from social networks; and (6) the nature of the relationship: whether secure or ambivalent, dependent or symmetrical.

Mode of Death

Sudden and unexpected death elicits more intense grief than a death for which a family has had time to prepare. AIDS death is seldom sudden; in many cases family members have had time to prepare and to make peace with the dying person. Even if the adult child has not disclosed the AIDS infection to parents when he or she becomes ill, most parents know or have guessed that the adult child is gay, a hemophiliac, a drug user, or the sexual partner of a person in one of the high-risk groups, and therefore at risk for AIDS.

In Chapter 12 we saw how Michaelangelo and Fiametta were finally able to discuss his dying and to make plans for the family's future, as were Jacob, his parents and friends (Chapter 13). Families who prepare as these families did – who feel they have done everything possible to give comfort throughout illness and remain close to the dying person during the last weeks, days, and hours of his life – will have an easier course of mourning than those who felt isolated from the dying person or unsatisfied with their medical decisions. The discussions between Jacob and his mother, Fiametta and her husband, were an artifact of therapy. For many families the pervasive denial of death precludes the exchange of emotion between the dying person and the family members, which is of critical importance in preparing the work of bereavement. Such families may seek therapy when grief seems inconsolable and reorganization fails to occur.

Synchronicity of Death With the Expected
Life Cycle

Even though AIDS deaths are most often anticipated, they remain out of synchrony with the patient's expected life cycle. Gorer (1965) has shown that the intensity of grief for parents who lose adult childen is even greater than for mothers who lose infants. Bowen (1978) has written of the emotional shock effect on families when children or parents die before their time. Perhaps the feelings of guilt and responsibility for the premature loss of a family member are implicated in this shock effect, which can cause a ripple of physical and psychological illnesses in other family members.

Often, for families who have sustained multiple losses, mourning is abbreviated, centered on the immediate post-death rituals, because sheer survival is at issue.

The Presence of Multiple Stressors

Studies by Parkes (1972) and others (Hauser, 1983) have suggested that widows who experience multiple stresses in addition to the deaths of their husbands tend to have a poorer recovery from bereavement. Families in which a member has died from AIDS often have been plagued by drug usage, the violence of inner-city life, poverty, unemployment, poor and overcrowded housing. While they have resources for survival, they are dealing with a mulitude of social problems, of which AIDS is but one.

Gay men live in a world of death and loss which, for many, affects everyone with whom they are close (Monette, 1990). At the same time they are constantly confronted with the social stigma of being openly gay or the psychological stress of remaining in the closet. Furthermore, many gays live with a real threat of physical violence ("gay bashing"), which has increased since gays have become more visible and assertive.

Socioeconomic Changes Resulting From Death

Socioeconomic changes following the loss of a partner may also complicate the grieving process. Gay men may lose economic status when their partner dies, just as they may lose housing if they do not share the lease. Women with young children are faced with the loss of income, and if they are HIV-positive, they must find family support in case infection converts to illness. They may already have an ill child who needs care and have no partner to share the burden. Survivors who are willing to take in orphaned children may be unable to find emergency housing to enable them to do so, without intolerably disrupting family life.

Support Available From Social Networks

Social networks can impede or disturb the bereavement process (Linde-mann, 1944). AIDS death can weaken normal familial and social net-works, causing the bereaved to keep secrets from schools, colleagues, relatives, neighbors, and co-workers. When pre-existing support systems are absent or damaged, it is critical that the client be introduced to AIDS-related networks such as survivor groups or to AIDS organizations that promote activism and mutual support.

A critical issue in the resolution of grief during the initial stages of loss is the availability of family and community rituals that memorialize the dead. Families from cultures of poverty where death is a familiar com-panion, such as the African-American and Latino communities, have available to them the strategies developed over time for dealing with the chronic loss endemic to urban poverty. In these cultures, spiritual support and religious rituals are central and kin systems are often skilled at giving comfort and solace (Boyd-Franklin, 1989; Garcia-Preto, 1982; Murphy, 1988). In the black community the gathering of a wide kin network to view the body and attend the church funeral, together with the often dramatic expression of grief and loss, is a critical ritual that not only expresses solidarity and the acceptance of loss but also symbolizes the continuing survival of the community. If the ill person has died at home, as is traditional in these cultures, a death ritual of kin and community initiates healing in the bereavement period that follows.

Unfortunately, the stigma of AIDS death may compromise traditional mourning rituals in African-American and Latino communities. Fre-quently, a family has sustained multiple losses and does not have the money for another funeral, with its attendant customs of providing food for the kin network. It may be difficult to find an undertaker willing to embalm the body, making the usual practice of viewing the dead impossible. Such a violation of normal practice can lead to the fear that the secret will be disclosed. Such fear further inhibits natural rituals of comfort.

The gay community has developed rituals that allow the public expression of feeling, alleviate spiritual discomfort, and give meaning to death from AIDS. These rituals create a transitional event, emphasize the continuity of life, and are emblematic of the struggle between the need to hold on and the need to let go. Since many gay people have been cut off from traditional religions of their youth by church attitudes toward their sexual orientation, new rituals, both communal and secular in nature, have been created: memorial services in which participants let loose balloons to celebrate the release of the soul of the dead; candlelight processions in memory of the deceased; the making of the great quilt, joining together thousands of lives with the sadness and gaiety. Each huge square contains scraps of memory of a living soul—a child, a father, a writer, a spouse or life partner. In an age that has lost touch with the importance of ritual, the rediscovery of its value in recovering from loss seems critical.

For the families of gay people who have died, the sharing of grief in hometown communities, which the gay person frequently had to leave because of homophobia, may be next to impossible. To counter community isolation, some telephone networks such as San Francisco's MAP have been established. These networks connect parents of gays who have died of AIDS from all over the country, allowing them to share their grief with one another.

If the family, whether of origin or of choice, is able to reorganize to provide support for the bereaved, grieving will be easier. Often, however, families are so angry at the dead partner on behalf of their relative whom he may have infected that, for instance, the widow can find no one in the family with whom she can share her grief. The gay lover may want to share memories and grief with the family of his dead partner, as he does the grief work of piecing together the life of the person he loved and lost. But family members may blame him for their son's infection and want no further contact. This ostracism after the death makes AIDS different from other illnesses: It leaves the bereaved partner with a legacy of infection and surrounded by a hostile family of origin.

Family schisms around a dead parent or silence around an AIDS death may be particularly difficult for children who have no outlet for mourning, have a sense of the presence of a secret concerning the death of the parent, but know that they cannot ask questions. Furthermore, many children who have lost parents to AIDS come from drug-using families. Drug users often medicate feelings with drugs, thus inhibiting their verbal expression except when "high." Their children may have seen violence and abuse, learning from their parents to keep silent and not share their feelings with outsiders. Not being able to share the complex feelings they carry about their parent's death, not being able to mourn the loss openly, makes them vulnerable to future drug use. This correlation between premature loss and drug use in a later generation has been documented in the literature (Stanton & Todd, 1982). For these children the only discharge of their grief and anger may be through acting out at school, becoming symptomatic, or identifying with problematic aspects of the dead parent.

The Nature of the Relationship

The nature of the relationship to the deceased will affect the process of bereavement. The loss of a dependent or ambivalent relationship can cause intense mourning that is difficult to resolve. Survivors of marriages, life partnerships, or parent-child relationships that were highly conflictual may have more difficulty completing the fundamental task of bereavement: that of letting go and internalizing valued aspects of the dead person so that durable connection can be created.

Parkes and Weiss (1983) believe that ambivalence during a relationship contaminates the grieving process with self-reproach for any negative feelings previously experienced toward the person who has now died. For example, parents and spouses of drug users may have been dedicated to rescuing the drug user, while still feeling angry, used, and powerless to save. AIDS illness intensifies family members' sense of helplessness and guilt, because it bears witness to the ultimate failure of their efforts. Helplessness and guilt in turn lead to rage, expressed overtly through ostracism of the dying person or covertly in the reaction formation of overly heroic efforts to preserve life. These complex and ambivalent feelings then infuse the grieving process with added pain, isolation, and self-recrimination.

One woman, who discovered that her husband knew he was bisexual when he married her but chose to conceal the knowledge, often wished him dead during the terminal period of his illness. However, her fury alternated with periods of intense grief. After his death she continued to fear that she was infected, despite the lapse of a significant period of time during which she tested negative. Her rage and bitterness seemed unabating and clearly masked an underlying attachment that could find no expression. By contrast, two other women who knew that their husbands were bisexual nonetheless had experienced caring and satisfying marriages. As a result both were able to remain close to their partners as they were dying; both were able to mourn and support other women through the grieving process, moving through it to lead productive post-bereavement lives.

Complementary relationships can result in intense, unresolvable grief after the loss of a partner. The lost relationship may have been overly reparative, providing a single experience of being loved and supported, or it may have fostered dependency as a substitute for missed early experiences of parenting. Gay men often have had difficult times growing up in their families of origin, where a sense of being different, the harboring of a stigmatized secret, or actual parental discovery and disapproval gravely injured the parent-child relationship. Drug users have higher than average experiences of early loss and therefore tend to have difficulty separating from their families of origin. This lack of adult separation results in conflictual relationships with their partners or spouses, in which the need to satisfy dependency needs outweighs the ability to seek and provide personal autonomy.

The death of the partner in a complementary relationship may disrupt a sense of personal security which depends on the relationship and the role that the partner has played: "Any movement away from grief among the dependent bereaved exposed them to a dangerous world with which they could not cope. They turned to the partner to protect them but doing so faced them with endless grief" (Parkes & Weiss, 1983, p. 97). Dependency in life thus is converted to a dependency on grief after death – an endless yearning for the missing part of oneself that the dead person seemed to represent. For example, Frank had been extremely shy and socially reclusive until he met his lover, Jay, who had a great zest for life. Jay was searching for someone who would care for him and the fit was perfect, since each admirably complemented the other. Jay's ability to build a world of friends reflected how he had survived a difficult family; Frank had derived his sense of self-worth from caring for others.

In some ways the arrangement even suited the requirements of illness although, as we saw in Chapter 11, Jay's need to be cared for made it more difficult for him to fight his illness. When Jay died, Frank experienced his world as shattered. Despite friends, he no longer had Jay to make him feel comfortable and loved and he had lost the role of caretaker that was fundamental to his self-esteem. Furthermore, it was difficult for Frank to make use of therapy, since he was not accustomed to seeking help and being cared for, except in the context of helping his lover. Shortly after Jay's death, Frank became ill for the first time. To his surprise friends emerged who devotedly cared for him as he had cared for Jay. Unfortunately, it was too late and three months later he died.

STAGES OF GRIEF

Parkes and Weiss (1983) describe at length the stages of normal grief, noting that the person may go through one or more of them and also may oscillate from stage to stage. The stages they identify are: numbness, pining, disorganization and depression, recovery (forming a post-bereavement identity).

After the initial shock of death and the rituals of the funeral or memorial service—which may be accompanied by a psychic numbness, a measure of denial, or intense grief—the bereaved person enters upon the work of grieving. Initially, the work must contain a ruminative preoccupation with thoughts of the lost person, a tireless examination of the events preceding illness or of the last weeks or the last day, when the cause was lost. It is as if remembering the bereaved could reverse the flow of times and redo the events. This period of obsessive remembering may also contain dream phenomena wherein the dead person appears in different circumstances, hallucinatory-like experiences of the dead person's presence, as well as impulses to join the person in death. Parkes and Weiss (1983) have noted that the work of grieving is a struggle between opposing impulses: one tending toward realization of loss, the other toward retention of the lost object.

The seeds for this concept of joining can be found in Freud's brilliant work, *Mourning and Melancholia* (1917), which describes how the ambivalent love or libido, which was attached to the disappointing object, is drawn into the ego and then becomes identified with it. Freud's idea of incorporation (which has pathological consequences in melancholia) was based on a far more ancient notion, whereby the powers of the dead are received into the living through rituals and sacraments of incorporation. The resolution of grief requires identification of experiences that allow the relationship to be completed: The living are able to let go of the dead, knowing that they both *have* and *have not* lost them. The idea that the process of mourning should end in connection to rather than decathection from the loved object is a crucial one for therapeutic intervention. Michael White's paper, "Saying Hello Again: The Incorporation of the Lost Relationship in the Resolution of Grief," lists clinical questions that are useful in helping the bereaved create a new identity that reclaims those aspects of the self which had been projected onto the dead person.

How might this process of grieving and reclamation actually manifest clinically? Let us assume that the survivor played a subordinate role in the relationship. In the early stages of grieving he pines for the lost person, believing that only with the restitution of the beloved (the lost object) will his pain diminish. As part of the process, he begins to review ways in which he depended on his partner. During this time his grieving is eased by the presence of friends, although typically they become impatient over time with his need to obsessively review the relationship. This painstaking review, this "filagree" of mourning, as Parkes and Weiss (1983) have called it, is essential if the survivor is to internalize the relationship and eventually let go of the deceased.

If mourning goes badly, the bereaved person becomes fixated on what has been lost, fearing that he will never be able to supply for himself those attributes so valued in his departed partner. The more the therapist tries to reason him toward acceptance of loss, the more he resists, because acceptance of loss to him means psychological devastation. For this person, once the partner vanishes from continual remembrance and awareness, critical support systems vanish as well.

If mourning goes well, remembering gradually becomes a celebration of cherished aspects of the relationship. The bereaved person begins to believe that he can learn from the warm memories of his relationship to his partner and discover in himself the projected attributes. Little by little, such self-acceptance allows the formation of a post-bereavement identity, as the person begins to shape a new life, often taking over the roles played by the dead person. An exquisite example of "saying hello" can be found in Milton H. Erickson's lovely parable of the woman who, childless for many years, finally gave birth to a baby girl who died a crib death at six months. Instead of focusing on the woman's inconsolable sense of loss, Erickson asked her to remember the nine long months when the child was growing within her body and the long and pleasurable six months of the baby's life. Using rich images of growth, incorporation, and pleasure, he then suggested that she plant a tree in memory of her daughter's life, so that she could one day take pleasure in its shade—a ritual act that would transform the loss symbolically. After the session the woman, who could have no more children, seemed much helped in resolving her mourning. Ultimately she paid tribute to her daughter's life by becoming involved in growing rare and beautiful plants (Zeig, 1980).

RITUALS OF MOURNING

The essence of grieving and incorporating ritual and symbol to facilitate letting go is exquisitely illustrated by Joe, who went to a gay pride march to begin to say goodbye to Herbie, the man he had loved.

"I went down to Washington, you know, for the names project. I had a panel made for Herbie. I was there at six in the morning when they were setting up the quilt and I was there at sunrise when they started reading the names. It was very, very emotional. When I was leaving Washington, when I was walking away from the rally to go toward the train station, I felt sad because I felt like I was leaving a lot of that love behind. It was a loving weekend; it was really beautiful. But I also felt like I was leaving Herbie behind. And part of me wanted to and part of me didn't. I had a piece of cardboard with his picture on it and his name and birth and date of death and a little message. I had pinned it on my backpack when I marched. As I was walking away from the rally, I put it in my bag. I wanted to keep it, but there was a part of me that wanted to let go of it. And I, ah, I looked around and I went like this [*demonstrates looking over his shoulder*] and, sure enough, there was a nail sticking out of a tree right there—you know, no coincidence—so I just left his picture hanging on the tree. I've even—I've talked to him, you know, and I've said, 'I don't want to let go, and I do.'"

The following case translates the principles of grief work discussed above into therapy practice. It illustrates the impact of AIDS secrecy on mourning and offers interventive techniques that permit the mourner to begin the process of incorporating valued aspects of the dead person and enable the family to heal splits rigidified by the loss of a family member to AIDS. While the case begins with only one family member in therapy, it demonstrates how the working of family themes, as well as the eventual addition of a second family member to the therapy, facilitates the process of mourning.

CASE EXAMPLE

Mathilda, an Irish woman in her late fifties, came to us a year after her daughter Sara, an IV drug user, died of AIDS. Sara's daughter Michelle, aged four, also died of AIDS, six months after her mother. For Mathilda the bereavement process has been interrupted by memories of an ambivalent relationship with Sara; also, Sara's death has evoked the unmourned loss of her own mother, whom Mathilda feels she failed to save. Furthermore, Mathilda is isolated from emotional contact with her nuclear family. She lacks a social network and she observes cultural restrictions against displaying emotions. As a result, she is almost paralyzed by grief that seems to have no end. When family members see her grieving, they remain fixed in silence, watching television, distracting themselves from her evident pain. When she first comes to the institute, the very act of sitting in the waiting room watching other families converse fills her with grief and envy.

On meeting Mathilda we asked ourselves, "Why has there been no easing of her grief? Why can't she share her grief with another family member?" In the first session, the therapist, Laurie Kaplan, constructed a genogram with Mathilda, which gave some answers to these questions that would form the basis for a hypothesis to guide our work.

Both Mathilda and her husband, Brian, come from working-class families in which the spouses had severely conflictual relationships. Brian's father was an alcoholic and Mathilda's father had two other "secret families," including children. Mathilda's mother was described as always depressed and often suicidal. Mathilda and her sister were her caretakers and would often have to stay home from school to prevent mother from taking her life. Mathilda was the favored child but never felt, try as she might, that she took as good care of her mother as her status as "favored child" merited. Brian was close to his mother, her "man" in the face of desertions by her alcoholic husband, who died when Brian was 16.

In both Mathilda's and Brian's families of origin, the primary marriage was between a parent and a child. Brian's mother leaned on her son, as Mathilda's mother leaned on her daughter. These significant relationships ended at critical times in the life cycle of Brian and Mathilda's marriage. Brian's mother died when Brian's oldest son, Matt, was born. Brian never grieved, according to Mathilda, as he is just "not that kind of man." The men in Brian's family are stoic and turn to alcohol instead of expressing emotion. To replace his lost attachment to his mother and his partial loss of Mathilda (who also mothered him) to the new baby, Brian followed the tradition of his family and made the relationship with his son his primary marriage. His attachment to his son was overdetermined by his longing for a relationship with his own father, which the intensity of his connection to Matt to some extent repaired.

Mathilda's mother died when Mathilda's oldest daughter Sara was 12, just approaching adolescence. As a child, Mathilda had received little attention from her depressed mother; consequently, she tended to harbor feelings of insecurity and worthlessness under a busy exterior as a "strong caretaker." "I didn't amount to much," she says of herself later in therapy. Burdened by the difficulty of caring for a depressed mother, Mathilda learned early that there was no room for the expression of her feelings. Mathilda's ambivalence about her mother, together with familial and cultural injunctions about mourning, drove her grief underground. She said of her mother's death, "I never grieved. I developed food allergies instead. I felt so guilty because I don't think I took care of her as well as I should have."

As mentioned, at the time of her mother's death, Mathilda's favorite child, Sara, was entering adolescence. This confluence of events – the threatened separation from a daughter as she matured, the loss of a mother, the inability to express grief, the guilt about her mother's death – set in motion a process in which Mathilda would ask Sara to be as close to her as she had been to her own mother and Sara would outwardly comply but inwardly resist. Difficult as her life with Sara was, Mathilda now says tearfully to Laurie, "She was absolutely great. She was the only one in the family who treated me like a person."

Drug use proved a solution to Sara's conflicting wishes to grow up and become independent and to stay at home with a needy mother. Family research on drug addiction indicates that an unresolved death in a prior generation which carries residues of guilt makes families vulnerable to separation. At the same time, if the young person becomes involved with drugs, unresolved mourning fuels the parents' determination to rescue him or her no matter what the cost. The rescue of a drug-using child becomes identified with the failed rescue of the dead parent. This attempt to symbolically undo the previous loss becomes an attempt to retrieve the lost object and substitutes for the original mourning (Stanton & Todd, 1982).

The work of the therapy seemed clear. Mathilda needed to connect with other members of her nuclear family, most particularly her husband, in order to share her mourning. She must also begin the work of incorporating valued aspects of the people she has lost. Until now, she has been preoccupied with controlling her tears in the presence of her family and trying to overcome her grief. Pain connects her to Sara and Michelle, and she dare not give up this connection, because after all, as she sees it, Sara was the only person who really valued her. But Mathilda is also angry at Sara. She cannot talk about the conflictual relationship with her daughter for fear of being disloyal to her daughter's memory in this deeply divided family. Her buried anger, in a classical sense, takes the form of melancholia and must be addressed during the therapy. Finally, Mathilda must see the connection between the unresolved mourning for her mother and her unrelenting mourning for Sara, who took her mother's place in her life.

Mathilda and Brian have a younger daughter, Carolyn, who was somewhat neglected in the passionate partisan relationships of father with Matt and mother with Sara. Because Sara's death has destabilized a longstanding family structure, which depends on the marriage of each parent to a problematic child, there is a danger that the family will restabilize with Carolyn replacing Sara as Mathilda's problem child. In that way, rescue will once again become a substitute for mourning and will prevent Mathilda from "letting go" of Sara, Michelle, and her mother.

A critical task in grief resolution is to build a network of people with whom the mourner can share her grief. Isolation is common among parents of people who have died of AIDS. As with suicide, secrecy, which conceals the stigma of AIDS death and the behaviors that it represented, may isolate the mourner even from close family. Furthermore, as we have seen, drug use, gayness and AIDS often create rigid family coalitions and split or solidify pre-exisiting ones.

From Laurie's opening exploration, "Who else is mourning for Sara and Michelle?" we learn (1) that, while Mathilda thinks her daughter Carolyn is mourning her sister's death, she would not speak to her about it because she would be afraid to burden her further; and (2) that Mathilda will not speak to her son Matt or to her husband because she believes "they are not grieving." Two premises organize Mathilda's family: "A parent only shares his/her intimate life with the children," and "Women carry the burden of caretaking and cannot count on men for help." Mathilda, for the most part, hides her pain from her family, but when she does cry, neither her son nor her husband notices. Challenging the governing premises, the therapist starts to weave connections between Brian and Mathilda. She asks Mathilda to describe Brian. Mathilda sums him up as "uncommunicative." The therapist suggests an alternative story about Brian.

Therapist: So he might be *secretly* grieving. How would you know if he were in pain? How could you tell?

Mathilda: I guess I couldn't really, because he doesn't really show his feelings . . . . He goes to church all the time. He's a hypocrite. He goes to church and wouldn't visit his daughter in the hospital.

Therapist: Perhaps church is a place where he secretly grieves.

Mathilda: [*Relenting*] He did say he lit a candle for Sara.

Therapist: [*Underlining the connection that Mathilda has made*] So, in some sense, you're doing your private grieving and Brian may be doing his, but you wish that he would notice your need a little more. But he may not be the kind of man who knows how to help when he sees someone else in pain. You told me he lost his Dad when he was 16 and had a mother who had ten children to raise and who was always in great pain. As a little kid he must have felt pretty powerless to help. He probably found in you a strong, competent woman, who would take care of him. Now, when he sees you in trouble, he has a hard time shifting. So you may be wise not to ask for help.

Having seeded the idea that the spouses may be able to share their mourning, Laurie begins by reviewing Mathilda's memories of Sara's and Michelle's deaths, of their funerals, of who joined her in mourning her losses. Mathilda needs to share her memories with other people, but she feels hopeless about sharing her mourning with family members. The men in her family are uncaring, Carolyn has too many problems and shouldn't be burdened, and other relatives would ask embarrassing questions. At this point Laurie stands for the family; later she will press Mathilda harder to bring another family member with her.

As they review the past, Laurie begins the process of helping Mathilda incorporate positive aspects of her daughter and granddaughter. She asks what was special about Sara and Michelle. Mathilda says they were the most outgoing and open people in her family.

Therapist: Both Sara and Michelle were outgoing and shared their feelings and brought joy to your life. That's a special thing. I am wondering if in some way you can pay tribute to that, so that you honor that memory in a special way.

Mathilda: I would like to but I don't know how.

Therapist: What was special?

Mathilda: [*Crying*] Sara was more of a person than anyone else in the family, more of a human being than the others. She was accepting of people for what they were. She made you feel you really mattered.

Therapist: Are you like Sara?

Mathilda: I think I accept people for what they are. I don't judge them for what kind of a job they have and how much they make. But she was the only one who treated me like a person and now she's gone. [*Crying throughout*]

Therapist: Tell me, Mathilda, from whom do you think Sara and Michelle inherited that ability to be generous and not judging?

Mathilda: [*Long pause*] I think my mother was like that and I feel guilty for not doing more for her.

The two mournings are now linked: the unresolved loss of Mathilda's mother and the loss of the daughter who replaced Mathilda's mother in her life.

Therapist: You think your mother, too, was generous and not judgmen-
      tal?
Mathilda: I think she was a lot like Sara.

Laurie makes a delicate connection betwen the three generations as
she begins the process of helping Mathilda incorporate valued aspects of
her daughter.

Therapist: In your own way you did pay tribute to your mother. You say
      you felt guilty, but in your own way you took qualities you valued
      in your mother and made them your own and passed them on to
      your daughter and to your granddaughter. You created a testimony
      to your mom by passing something of her on to your children.
Mathilda: [*Crying*] But Sara and Michelle are no longer here.
Therapist: Right. Your mom isn't either, but look what you took from
      her. You said, perhaps not consciously, "This is something beautiful
      about my mother and I want her memory to be alive in me and in
      my children." And you passed it on to your child and your
      grandchild. It is something for you to think about. How can you
      keep their memory alive, too, in a way that reminds you of what
      they brought to this world? It is hard for you, because if Brian and
      Matt are mourning, they do not show it, so you feel you are the
      only one keeping the memory alive. But perhaps as a beginning you
      could begin to share some memories of your mother with your
      children, who know very little about her.
Mathilda: I suppose I could do that

This first task is more neutral than sharing mourning for Sara and
Michelle. Laurie asks Mathilda if she is ready to look at pictures of Sara
and Michelle. She says perhaps she can start to look at pictures of Sara
and offers to bring them to the next session. Laurie suggests that perhaps
she could even look at them with Carolyn. Mathilda agrees to try.

In the third session she and Laurie share the photographs of her
daughter and grandaughter. Laurie uses the photographs to get to know
the family and to begin to construct a lighter, more positive image of
family members, so that Mathilda's belief that she has "no family" can be
challenged just a little. Because Mathilda's grief seems without relief and
unattached to family, social network, or the ritualized comfort of religious practice, Laurie asks her how she would like to shape her mourning. She describes different customs of mourning; for example, Jewish
people sit Shiva for a week and mourn for a year. She asks Mathilda to

construct a grieving map by thinking about the kinds of things she would need to do to mourn her daughter's death. This map, consisting of specific "mourning tasks and rituals," will allow her to do fully what she needs to do.

By the fourth session Mathilda's grief seems to have abated somewhat. She feels that one result of the session in which she discussed her mother's death with Laurie and the connection between her mother and Sara and Michelle is that she has begun to grieve her mother's death. But she has begun to worry about Carolyn's depressions. She does not know how she will get her surviving daughter to therapy.

Therapist: You said this week you felt a little better. How much time would you say you gave to grieving about Sara and Michelle, worrying about Carolyn, or thinking about Mathilda?

Mathilda: Well, I guess probably grieving about Sara and Michelle half the time [*crying*], and worrying about Carolyn maybe a fourth of the time, and thinking about myself a fourth, something like that.

Therapist: OK, so we'll stick with the bigger chunk. Last week I suggested we give some shape and form to your grieving, in order to give it the respect that it deserves. So I wondered what you thought about that. Did you think about it during the week?

Mathilda: Well, I started going to church. I haven't been going to church for a long time.

Therapist: What meaning does church have for you, Mathilda?

Mathilda: Well, it's like spiritual values, you know. So it would be praying for her and Michelle. It's kind of uplifting to go. It makes you feel better.

Laurie asks her to think once again about her grieving map. What would be the task of the beginning, of the middle, of the end? How long would grieving last? The suggestion that mourning is time-limited is both comforting and frightening to the mourner.

Mathilda: What if you can't stop after a year?

Therapist: Then you can extend it, as students do if they have not finished college; they extend the time it takes to learn the things they need to learn. [*A positive redescription of grief as a learning process, suggesting growth and continuation of life*]

Rituals memorialize the dead and provide a framework for maintaining connection. They provide a calm and ordering punctuation to the disordered time that follows death. They are a counterbalance to the disorder of obsessive thoughts about the dead that preoccupy the mourner. If rituals are performed with another person, they create a metaphor with private and communal meaning. Here Mathilda begins to identify her own rituals. She has started to go to church and to meditate, which helps her focus on what she wants to do. Laurie says that, to give some shape to her grieving, she might plan to do those two rituals regularly.

Mathilda: It seems that the pain is getting less, but when I start thinking about the pain getting less, I start crying. I don't know why it's so painful. All I know about grieving is that it's very painful.

Therapist: It's painful for you even to think about putting an end to grieving. Remember last time when we talked about Handel's *Messiah*, about birth and death, joy and sadness? Grieving is a way both of feeling pain about the people you have lost and of immortalizing the people you love.

Mathilda: After that session I thought about bringing my photo album of Sara and Michelle up to date. I also thought that maybe I might give gifts in their names at Christmas time.

Therapist: That's a beautiful idea. To whom?

Mathilda: To needy families. You know, you spend so much during the year on unimportant things, you could save it for Christmas.

Therapist: That's a beautiful idea for the future. What could you do *now* that would make you think about the joy they brought to your life?

Mathilda: You mean, instead of just thinking about the pain, could I begin to think about the happy times?

Therapist: What would be a ritual to bring back the joy?

Mathilda: Just to do something enjoyable. Like Sara, she always liked to do something enjoyable.

Therapist: So that would be another ritual you could add to your week: to do one fun thing that would remind you of Sara, a thing she would have enjoyed doing and seeing her mom do.

Laurie asks Mathilda again how long she sees grief lasting. Mathilda guesses about a year, but says with some relief that if a year were not a long enough time, she could prolong it.

Therapist: I suppose that, in a way, the scariest thing for you is the thought of stopping grieving, because the grieving is the way of feeling connected with them.

Mathilda: It seems like, if you stop grieving, you just stop thinking about them. They would be out of your life.

Therapist: It is important to stay connected to them. We were thinking that it would be very helpful for you to have a daily ritual right now. But you also need to know that grieving is a process that will change over time. And rituals will be part of the process and will also change as mourning changes. Ritual will help you stay connected to Sara and express your feelings and thoughts to Sara and Michelle. What is a ritual that you would be comfortable with?

Mathilda: Well, maybe praying.

Therapist: So, what if you were to commit for the next week to get up a little earlier and go to church each morning and light a candle for Michelle and Sara?

Mathilda: [*Sounding alarmed*] It seems like once a week is enough.

Therapist: We felt that it was really important that you spend a certain period of time every day focused on your grieving, performing a ritual of mourning, focusing specifically on Sara and Michelle. Not necessarily focusing on your grieving but making the connection.

Mathilda: But it wouldn't be going to church every day, 'cause I don't think I could fit that in.

Therapist: How come?

Mathilda: I'd have to get up earlier . . . that would really be a project.

Therapist: Not to go to Mass, but just to go to church and light a candle. A private time just to grieve for Michelle and Sara.

Mathilda: There's a church right on our block, the block near where I work. When I'm at work, I could stop in at lunchtime and light a candle. Or maybe on my way home from work. Then I wouldn't have to rush to get my lunch and get back.

Therapist: So you will make a commitment to spend 15 minutes with Michelle and Sara every day.

In order to get information about the times that the church is open evenings and weekends, Mathilda has to ask her husband, who is a regular churchgoer. Her inquiry begins to bring them together around the rituals of mourning because, by stopping at church each day, she is doing something that means a great deal to him. He has often begged her to go to church and she has resisted. As we know, lighting a candle is his mute way of expressing his mourning for his daughter and granddaughter.

At the end of the session Laurie asks Mathilda to describe a trip to a museum, which she had made the previous Sunday with her daughter

Carolyn, and which she had mentioned earlier in the session. The therapist asks her to think about what it would have been like with Sara and Michelle. Mathilda describes how a trip to the museum or a stop at a toy store brought back memories of Sara and Michelle that were both enjoyable and painful. During the discussion Laurie suggests that eventually she might share some of her memories with Carolyn on these trips. Mathilda says that, in fact, in the past week they have been able to talk a little about Michelle and Sara.

By the fifth session Mathilda has done the ritual and feels better. She begins by expressing her sadness that no one else in her family would come to therapy.

Mathilda: Actually I do feel better since you told me to go to church. I spend ten minutes a day with Sara and Michelle. I did that and it does feel better. [*Crying*] It's still very hard to accept that they're really gone. I just can't get used to it. When I went every day, it seemed to drive home to me the fact that they were gone.

Therapist: What did you do when you were in church?

Mathilda: I lit a candle to Sara and Michele and tried to make myself feel I was in their presence.

Therapist: Did you talk to them?

Mathilda: Yes.

Therapist: What did you say to them?

Mathilda: Well, with Sara it seemed as if she got sick so fast, went so fast. I was wishing that I could have spent more time talking to her about really being terminal, and I didn't do that because I always kept hoping she wouldn't die. I suppose if I had to do it over again, I would have done the same thing, because you would hate to bring up that someone is really dying.

Therapist: How would it have been different for you and Sara if you had talked?

Mathilda: I don't know. When she went into the hospital the last time I couldn't believe she wouldn't come out. I just kept hoping she would get better.

Therapist: I suppose you feel you would have liked to have had a chance to say goodbye. Tell me, when you go to church and light a candle, is that a way of saying the goodbyes?

Mathilda: I guess so, because when I went every day, I seemed to accept it better. But if I accept it better, why am I crying?

Therapist: I wonder if when you began to feel better, you began to feel less connected to Sara and Michelle. Mourning, feeling pain about their death, has until now been the way you have remained connected to them. In the old way you felt connected through the pain and sadness. Going to church and talking to Sara and Michelle is a different way of being connected. And maybe you are not totally ready to give up the old way, which isn't crazy because most of us don't give up our old shoes until we are sure we like the new ones and have broken them in and feel comfortable in them.

Mathilda: I guess I wouldn't know unless I kept it up longer. But when I went every day I seemed to feel better and to really accept that they are really gone [*crying*].

Therapist: Maybe your tears are really saying just that. You are really negotiating saying goodbye in a different way. And those breaks from the ritual are a way of slowing it down.

Laurie pursues the theme of Mathilda's isolation. Without Sara she feels terribly alone. She is angry that her husband and son abandoned her daughter and did not try to help her out during the long years when she alone struggled to help her daughter with her drug problem. Mathilda feels hopeless about ever connecting to her husband, who seems to have no wish to be connected to her. She sees him as hysterical, using emotion and rage as a way of controlling people. He will never change. Only Carolyn had some feeling for Sara's problems. Recently Mathilda has become more aware of Carolyn's grief.

In the intervention at the end of the session, Laurie asks Mathilda if she has ever thought of asking her husband to go church with her. She says she would like it he went peacefully, but she makes it clear that if he does not ask her, she will not ask him. She knows that he will just attack her for not going to church for all those years. Laurie drops the subject for now and asks Mathilda to continue to do the ritual but to be comfortable with those times when she does not do it and then feels worse. The ritual is a new way of being connected; the pain and the grief are the old way. At this time she still needs the old way because it is familiar and reassuring. Mathilda says that going to church is surprisingly helpful, and for a long time she had felt that nothing was going to be helpful.

Perhaps because of the pressure that Laurie has put on Mathilda to connect with her husband, Mathilda comes up with an alternative. She begins to make a better connection with her daughter Carolyn. Without warning, Carolyn decides to come to therapy. With Carolyn present, Mathilda at last can see herself as having a family. Carolyn is simple, extremely plain, a woman who has lived her life in the shadow of a flamboyant though troubled sister. Mathilda voices her worries about Carolyn's depressions, but Carolyn refuses to be seen as ill – she is not her sister. As the two women converse, we realize that this exchange of simple revelations about how each interprets the family history is a landmark in a family in which emotional isolation and silence have been the rule.

Carolyn says she has worried about her mother but could not talk to her about her grief. She has seen a marked improvement in her mother since she has been coming to therapy, which made her curious about what went on here. Mathilda complains that Carolyn has refused to join her in the ritual of lighting candles. She adds sympathetically that Sara's death from AIDS has alienated a number of old school friends of Carolyn's and that Carolyn has a right to feel resentful of her sister's illness.

Carolyn talks about the intensity of Sara's relationship with her mother. Sara was always a rebel at school, always in trouble; mother was always in court trying to save her. Carolyn doesn't know how her mother put up with it. Carolyn's presence opens the way for Mathilda to touch on some of her frustration and anger at Sara. This unexpressed anger is part of Mathilda's hidden ambivalence towards Sara, which blocks resolution of her mourning.

Mathilda cries heavily as she wonders why Sara had to go through so much. Having a daughter on drugs was like leading a double life: on the one hand, going to work, trying to act as if she were leading a normal life; on the other, always in court and cringing when the phone rang at night, dreading that she would learn that Sara was suicidal again or had taken an overdose of drugs or had been picked up by the police. The terror is still in her voice. One recalls Mathilda's account of the two little girls, Mathilda and her sister Nell, staying home from school to keep their mother from committing suicide.

Laurie explains to Carolyn, as Mathilda listens, that her mother was raised to be a rescuer in a family with a suicidal mother and men to whom she could not turn for help. She says, "She couldn't count on her dad to help, so she couldn't turn to your father and your brother. In your family the women were the only people to be counted on. And I'm sure that at times your mother got angry at her mother for not being able to deal better with the problems of her life, just as you may be angry at your mother for not managing her life with Sara better and for dedicating so much time to her."

The parallel builds a connection between Carolyn and her mother. Carolyn is like Mathilda, worrying about and angry at her mother.

Carolyn admits that she felt hurt after her sister's death when her mother, instead of talking to her, went to therapy. She says, "I'm not a judgmental person. Why couldn't she say those things to me?"

Laurie explains that Mathilda, having grown up in a family where her own mother burdened her so much with her sadness, would never want to burden her daughters with her suffering. As a result, she determined to be the strong one who kept her grief to herself or sought therapy rather than placing that load on Carolyn's shoulders. Carolyn is moved by this explanation, which softens her feelings towards her mother.

Laurie then works on Carolyn's mourning for her sister, asking her what remained unsaid between them. Carolyn answers that before her illness Sara was in so much trouble that talking was impossible. Just as she began to recover from drugs, so they could have become closer, Sara got sick. Laurie asks Carolyn if she ever felt anger at her sister for using drugs and taking so much of her mother's care. She answers, "If I did, I would not have mentioned it."

Laurie suspects that the family is vulnerable to re-establishing its old structure, with Carolyn becoming mother's new problem bearer. Carolyn is subject to depression, she is fairly isolated, and she has little idea which direction her life will take. Laurie wants to block this possibility by predicting it. Her prediction becomes a leitmotif of the therapy.

Therapist: Do you think that you and your mom are going to become more like companions or do you think your mom might be tempted to try to take care of you with your problems?

Carolyn: [*Laughs*] I hope that we will become more like companions. I don't want her thinking about my problems.

The therapy has ritualized Mathilda's grieving and involved Carolyn in the process. The next step is to widen family involvement. In a serious and yet playful way, Laurie plots with Carolyn how the women could persuade Brian and Matt to go with them to pick out a headstone for Sara and Michelle. Since neither woman drives, it is framed as a necessary and practical task, not as an emotional one. The split in the family is described in a lighter vein—as something to be resolved with strategies to get the cooperation of the two TV-watching men.

With her daughter present, Mathilda is able to rework aspects of mourning that have been the subject of earlier sessions. Laurie asks her to tell Carolyn what she would have liked to say to Sara in that last week. In response to her mother's expression of grief, Carolyn for the first time begins to share her sadness with her mother, most particularly that she had not known her sister, that she had missed the opportunity of sharing their adult lives together, and that her sister had not had a better life. "There's a whole big question mark between us," she says. Laurie gives the women two tasks: to succeed in getting father to drive them to choose a headstone for Sara, and to finish the photo album of Sara and Nicole. As the two women cry together, share memories, and think about ways of involving the men in remembering Sara and Michelle, the rigid family structure, engendered by drug usage and reinforced by AIDS, begins to dissolve.

In the next session the two women share with Laurie the photo album they have made together and tell her that they have been able to get father and Matt to go with them to choose a monument by bribing them with a "nice lunch." Mathilda seems lighter and less tearful. She says to Carolyn, "That last session was the first time I saw you really crying. Because on the anniversary of her death, I was really crying and you just walked out of the room." Turning to Laurie she adds, "She doesn't like to get too emotional–like her father."

During the past week Mathilda was able to cry with Carolyn. She also went regularly to church and talked to Sara about her grief. Carolyn adds perceptively that the death of Sara is also the death of the way that the family was organized around Sara's problems. So her mother is mourning the end of the way her life was organized and perhaps as a result, she feels purposeless and empty.

Therapist: Mathilda, perhaps some of the things you said last time were hard for you to say. You said that one of the things you would have liked to have said to Sara was that you wished you had been in her place and that it was very hard for you to accept the death of your child. That's what many mothers would feel, that they would do anything to take away a child's pain. You don't want to see them suffer. And at the same time, you said that, as much as you want to lay down your life for this daughter whom you loved, you somehow feel angry at Sara for not having gotten rid of that drug problem before. You're really mad at her and that's a tough one to admit, that you can love somebody and be angry at them at the same time.

Mathilda: Yeah, I suppose I never really told Sara how angry I was about her drug problem.

Mathilda speaks of having felt so alone with Sara's problems. Her husband was indifferent, as was her son. If she were the only one who cared about her daughter and tried to help her, how could she be angry with her? Anger would have been a terrible betrayal. Sara had to count on her mother. There was no one else. The split in the family made loyalty to Sara paramount and prohibited Mathilda from expressing anger at her daughter while she was alive. She had to marshall all her strength to sustain her lonely fight for her child.

In the next session Mathilda tells Laurie that they have just found out that Matt has been using drugs for many years. He told his father and asked to go into a rehab program. Brian became immediately involved with his son, which infuriated Mathilda. After all, he did nothing for Sara, just let her die. Laurie and the team worry that Mathilda's bitterness will reopen the split and that Matt's treatment will be sabotaged by Mathilda, as Sara's was by Brian. We know that it is critical for Matt that the parents work together to support his becoming drug-free (Stanton, 1985). When Mathilda talks about her anger that Matt never helped his sister (*her* child), Laurie offers a different explanation.

Therapist: Your anger is also about the ways that perhaps you and your husband have not worked together with Sara's problems. You feel angry that Matt had a great deal of difficulty in dealing with Sara's dying, didn't attend her funeral, probably because he was using drugs and may have had some fears himself about seeing what had happened to Sara. It doesn't stop your being angry, but you can realize that his silence around Sara's death might have been his difficulty in dealing with the pain of her dying. It wasn't so much that he didn't love her, but he was locked in his own world....Because you and Carolyn have been courageous enough to come here, to talk about your daughter's death, the problems with drugs in your family, the way it affected Carolyn, you gave Matt permission to say, "I've gotta own up. I can't keep silent anymore about my sister's death, about my problem." You have made a beginning for your family. I think it might be a good idea if you continue to go to church and talk to Sara about Matt's problem, because she was an expert. Try to hear from her advice on how to handle Matt's problem.

Mathilda: Yeah, I went to church at lunchtime a couple times last week. I think her advice would be just to try and talk about your feelings and deal with them rather than to run away from them. And Brian, when we went to that family meeting in the drug program, he did say to Matt (it was really a first), "If you ever want to talk, I'll be

there for you." That was the first time he ever said that to anyone in
his life.

Therapist: What advice would Sara give you about Matt?

Mathilda: Well when it comes to Matt, she would probably tell me to
detach myself, help him to take responsibility for himself. I imagine
she would say that, because if you're too attached to the person,
then it doesn't work so well.

Therapist: She'd tell you, "Mom, don't get so involved." What would she
say to her father?

Mathilda: I don't think she would have any advice for him, because I
don't think he's ever gonna change.

Therapist: Carolyn, since you've had a little bit easier time dealing with
your dad, if you were giving your father advice, what would it be?

Carolyn: Well, he really tries to baby my brother. It's like he is his
mother, more or less. You know mothers overmother their sons. It's
like my father overfathers my brother. He watches every move my
brother makes.

Therapist: You and Sara are on exactly the same wavelength, because
Sara would say, "Don't overmother" and you would say, "Don't
overfather."

Carolyn: Maybe that's why my brother has had difficulty standing on
his own two feet. Maybe he's just too dependent on his father.

This session consolidates the family's relationship with the dead in a
positive way. As Laurie works on helping Mathilda imagine Sara's
understanding of her brother's problems and her wish that he be rescued
from a life she knew all too well, Mathilda is forced to join with her
daughter in making a commitment to help Matt. She is even able to
recognize a change in her husband and to accept his initiative in
attending a drug treatment program with their son. Carolyn is no longer
in danger of replacing Sara as her mother's problem child. She begins to
play an adult role with her mother, supporting her but not engaging her
inappropriately in her problems. A year later she sought individual
therapy, on her own, for issues in her adult life. Mathilda's grief seemed
to be resolved and the family had managed to achieve a new organization, which to some extent reconciled longstanding divisions.

PART IV

The Inner-City Experience

CHAPTER 16

AIDS in the Inner City

THIS CHAPTER EXPLORES AIDS as it affects poor families and people of color and examines the impact of poverty, drugs, and racism in the urban ghettos on the spread of AIDS.

THE ENVIRONMENTAL NICHE
FOR AIDS

The inner cities, shaped during the 1960s and 1970s by the middle class' emigration and the influx of the poorest African-American and Latino families into already overpopulated areas (Inclan & Ferran, 1990), provided the perfect ecological niche for the spread of HIV infection. The general economic crisis of the seventies—the conservative resurgence with its emphasis on vastly expanded military budgets—led to drastic cutbacks in social services. Community centers that had provided centralized care—places where a whole family was known by the workers, received health and dental care, socialized with other families, and had recreation programs for their children—became early and tragic casualties. Housing programs and even preventive services such as fire and police forces were cut back, even as the urban infrastructure was deteriorating. Housing was rapidly abandoned or burned down as repairs were too costly for landlords; school buildings were dangerously overcrowded and understaffed, as were the hospitals that must serve the urban poor. Job opportunities decreased as manufacturing was ceded to foreign countries and the urban poor were educationally ill-prepared to assume jobs requiring technological skills.

The failure of traditional structures, compounded by the denial of access to additional resources, prevented the acquisition of education and job skills that would have provided an exit from the cycle of persistent poverty. As the cycle of poverty amplified, so did the critical experience of powerlessness. As the inner cities deteriorated, the physical isolation of inner-city populations from the mainstream increased. In many cases the inner cities were a war zone that outsiders entered at their peril. In systems terms, inner cities and their families were becoming closed systems, cut off from an outside world that could support growth, change, and aspiration (Hartman & Laird, 1983). Inner-city boundaries neither permitted the importation of necessary supplies for internal health nor allowed the inhabitants a meaningful exchange of information with the outside environment.

What does permeate the boundaries of the community are drugs, and with them, the means of transmitting AIDS. Heroin use spreads AIDS through needle-sharing, which is done as a drug-taking ritual symbolizing community, as well as a necessity when the purchase of hypodermic needles is illegal. HIV infection is also spread by crack users who are frequently polydrug users of heroin or methadone to mediate the crash that follows the crack high. Since crack and sex are inextricably linked, the pathway of HIV transmission is complete. During a crack high, addicts report that they think of nothing but obtaining the drug. Condom use requires thoughtfulness and preparation, qualities that are simply not present when the person is using crack. As a result, sexually transmitted diseases are at a record high in inner-city communities, and the sores caused by sexually transmitted diseases make the perfect entry point for HIV.

THE AIDS EPIDEMIC IN THE
INNER CITIES

In the late 1970s intravenous drug users began to be infected with a new virus, which was identified as HIV in 1985. While in the early years of the epidemic the majority of AIDS-infected people were gay men, massive safer-sex education programs in the gay community dramatically reduced the new infection rate. By contrast, the number of infected persons among drug users and their partners continued to climb: by 1989, in some urban areas such as New York and New Jersey it was estimated that 50 percent of the IV-drug-using community was infected (Osborn, 1989), as well as 50 percent of non-drug-using heterosexual partners. The infection rate of sexual partners of IV drug users is substantially higher than the infection rate of the partners of bisexual men and drug-product users. This inequality probably reflects the rates of untreated sexually transmitted diseases in populations of poverty.

Public identification of the AIDS epidemic first with homosexuality and then with heroin use lessened awareness of the risk of spread through heterosexual sex and injectable cocaine. Intravenous cocaine is particularly dangerous, since maintaining the cocaine high is such a driving need that cocaine users are the least likely among drug users to spend the time cleaning apparatus. Furthermore, while there was a public outcry for more methadone slots to help heroin users, there was little recognition that heroin users are usually polydrug abusers who may shoot IV cocaine or smoke crack as well as use methadone. Clean needle programs, which have been proven effective in reducing HIV infection in heroin users in Amsterdam and Liverpool, were too politically controversial in the United States.

In the punitive climate of the 1980s, spending money on treatment slots for cocaine users in the absence of the cheap solution – a drug that blocked the effects of cocaine, as methadone does with heroin – seemed less appealing than building more prisons. In effect, the drug-HIV link went unaddressed and the rate of infection of cocaine users and their sexual partners continued to climb.

It is important to add that the spread of HIV infection in communities where people of color live may be exacerbated by the secrecy surrounding homosexual activity. While the great majority of men in these communities think of themselves as heterosexual in orientation, and most have female sexual partners and children, many routinely engage in sexual activity with males without considering themselves to be bisexual or gay (Osborn, 1989).

The predominantly heterosexual orientation of communities of people of color means that women and children are at particular risk for AIDS infection. Indeed, AIDS in inner-city communities becomes a family disease where multiple family members may be infected. It is common in treatment to see families in which both parents and one or more children are ill or infected; it is equally common to see families in which several adult family members are dying and a single sibling or grandparent is left with the burden of raising numbers of orphaned children. If the gunfire of the crack epidemic makes the urban ghettos seem like a war zone, then the quiet destruction of whole families by the virus is like a silent, invisible, lethal gas that is invading ghetto households.

In many cases the word *AIDS* is not mentioned and the nature of the deaths remains shrouded in secrecy. There exists a pervasive shame that has no words. While secrecy may freeze family mourning processes and create an atmosphere of fear and watchfulness, it may also offer protection at the most primitive level. As we have seen, revelation may bring social ostracism, discrimination in schools against healthy children of an AIDS-infected parent, and even loss of housing and loss of employment, leading to homelessness. A mother coping with her own sickness, the illness of a baby, and the raising of other children may find it impossible to obtain the homemaking and child-care services that would keep her family together. In addition, she must negotiate the shame and stigma of AIDS. She must live with the fear that a school, a neighbor, a landlord will find out about her illness or that of her child and that her family will suffer the consequences. Given the risk to the family of embracing the person with AIDS, it is remarkable that most families of drug users do continue to care for the ill person throughout the course of the illness.

For families of people with AIDS, feelings about the illness are inextricably mixed with the history of the preceding sexual or drug-using behaviors. For example, families of drug users share community anger at their deviant members. The families are the first to fall victim to the user's need to obtain money for drugs and the parents' fear that their other children will follow the example. Shame on several levels is associated with drug use: for the drug user during lucid moments, for family members wrestling with the sense of having failed to save the user from drugs, and for the community fearing it will be identified with the "junkie."

The epidemic of AIDS piles stigma onto a community already stigmatized by racism and prejudice against poor people. The popular belief that AIDS originated in Africa is experienced by African-Americans as another attempt to blame their community for social ills. As Dalton (1989) has written, "More than insult and affront are at issue here. So long as we African-Americans continue to worry that any hint of connection with AIDS will be turned against us, we will remain leery of accepting responsibility for its impact on our community" (p. 212).

WOMEN AND HIV INFECTION

HIV-infected women who were not drug users were conspicuously missing from the early statistics, subsumed in a category called "Other." This popular association of AIDS with what is considered to be social deviance continues to be particularly dangerous to non-drug-using women who are the sexual partners of infected men. Women are in fact more at risk than men in the heterosexual exposure category, both because of the high concentration of virus in sperm and the permeability of the vaginal mucosa and because, since more men are infected than women, women living in highly impacted communities have a significant chance of having sex with an infected man. Since a recent study (Wyatt, 1988) shows that a third of white women and almost half of African-American women studied had their first experience of intercourse before age 16, and three-quarters of all white women studied and one-fourth of African-American women reported 13 or more sexual partners since the age of 18, it is clear that women living in communities where the majority of men are infected are at high risk for having an infected partner.

Even if a woman suspects she is at risk, she may take no steps to protect herself from sexually transmitted infection because she has been gendered to acquiesce to male sexual demands. Fatalism, passivity, and denial are more familiar and, in the short run, appear less dangerous than sexual assertiveness. Sexual assertiveness may result in male violence or abandonment. For most women, identity is rooted in the ability to achieve and maintain primary relationships, even though the relationship may constitute a danger to themselves (Goldner, Penn, Sheinberg, & Walker, 1990). While losing a primary relationship is for all women extremely painful, for poor women the loss of a relationship may also result in devastating economic hardship for themselves and their children. Although women are counseled to protect themselves, programs seldom reach out to their men or provide couples counseling to engage the men in protective behaviors.

TREATMENT PROGRAMS IN
POOR COMMUNITIES

The development of effective AIDS prevention, education, and social service treatment programs in poor communities has been remarkably difficult and is in strong contrast to the effective response to AIDS authored by gay activists. While the gay community was able to finance its own AIDS prevention and education programs in the face of government neglect, poor communities were dependent for financing on a government that was indifferent to the spread of AIDS in the early years of the epidemic. Gay communities in the urban centers where AIDS initially surfaced—as, for example, San Francisco and New York—had a strong middle-class base, which gave them access to money, existing organizations, formal and informal community centers (including bars and even baths), newspapers and other publications, and social networks. All of these resources were utilized for disseminating prevention and safer-sex information and for creating a climate in which the practice of safer sex became the sexual norm rather than the exception. The implementation of safer-sex education programs was further facilitated by the fact that open discussion of sexuality was part of the social discourse of gay men and there were no complicating issues of child-bearing to prevent condom use.

In poor communities, urban neglect and dislocation, the spread of drugs, and the curtailment of basic services had destroyed many community organizations. The crucial remaining organizations—churches and schools—have had enormous difficulty in dealing with sexuality in any way that is in accord with the reality of human sexual practice. Needless to say, government preaching about the need for monogamous heterosexual relationships, with the implication that if one adhered to this moral code one would not become infected, did not help in communities where it was highly likely that one's monogamous partner was carrying the infection from a previous drug or sexual life. At the same time, the association of AIDS with morality created a climate of shame and secrecy, as well as reinforcing primitive beliefs that contagion could spread like sin or temptation.

In the gay community AIDS was seen as a political issue threatening the very life of the community and therefore requiring political action. By contrast, the late sixties and seventies in urban ghettos saw a destruction of the emerging radical African-American leadership, with the assassination of national leaders and the destruction of the Black Panther Party. Hopelessness had replaced the political activism of the sixties. Drugs (especially cocaine and crack) had become the economic infrastructure for many poor communities, simultaneously destroying a generation of the young by placing drug users and their families at high risk for AIDS infection. All these factors resulted in communities that were gapingly vulnerable to the spread of an epidemic—communities already burdened by a thousand threats to survival more tangible than an invisible virus, communities without the will or resources to combat it.

CHAPTER 17
Pediatric AIDS

IN THIS CHAPTER we will look at the epidemiology and medical aspects of pediatric AIDS and describe an interdisciplinary, systems-oriented training program for a pediatric AIDS unit.

DRUG USE, REPRODUCTIVE DECISION-MAKING, AND THE SPREAD OF HIV INFECTION IN CHILDREN

The infection of newborns with the HIV virus continues to grow as the epidemic spreads through vulnerable, impoverished, IV-drug-using communities, where an increasing number of the infected are women. Advances in maternal treatment have reduced babies' chances of acquiring HIV infection from 20–30 percent to 8–15 percent if the mother uses AZT in pregnancy. However many mothers refuse to be tested for HIV and many others do not seek prenatal care.

Even if the baby is not HIV-infected, there is almost no chance that an HIV-infected mother will live to raise her child. It is estimated that by 1995 45,000 children and teenagers will lose their mother to AIDS. By the year 2000, that number could rise to 80,000, 80 percent of whom come from poor communities (Michaels & Levine, 1993). This social disaster will be addressed in Chapter 18.

In poor inner-city communities, the few existing drug prevention programs discourage mothers from seeking treatment since they neither provide for day-care for children nor permit them to reside with the mother in treatment. New York City reported a 400 percent increase in maternal drug use in the period 1984–1989, with most of it accounted for by a sharp rise in maternal crack/cocaine use. And if the women herself is not a drug user, the majority of available men have used drugs at some point in their lives and as a result are at risk for carrying and sexually spreading HIV. When one considers the ever-increasing rate of drug addiction in urban cities, together with the dramatic rise in crack use, in which drug is frequently acquired in exchange for sex, the potential reservoir of infection is enormous.

In the culture of poverty, halting the spread of pediatric AIDS is made more complex by the crucial role that childbearing plays in a community where there is little access to money, educational opportunity, or property. For both men and women of poverty, childbearing may be essential to self-respect and self-definition: Dreams for the children's future become crucial in a culture where success and recognition in the present are blocked. As a result, birth control is regarded with suspicion: it is seen either as a ruling-class attempt to control minority population growth or as religiously discrepant. Abortion becomes another difficult option—one that may destroy a woman's relationship with a man she either loves or needs.

In a culture of poverty, where infant mortality is already high, 70–80 percent odds that a baby will *not* be infected with HIV even if the mother has been identified as infected seem reasonable enough to leave to chance. In a culture where both adolescent pregnancy and drug use go hand in hand, the difficulty of providing effective prevention becomes enormous.

Drug-using women who are most at risk for bearing infected children often look to childbearing as the route to a "clean" future. But while childbearing may provide the motivation to enter a treatment program and attempt to "go straight," most drug free treatment programs demand separation from the family so that the woman can "focus on herself"—a goal that is gender discrepant although popular in the parlance of drug programs and psychotherapy.

Such enforced separation is intolerable for most women, all the more so for the emotionally vulnerable drug user. Women construct a positive sense of adult identity around their ability to form and maintain relationships (Gilligan et al., 1988). The drug user is asked to exchange these building blocks of identity for drug treatment. Ironically, feelings of guilt and grief for the children who must be given up to foster care if a woman is to find "help" will often drive her back to drugs. The attempt to cure the problem creates another problem in an endless cycle that leaves its legacy through generations, as another child is often conceived to replace those lost to the system.

One drug-using mother with AIDS came to our project shortly after the birth of her youngest and AIDS-infected baby. She was 30 and had ten children, all in foster care. Many attempts at treatment had been unsuccessful in helping her go straight as will as become reunited with her children. Despite the fact that she saw herself as a lesbian woman, a new pregnancy with the father of all of her children was her way of comforting herself and the children's father for their devastating losses. Only when her lover, with the help of her therapists, Sippio Small and Joan Gilbert, were able to help her fight for the return of her children did she feel that she had the motivation to remain drug free. In Chapter 19 we will propose a gender-sensitive program to help drug-using women stay with their children as they handle their drug use and learn strategies for preventing HIV infection.

MEDICAL OVERVIEW OF PEDIATRIC AIDS

As of December 1988, there are relatively few reported pediatric AIDS cases in New York State (422). However, studies of the rate of HIV infection in children revealed that less than half the infected children had developed symptoms (Giaquinto et al., 1989; Mofenson, Hoff, & Grady, 1989). We may therefore assume that there exist many school-age infected but asymptomatic children who will become ill later in childhood.

The majority of children have been infected perinatally, but the high rate of sexual abuse in families with alcohol and drug-addicted members bodes ill for the prevention of transmission of HIV to young children not infected at birth. The efficiency of perinatal transmission from an HIV-infected mother who does not use AZT during pregnancy is estimated at between 25 and 30 percent. AZT use during pregnancy or even shortly before birth dramatically reduces these odds (Altman, 1994). The factors predisposing the fetus to infection and those which trigger disease onset are not known. Anomalies occur. For example, there has been a case where only one of a pair of monozygotic twins was infected in utero (Falloon, Eddy, Weiner, & Pizzo, 1989).

Because antibody testing may not accurately determine infection in children during the first 18 months of life (see Chapter 6), diagnosis of HIV disease may depend on the appearance of clinical symptoms. The

Centers for Disease Control criteria for a child being diagnosed with AIDS were broadened in 1987 to include a wider range of clinical manifestations: candidiasis of the esophagus, trachea, bronchi and lungs; cytomegalovirus disease; Kaposi's sarcoma; lymphocytic interstitial pneumonia; pneumocystis carinii pneumonia; progressive multifocal leukoencephalopathy; toxoplasmosis of the brain (Falloon, Eddy, Weiner, & Pizzo, 1989). Of these syndromes the most common is lymphocytic interstitial pneumonia, which occurs in about half of all children with AIDS (Rogers et al., 1987) and causes irreversible damage to the lungs. Children who have had this disease may have increased trouble breathing and be unable to gain weight. Pneumocystis pneumonia is a common opportunistic infection and one which is associated with high morbidity. Children with AIDS may suffer from persistent high fevers and have trouble eating and retaining food. Chronic herpes or thrush (candida) may make eating and drinking painful. Also, common to these children are multiple or recurrent bacterial infections, including septicemia, bone and joint infections, internal abscesses, meningitis, wasting syndrome, HIV encephalopathy, tuberculosis involving one other site than the lungs, and recurrent non-typhoid salmonella bacteria. Although infections can be subclinical, ranging from mild to severe, once the child has shown disease symptoms, in general the course is one of progressive immune dysfunction and clinical deterioration despite some asymptomatic periods (Falloon, Eddy, Weiner, & Pizzo, 1989).

The HIV virus frequently attacks the brain and central nervous system. A tragically difficult experience for a young mother with an HIV-infected baby is to watch a progressive encephalopathy result in the loss of developmental milestones, deterioration of motor skills and intellectual abilities, and behavioral abnormalities. To nurture and care for an unresponsive baby is extraordinarily difficult at best, the more so because the mother knows that it was her actions that have caused this condition. Nursing staff also find the care of such babies to be emotionally draining and without the rewards that responsive infants give; frustrated nurses may inadvertently project their feelings of anger and helplessness onto the mothers.

The vulnerability of these children to life-threatening infections is painful to witness and immensely disruptive to family life. Management issues are complex, involving the procurement of special equipment, many medications, and special diets. The needs of these children put terrible strains on families already strained by drug use, poverty, and other psychosocial problems. The mother's guilt over her role in what has happened to the HIV-infected baby may influence the frequency of her visits. She may avoid the hospital altogether because she feels that the staff members blame her, or she may devote all her time to saving the baby, thus neglecting the needs of her other well children. Siblings are often frightened for their ill sibling and scared because their mother does not look well. Often, a father is also ill or has died.

Parents must make difficult decisions about the degree of normal life their immuno-compromised child can lead. For example, exposure to varicella (chicken pox) can have disastrous consequences. If the child is well enough to attend school and the parent learns of an outbreak of varicella, immunoglobulin should be administered. One complicating factor is that mothers of HIV-infected children who attend school often avoid other mothers, because they fear that somehow the secret of their children's sickness will be revealed. Since children are not identified to school personnel as having HIV infection, mothers may not be aware that there has been an outbreak of varicella until their children have already become ill.

Normal childhood immunizations are another area of concern for parents of HIV-infected children. Exposure to live vaccine was originally thought to be dangerous, but current thinking is that it is less dangerous to give the children regular immunizations against measles, mumps and rubella than to have them exposed to those diseases, which could be fatal.

However, HIV-infected children and their siblings should *not* be given live polio vaccine but inactivated vaccine. Often, pediatricians do not realize that there are a number of other siblings living in a household who are receiving live vaccines—vaccines that could infect the HIV-infected sibling. In poor families it is common for many family groups to share common housing or for various relatives and non-kin children to move in and out of the household. Mothers may not wish to inform other family members of the nature of their child's illness; this unwillingness precludes ensuring that the ill child is not exposed to potentially life-threatening situations.

PEDIATRIC AIDS PROGRAM IN AN INNER-CITY HOSPITAL

AIDS has put enormous stress on medical professionals in all communities. In poor communities the burden is intensified, as physicians barely have time to write prescriptions, much less attend to their patients' narratives of illness experience. Providers are overburdened and medical staffs are depleted, as workers flee from the low pay and impossible demands of inner-city medical centers. One physician in a city hospital came to see me because she had lost half her nursing staff and the other infectious disease doctor, who shared all AIDS-patient responsibilities with her. She was exhausted and demoralized about the possibility of providing the kind of care she sought for her patients. A totally dedicated professional who had worked for four years with AIDS patients, she knew that she had to choose between the destruction of her personal and professional life and her dedication to the patients she treated.

Given these circumstances, it is easy to see how the inexorable progress of illness in AIDS elicits provider helplessness at the same time that the opportunistic infections demand high-tech medical intervention. Add to this mix of helplessness the continual demand that physicians *do* something in a professional world that increasingly relies on medical technology to provide magic bullets. The complex loop between poor patients and physicians dehumanizes the disease and drives patients away from treatment. This medical-patient interface is a critical area for intervention.

Working with families in which there is pediatric AIDS in an ecosystemic model will alleviate staff burnout and stress by creating a more collaborative relationship between staff and family. The model we propose utilizes the strength of families to empower other families in breaking the rule of silence and shame. Developed in the gay community, the empowerment model, which encourages a positive attitude toward illness, is wedded to a nonblaming systemic approach.

We have had the opportunity to create new models of family-staff collaboration in various settings, including the pediatrics ward of a large city hospital. When the hospital social-work staff asked us (John Patten, Gillian Walker, and Lauren Kaplan) to create a weekly AIDS conference on family issues, we decided to focus on pediatrics. We knew from our interviews with pediatric social workers that only the mothers of ill children received counseling. We were interested in exploring the effectiveness of a family approach that would include as many members as possible. We felt that family members had untapped resources and could act as problem solvers for their families. Accurately identifying the problem context would lead to effective intervention. If, for example, a young woman were suffering from depression because her baby had AIDS, instead of prescribing individual therapy and medication, the grandmother could be brought to a session to help the mother deal with grief, isolation, and child-care tasks. In addition, the mother could be introduced to other mothers with similar problems.

The pediatrics department with which we consulted was relatively small and community-oriented, providing a warm environment for its patients and their families. The department had not treated many terminally ill children until the advent of AIDS. Severe pediatric illness cases were usually absorbed by hospitals who specialized in particular diseases. Becoming a designated center in a high-risk catchment area generated enormous stress for a staff unused to absorbing increasing numbers of terminally ill children and infants. We experienced the strengths of the staff members in their dedication, expertise, strong feelings of compassion for families, and determination to provide a sense of intimacy in the difficult world of the large institution. Furthermore, we were impressed by their flexibility and openness to different ways of intervening. Most important of all, the department was dedicated to continuity of care: Children moving from inpatient to outpatient status were treated by the same health-care professionals, so that we could ensure the implementation of treatment plans over time.

Pediatric staff members expressed concerns in three areas: the pain of bonding with terminally ill infants; the AIDS transmision route of drug use or sexual activity with a drug user; and the complexity of bridging vast cultural, ethnic, and economic differences. The mothers who present with AIDS babies tend to be poor, Latino, African-American, or Caribbean; staff members tend to be middle-class and white. Professional ignorance or nonacceptance of family structures and parenting practices that differ from accepted middle-class norms; negative client attitudes toward counseling by professionals; negative client perceptions of how social service systems view them and deliver services – all impede the creation of the positive bond between staff and family that is necessary for effective treatment.

In addition, for staff members the stigma of AIDS, fears of contamination, and the helplessness of witnessing the eventual deterioration of babies they have grown to love create a situation of enormous stress, leading to demoralization and burnout. Frequently these factors, intensified by feelings of helplessness to cure or ease pain, lead staff members to project their anger onto the parents.

The family interview was structured to accomplish several goals: (1) to give staff members a more positve view of the family's struggle with the disease by helping them "walk in each family member's shoes"; (2) to identify family resources (via the genogram) and useful family coping styles; and (3) to demonstrate strategies for creating a more cooperative loop between family and staff. To this end, we introduced techniques of reframing patient behaviors and circumventing patient "resistance" by utilizing whatever behavior the patient offered. We also asked families to teach staff members about their needs.

As we worked with the pediatrics staff, we began to structure a family case conference that had the following objectives: (1) to create a supportive atmosphere for family and staff; (2) to help staff view the family as a living system in which death was a part, rather than focusing solely on the dying patient; (3) to teach staff members to create alternative narratives and positive redescriptions for family members; (4) to help staff members identify family resources; (5) to help staff members create a collaborative relationship with the families; and (6) to eliminate redundancy of service.

Creating a Supportive Atmosphere

As a foundation for beginning this pioneering project, we wanted to create a supportive atmosphere for families and staff. Fortuitously, we were assigned a small and uncomfortable room that allowed no separation between the family interviewed and the attending staff. This spatial limitation permitted us to loosen the hierarchical boundaries between patient, family, and staff. Physical closeness served to bridge some of the distance that a frightening disease like AIDS can create—the us/them syndrome. When we interviewed family members, we could take advantage of the physical surroundings to bring staff and family together.

In order to foster a sense of interdisciplinary collaboration, we solicited the ideas of each staff member before the family arrived. We were interested in receiving as many descriptions as possible, emphasizing that multiple perspectives are more useful than any one person's view. We noticed that the descriptions of floor nurses were of particular value to us; they were likely to be practical and immediate. In the pre-session meeting with staff, we attempted to create a family of health-care professionals—a safe, nonhierarchical group in which each member could begin to feel empowered. We tactfully discouraged the use of professional jargon, wanting staff and family to share a common language.

Because AIDS is such an enormous stressor, we emphasized that people's human reactions were helpful, not harmful. Each staff member had a unique coping style that allowed him or her to get through the day and perform his or her tasks in this most painful of areas. For instance, one staff member was frequently very emotional about the clients and cases she saw; another, distant and coolly professional. We identified both of these behaviors as valid and useful: Families could sense the emotional caring and humanness of the one worker and could find a steadying calm in the other professional's matter-of-factness. The safety of the pre-session meeting also ensured that staff members would be able to get support from other staff when necessary, and encouraged them to share their feelings about the family without being judged as too emotional, too distant, or too inexperienced. We also began to ask questions about the patient-family context, as well as listening to the volunteered information about the individual patient. We recognized that staff members were expert in their understanding of developmental and personal issues for children. At the same time, we tried to suggest casually that introducing information about the structure and organization of family systems and family interactional patterns could widen the scope of the perceptions and increase the effectiveness of interventions.

The Family as a Living System

Another major goal was to shift the staff's thinking from the dying patient to the living system. Our belief was that if staff could become involved with the future of the family, they would become less death-focused and, in turn, feel less helpless as their relationship with the family became more collaborative in nature. We also felt that if staff members were able to have hope—even if it was for the future of another child—then they would experience less burnout. During the course of the year it was interesting how many discussions focused on the future of other family members rather than on the mother/ill-child dyad.

Creating Alternative Narratives

Women who are most at risk for AIDS are drug users or the sexual partners of drug users. When they bear children with AIDS, they are further stigmatized. A woman who uses drugs has probably known abuse most of her life. Drug use further defines her as contemptible. Professionals depersonalize her, seeing her as her habit. They seldom focus on the many times she has tried to go off drugs or enter programs. In some sense drug treatment programs are thought to be infallible; it is the drug user who didn't try hard enough. But drug treatment programs are not designed to meet women's needs. A woman repairs her life best in a positive context of care (Gilligan et al., 1988), where she can create a positive narrative about herself. In this narrative she begins to see herself as a woman competent to tend her children and able to create a rich tapestry of meaningful relationships.

Women who are sexual partners of drug users are also seen in a negative fashion. The AA term *enabler* is derogatory in that it puts the addicted person and the partner on the same level of "vice": If the addicted person is addicted to a substance, then the partner is addicted to the person's addiction. The non-drug-using partner may feel a personal sense of moral superiority to her partner, in that he does terrible things and she does not, but, nonetheless, when she enters the social and health-care system because of her baby's illness, she feels a sharp sense of shame. The implication is: had she been more courageous and independent, were she less addicted to her partner's addiction, she would not be in this mess with him.

As the mother enters a hospital system with an HIV-infected baby, she feels an overwhelming sense of shame and failure. She therefore expects staff to judge her harshly. And all too often they do. She may also be accustomed to professionals having immense power in her life and may become openly hostile or overtly submissive, while concealing important information about her situation. For example, the partner of a drug user might conceal the fact that she is still living with him; the drug-using mother may hide the fact that she still uses drugs. Both may conceal the fact that, because of the erosion of family life engendered by drug use, they have turned real decision-making power over to another family member. These concealments can critically affect the ability of the health-care team to help the mother provide optimal care for her child.

In the hospital, families were often referred for consultation because they had become "problems": Family behaviors and staff expectations about how the family should behave were discrepant. In the following case example, the pediatric staff had become increasingly frustrated with and alienated from the mother of one of their young patients.

CASE EXAMPLE*

Gladys was the 29-year-old mother of Michael, a six-year-old boy with AIDS who had been admitted because of another bout of pneumonia.

*The author was the therapist.

Michael had been a model patient who had been hospitalized many times before. He was well known to and well liked by the staff. This time, however, his behavior was startling different. He refused to have his IV unless his mother was present, repeatedly attempted to pull it out, would not allow staff to comfort him. He appeared angry, depressed, and refused to talk. Staff blamed Gladys for this change in behavior, feeling that she was cold and erratic in her manner with her son. They requested the consultation, hoping that the consultant might be able to convince Gladys to become softer and warmer to her son in a way that they had been unable to do.

In the pre-session meeting before the interview, we learned that three months prior to Michael's recent admission he had developed chicken pox. Instead of being admitted to our hospital, which Michael regarded as a second home, he was sent to a large city hospital that had facilities for handling highly infectious diseases. Pediatric staff were angry at this administrative decision, even though they understood its clinical validity. Michael was their child, too, and they had a helpless feeling of having abandoned him as he entered the huge, impersonal hospital, where he was put in isolation. After four days Gladys also developed chicken pox and could no longer visit him. Michael panicked. He tried to pull out his IV, perhaps thinking that if he were not tethered to the hospital, he could go home to his mother in safety. The staff at that hospital tried to hold him down; he became terribly angry, lashed out, tried to bite. He was then tied down and caged in a special restraining crib. He had to urinate and defecate in his bed. When he refused to eat, all his toys were removed from the room. His mother found him three weeks later in a bare room, restrained and caged, and he melted into her arms and clung to her. He was a good little boy in the hospital after that, but when he went home he was very angry with her.

When Michael returned to our hospital for his next admission, he was not only a very sick little boy, but he was also angry, mistrustful, and depressed.

Oddly enough, Michael's depression may have been worsened by the good intentions and caring of the hospital staff. When he returned, so hideously disfigured with chicken pox scars, depressed, and silent, the staff felt terribly guilty, especially the pediatrician who had taken care of him since he was a baby. The staff, unable to bear the reproach that Michael's misery represented, criticized the mother for not responding adequately to her son's depression. They wanted her to make up for the comfort they had not been able to give Michael when he had been sick, but their reproachfulness may have prompted the mother to visit her son a little less. Eventually this created a cycle in which staff members became even more angry, distressed, and helpless at the little boy's refusal to let them comfort him. Gladys had been coping with her son's illness since she was 23. This strong, proud, courageous woman told the interviewer: "People here think that I don't know Michael may die. I know very well that he may die, but if he dies, right up to the end, I want him to know that I, at least, believe that he was a normal little boy."

What the staff had come to see as her coldness was, to her, a refusal to indulge her son's manipulations. She was determined that he would be normal, and to be normal she had to be tough with him and not yield to pity.

"He is a very clever little boy," she continued. "He does what he needs to do to get what he wants, but sometimes it is not good for him and I will not tolerate that." At the end of the interview the interviewer remarked, "You know, you are training him to be a little soldier, and he needs to be a little soldier in fighting the big war he is facing. I think you have done very well in preparing him for that. But, as you know, every soldier needs a little R & R after a long battle, a time when women comfort, hold, and cuddle men. All men in wars need to be babied a little, because they have to do such super-human things. Babying them in that way does not turn them into babies—it turns them into brave men. Since your little boy has to be so brave, such a big soldier, I think he needs you to give him some R & R."

Gladys was not someone who talked to her son much about his emotions, but in her own rough way she knew how to comfort him. Because that way was alien to the more middle-class psychologically-minded members of the staff, they did not understand fully what she was doing or its effectiveness. After the interview, however, they more clearly recognized that under her apparent coldness was enormous determination to have her son live a normal life in a world that was hostile and increasingly stigmatizing to people with his illness. In fact, she drew on her own experiences as a black woman learning to survive in a world of poverty and racism. She was determined to give that courage, strength, and grit to her son. By the end of the interview, Gladys' articulation of her vision had deeply moved the staff. The therapist's reframing helped Gladys soften toward her son, while at the same time permitting her to see this softening as being merely a part of the battle that she knows he has to face. The reframe was done in Gladys' language and was an attempt to broach the difference between her determination to handle her son with toughness and love and the staff's wish for a gentler, softer, and more compensatory approach. This perceptual shift allowed Gladys and the staff to work together to help Michael and to comfort each other as well.

A year later Gladys is perceived by the staff as one of the most positive examples of how mothers can cope with AIDS and inspire their children with hope. When the newly evolved caretaking group was organized on the pediatrics unit, Gladys became a leader of the group and a source of strength to other mothers. She remains connected to the clinic even after the recent death of Michael.

Identifying Family Resources

We asked the staff to try to think of these families as multi-resource families who were dealing with complex social problems. This change of point of view allowed the staff to begin to look for underlying strengths. Workers are often not knowledgeable about the resources available to families as caregivers. Because workers are trained in a deficit model, the worker and parent will frequently end up in an antagonistic relationship as they covertly fight over the ill child's care. Staff was helped to understand that family members could lighten their work if they were encouraged to collaborate with staff in patient care.

Frequently, a worker would accept the client's first statement about family, "I don't have nobody," and go no further. He would not realize, for example, that in different cultures the establishment of a bonded, trusting relationship with the worker is a prerequisite for divulging family information. We encouraged staff to learn to do a genogram and an ecomap together with the family, so that they could understand the complex web of relationships which made up every family's social network. A systemic crisis intervention approach allowed these professionals to develop hypotheses necessary for devising a parsimonious, pragmatic treatment plan utilizing the resources of the natural unit.

Creating a Collaborative Relationship

A common scenario between hospital staff and worried mothers is one in which mother drives staff crazy by questioning every medical intervention they suggest. They then informally diagnose her as paranoid and attempt to be patient with her, but under their politeness she senses impatience and even concealed anger. Her perception of their attitude

increases her paranoia. As she becomes more suspicious, she also becomes more demanding; staff, in turn, become more evasive, and the
cycle escalates.

The family therapist, using the "resistance," would interrupt this
feedback loop by helping staff encourage rather than discourage her
behavior; her behavior would be reframed as a model for other mothers
in how to attend to their children, gather information, raise important
issues, and be assertive on their behalf. She might be directed to utilize
her skills to help professional staff by bringing to their attention new
information they might not have seen. These interventions would (1)
help staff members understand that all behaviors have an adaptive
function, (2) interrupt the staff-patient feedback loop labeled "paranoia,"
(3) turn her into a real collaborator or at least reduce her demands, and
(4) put staff in charge of their relationship with her.

At the end of the family interview, we often invite the family to join us
at a conference table and ask any questions the interview may have
aroused. We also ask them to give suggestions from their perspective
about how hospitals and families can develop better relationships and
what services they need. These interactions are designed to place the staff
and family on more equal footing as collaborators in care. An example of
a service that developed out of the conference was a caretakers group.
Families had repeatedly spoken to us about their isolation and the need
for networking with other families dealing with AIDS. This caretakers
group provided socialization for children with AIDS and relieved stress
on the social workers, as families provided resources for each other.

Another method of facilitating staff-family collaboration is to identify
natural family leaders who could advise the professionals regarding
specific family needs, orchestrate the relationship between professional
and family, and serve as family problem solvers and managers.

The effect of these case conferences was succinctly stated by a pediatrician: "I like my mothers better now." This positive view seems to have
permeated the pediatric staff.

Eliminating Redundancy of Service

That the family become the unit of service delivery and case management
for AIDS patients was an idea generated by the social work department
in response to an interview in the pediatric case conference. The interview was organized in response to a family crisis following the death of a
mother from AIDS. The case was a typical one for many city hospitals. It
concerned a four-year-old HIV-positive child and her father. The mother

had died of AIDS a few days prior to the consultation. Her death was sudden, but not unexpected by the patient herself. The mother was an ex-IV-drug user. The father, an IV heroin user, was now on methadone and had changed his drug of choice from heroin to crack.

The case was being followed by three workers from Gay Men's Health Crisis and by approximately eight workers from our hospital; however, there was no communication among these eleven workers. The methadone worker was barely aware of the marriage and had little knowledge of the child who was at risk. The mother's methadone worker had never seen her husband and had sketchy details about the marriage, which now appeared to have been violent and abusive. Pediatric workers had no access to any information about the drug use of the parents and were not aware that the mother was dying until the very end. From careful observation pediatrics workers had deduced that as long as the mother was alive, the child was relatively well cared for. There was concern, however, because Child Welfare had been brought in twice during the mother's hospitalization for AIDS. The inpatient service AIDS worker saw the mother concerning her depression, but did not have the authority to help the mother plan for her daughter's future if she were to die. The worker did not know the husband or have much knowledge of the marriage until after the mother's death, when she was confronted with stormy, violent scenes between the father and the mother's frightened mother.

Numerous other workers were also involved with the family, but no one person was following the family's history and no one person had the responsibility of helping the family plan for the illness and possible death of the parent. As a result, after the mother's death the child was left in the custody of the father—a crack abuser who could not in any way provide a suitable home for a young child who had an illness of which he was only dimly aware. Following the family consultation in the pediatrics case conference, the social work department made an immediate decision to take the child into the hospital's protective custody.

This case dramatically demonstrated to everyone present that redundancy of service, in fact, made matters worse. It became clear that there was a compelling need for unified care delivery and for skillful, systemic assessment of families in which there is an HIV-infected person. In addition, in order to implement a family case management approach, specialized training in the understanding of family systems and in basic family intervention techniques would be necessary. In Chapter 19 we will re-examine this case example from an ecosystemic perspective.

CHAPTER 18
Dislocations: Children in the Aftermath of AIDS

AKISHA HAS TWO children, Jose, six, and Stefanie, four.* After her second bout of PCP, she knew she was too weak to care for her children. Her drug-using husband, Pedro, had also been sick. Besides, although he loved the children, she couldn't count on him. She asked her mother for help. Her mother was tired. She had been in poor health for years. Her last child was grown and all her children, except Akisha, were doing well. It was her turn to rest and enjoy things a bit, but she couldn't turn her daughter down. She agreed to provide care on one condition: that Akisha leave the drug-using husband and return home. Akisha swallowed her anger at her mother's command and returned home with her children. Jose cried a lot. He drew obsessively, always pictures of himself rescuing his parents from the alien bugs that were killing them. Akisha says, "He does not know his parents have AIDS, just that I'm sick sometimes."

Akisha's mother wanted nothing to do with the children's father. He used drugs and alcohol and sometimes beat Akisha. Soon her daughter would die from a virus he had given her. Grandmother went to court to prevent his visiting his children. She wanted the children to settle down, for her daughter to get her strength back. Akisha is caught in the middle, in a bad dream which repeats itself. When she was a child she was dragged into court to testify in her mother's behalf against her father. Akisha loved her father, but she did not see him for eight years after that

*The therapists in this case were Joan Gilbert and Sippio Small.

because she was afraid that if she did, her mother's heart condition would act up and her mother would die. She used to try to pretend to herself and to her mother that she had forgotten her father, that she no longer cared. She explained, "I won't have too much of an opinion around her. She can silence you with her voice. Always could. She kept my dad away, too. He was scared of her." But when she met Pedro, and her mother wanted her to stop seeing him, her anger flared up and she married him out of spite.

Now she does not want to cut her children off from their father. But she loves her mother and is afraid of her anger: "I'm just like my mother. Our ideas are so close, you can't tell us apart, except that she's stricter." Part of her is lonely for Pedro and for the parenting they shared. Stefanie speaks to that voice in her, "Mommy, you should let Daddy tell you he's sorry and then you can say back, 'I love you,' because you do love him, even if you fight." Jose's anger hurts her the most. He was her companion during the bad times in her marriage: "Jose helped me keep my sanity. I talked to him constantly. He was my company. We did everything together." Now he turns on her. "You like grandma better than you like my father. I'm not your mate, Mom, I'm your son, and I wanna go to the Bronx and see my dad and live with him. I'm just like him. I gotta be just like him. If he went to jail, I gotta go to jail, Mom, 'cause I'm just like him and I gotta be just like him." Grandmother hates Jose's feisty devotion to his father. He is just like him, she says—bad, rude, headed for trouble.

Akisha is conflicted about Pedro. "I want an apology for what he did in *The New York Times*, so that all the world can see. I want to stop the world in shock. I won't be satisfied until I get that." But like most people in abusive relationships, Akisha and Pedro once had profound bonds. At other moments she cries and says, "He's so thin. He's going fast. If the court doesn't let him see them, he'll die right then and there."

The court takes things out of Akisha's hands and grants Pedro visitation. The visits are a nightmare. Pedro is late, forgets, or causes a fight. The children are disappointed and confused as to whose fault it is that they don't see their father.

Akisha dies. Grandmother is left with the task of raising the children. She wants to forget the man who killed her daughter. Jose has nightmares and begins to have trouble in school. The therapist, Sippio Small, empathizes with grandmother's anger, her devotion to the children, and her fear for the little boy who looks like her daughter. But he tells her gently, over and over, "You have to arrange a visit before he dies. Jose can't think you kept his father away. He will fill in the empty space by idealizing him, by being like him, by rebelling against you." The grand-mother lets Jose visit his father before he dies.

For families of poverty, the spreading epidemic is leaving a generation of orphans. Family members, most often grandparents, assume the burden of caring for the children. In one family we consulted, five adult siblings died of AIDS, leaving a dozen orphaned children to be cared for by the surviving sister and the grandmother. These children had all grown up in drug-using families; some had been well parented, others had suffered not only abuse and neglect but also previous dislocations and losses. Some of the children had severe learning and behavior problems; two had AIDS. Grandmother barely had the strength to manage; she was ravaged by grief at the loss of her children. But there was no time for mourning. She and her daughter had to make do and go on if they were to hold the family together. Then there was the cost to the surviving sister's two children, who had their lives turned upside down by this influx of refugees. Her son became depressed, even suicidal, expressing perhaps the feelings his mother felt she could not show. After all, it had been hard enough to raise her kids when there were just two of them, to keep them off drugs, in school. They were doing reasonably well. Then the deaths began.

The children of people with AIDS and the people who care for them after the parents' death are in need of support to help them with enormous dislocations. Unresolved feelings like Jose's about the extru-sion of a parent, mystification about what has happened to the family, fears of impermanence or even of the death of the caregiver may be represented in children as behavior problems at school or at home or as trouble with the law. Since silence has been the rule where there is AIDS, and life is unbearably precarious, children learn to be silent about their deepest fears and not to ask the questions about matters that terrify them most.

Caregivers in turn are ambivalent about taking on this additional responsibility. Grandparents may have been looking forward to a more relaxed life; older siblings of the AIDS orphans may be starting families of their own or entering careers or college. One older sibling, who had planned to have her younger brother live with her when she married, found her engagement breaking up because her husband-to-be did not want an additional responsibility as he was starting out with his new wife.

Children orphaned or uprooted by AIDS demand much healing and care. Life is often not easy for the caregiver, as many children constantly test the stability of the situation. Bobby, whom we met in Chapter 3, did well with his aunt until she and her husband had a child of their own. This displacement by a new and adored baby who had a far greater claim on the aunt's attention triggered enormous anxiety in Bobby. After all, Bobby's short life included being the scapegoat child who had been brutally abused by his drug-using father, being subject to the family belief that he was too much like his father to amount to anything, losing the mother he adored and the father he secretly loved, and being separated from his siblings. Bobby sensed that the baby had replaced him in his new family's affections. He thought that he was nothing but trouble to these new parents, whose young professional lives simply could not accommodate the demands of a new baby and the intense supervision Bobby demanded. He would not speak about what was wrong; instead he began to act out so badly that his aunt, to save her own family, felt justified in sending him to live with another relative. This solution, which was experienced by Bobby as a rejection, but one which could not be discussed, only made matters worse, and soon the family was considering placement as the only option. In retrospect, the AIDS team should have framed the ending of therapy differently, encouraging family members to come for a follow-up whenever a major change took place in the family. Instead we and the family were too quick to believe that we had come out from under the shadow of AIDS. Children who have lost parents to AIDS are likely to remain extremely vulnerable to events that threaten dislocation and families need to be able to predict behavioral relapse and to weather the storm.

CASE EXAMPLE*

The following case shows brief therapy with two children who come to live with their grandparents. In some ways, it is a case about the formation of a new family, about normal adjustments and conflicts, but this adjustment takes place in the context of a history of wrenching separations, of violence and abuse. The children's mother, who neglected the children, is a crack user, living in the streets, dying of AIDS. Their father is a drug user and dealer who abused them. The children have watched their mother hurled from a roof by drug dealers. They have been kidnapped by her from their grandparents, who had custody, and taken to live in welfare hotels and crack houses. They were rescued again

*The therapist was Ruth Mohr; the consultant was Gillian Walker.

by their grandmother, who then impetuously gave them back to her son, who abused them. Removed from their father's care by Child Welfare Association (CWA), the children are back with their grandparents. It is the safest home they have known, but experience tells them that it may not last. The children have some half-siblings, all of whom have been given up for adoption, and a half-sister with AIDS. Rumor has it that their mother tried to sell the baby and the baby is now in foster care.

The grandparents are in their late fifties. It is a time when they should have lessened responsibility, with the children grown. Financially it should be easier. But here they are again burdened with responsibility for young children—children with school problems, developmental problems, problems that they don't really understand. There's a generation gap between these grandparents, who grew up in the forties and fifties, and their children. They feel betrayed by their own children's values and behavior, their involvement in drugs and crime. They are ashamed and guilty about having failed as parents. They wonder if it will be any different this time around. The social service workers they encounter treat them as though they're failures.

Yet somehow these grandparents understand better than mental health professionals what their grandchildren have learned: that if they are to survive in the inner city, in the violent circumstances of their small lives, they must learn to fight and lie and steal. These adaptive responses are hard enough to live with, harder still to change so that the kids have a fighting chance at a decent life, but the grandparents remain determined, understanding, and patient. What is delightful about this case is the sturdy courage and humor of the family. In the midst of the tragedy of AIDS and urban violence, the love and laughter of this family are a beacon of light.

The family consists of the grandfather Robert (Grandpa), grandmother Teresa (Mama), Billy, age nine, and Betty, age eight. The grandparents reared six children in the inner city. Some of them prospered; some have been swept up in the drug epidemic. Betty and Billy's father, Mama's oldest son, Robert Jr., is a drug dealer, who has had three relationships. His first relationship, which ended in divorce, produced three children now in their middle to late teens, all of whom have spent most of their lives in placement. Robert Jr.'s second marriage was to Betty and Billy's mother, who abandoned the children. Mama keeps in contact with her. "I know it's crazy," she says, "But I can't help it. I love her. She's their mother." After Child Welfare discovered that Robert Jr. was abusing the children, Mama got a court order and now has perma-

nent custody of the children. The children have been with their grandparents for two months and came to Ackerman as a result of a school
referral because of Billy's fighting at school and disrespect for his teachers. The grandparents say that Betty lies and steals but that they are more
concerned about Billy. Our goals are (1) to help the grandparents
establish a functioning and secure family and (2) to bind this family
together by building experiences of approval and success rather than
failure and despair.

These grandparents are proud, private people, who have a healthy
distrust of social service systems, but obey their mandates because they
want their children to get on in the world. They have strong and vital
supports in their community, friendship networks, and particularly their
church. They are sensitive people, with decent values. They know that
their grandchildren have many fears. Will they adjust to the neighbor-
hood? How are they supposed to behave? How are they supposed to fit
in? Will their grandparents be able to keep them safe from the violence all
around? Will this home last? The grandparents also wonder if these
children have been so damaged by what they have experienced that they
will not be able to turn them around.

Mama brings two impeccably dressed children to therapy. Billy wears
a neatly pressed shirt and tie. Both children sit quietly, somewhat
impassively. They answer politely but without much affect. They have
learned to put on their best behavior when they think a great deal is at
stake. Mama is an exuberantly dressed woman, in her version of an
African gypsy. Her hair is wrapped in scarves and she has a sartorial
colorfulness. Grandpa declines to join the session and waits in the
waiting room while Mama "does her thing." Mama tells us enough about
him for us to know that in some way we must involve him in the therapy.
She tells us that he's a supervisor, which means both that he is a
respectable man and that he has some power in the family. It's not that
he's not interested – he communicates with her about the children – but
he's involved from a supervisory distance. He makes his own choices and
cannot be pushed, but above all, he's "beautiful people." Mama tells the
therapist of the children's difficult history. She also announces in a loud
whisper that their mother has HIV but that she does not want the
children to know. As the children are sitting next to her it is clear that
they know, but they are skilled at looking impassive; not a flicker of
emotion crosses their faces as Mama tells their story.

Therapist: What kind of help do you need?
Billy: Help in school.

Therapist: Anything else?

Billy tells the therapist rapidly the story of the abuse they suffered at their father's house and how much both children want to remain with their grandparents.

Therapist: What's to worry about in school?

Billy: I have fights in school. And the teachers don't like me.

Therapist: So Mama's concerned about that because she wants you to have a good experience in school. Anything else she's worried about you? [*Billy remains silent.*] Betty, why is Grandma worried about Billy?

Betty: Because she wanted to see if there was anything wrong with us, and if Daddy made anything worse on us or made us different than we were before.

Therapist: Like what? Can you explain that?

Betty: Like if we were bad over here, she wants to find out what were they doing, beating us or anything that would make us any badder.

Billy: And when we lie. Mostly Betty, but I lie sometimes, too.

Mama: I wonder if what they did made the children crazy. Sometimes I think that. Only sometimes.

The therapist asks Mama whether she thinks that, if the children were to wait in the waiting room, Grandpa would join the session. She invites him and he agrees. He is good-looking, serious, and conservative in comparison with Mama's flamboyance.

Therapist: I've been talking to your lovely grandchildren and Mama. We were talking a little bit about your son Robert Jr. and some of the problems for the children. I know that must be painful for both of you. So I'll just take this opportunity to find out from both of you what your major concerns are and how you think we may be able to help you here.

Grandpa: Our major concern is for those two kids. That's the bottom line. Getting them into a position where they can function in school and in church and in life generally. It's an uphill climb. They don't want him in church. He's very disruptive.

Mama: Billy was thrown out of church. Last week it was school. Like I told you, he fights back. You see, their mother is a prostitute. What has she got, Daddy?

Grandpa: HIV.

Mama: The HIV, OK? I have to help her clean up, because when she comes to my house, she comes so dirty. So when she first tried to come there, I, you know, would clean her up before the children would see her because I don't want the children to see her like that. I want the children to know their Mama as she is; they don't need to know anything about her disease or that she's a prostitute or whatever. Sometimes she says things that she shouldn't say around the children. So now I have her programmed. I say, "When you come, just be happy with the kids, be nice." I make her clean her hands with Clorox or whatever; I'm not saying it's contaminated or whatever but. . . . And when she uses the bathroom, I clean behind her and everything. Besides that, she has some syphilis. At Christmas time she had open sores and she was leaking.

Grandpa: [*Embarrassed*] What does how she was acting have to do with the kids?

Mama: [*Defensively*] I was just saying all this is why I'm so protective. Because I don't want them to know any of these things about their mother.

The therapist wonders what the children must think of Mama's rather unusual behavior with the Clorox bottle. Mama has used the word HIV in a loud whisper in their presence, so clearly Betty and Billy are shrewd enough not to reveal what they know.

Mama: God forbid she should die or whatever. I want them only to know her as their Mama. You see, these children had no feelings for their mother.

Grandpa: That was all washed out of them by my son. He talked badly about her. "She's no good," he said. He told them she was dead.

Therapist: I guess it's more Billy that you're worried about in terms of behavior. Why do you think that he is lying and fighting and getting thrown out of places?

Grandpa: He was doing these things with his father. You know, this is a continuation. Then he came to us. We're getting the same reactions that this father received. I have no idea whether there's something bothering him, but he's not acting normal.

Therapist: He's not acting the way you would like him to. [*Introducing a new idea about Billy.*] You know, he could have gone the other way. He could have gotten the life beaten out of him, just have been an apathetic kid. Then you would be worried about him for different reasons. At least he still has some fight left in him.

Grandpa: Too much.

Therapist: [*Having seeded the idea, she allows the grandfather's view to prevail for now.*] But unfortunately too much and at the wrong time. Do you have any specific concerns about Betty?

Grandpa: I can't say that I do.

Mama: What about the lying?

Grandpa: Oh, yeah, the lying and the stealing. She's a compulsive person.

Therapist: She's compulsive about stealing—she'll steal anything, anytime.

Mama: They dominated them so drastically.

Therapist: They dominated who?

Mama: Billy. He's not under their regime anymore, so he tries to dominate everything that's around him. This is what I picked up. I told him, I said, "You can't live like this. Somebody's gonna hurt you."

Therapist: So he tries to dominate in school?

Mama: Yes. He has no respect for his teachers. And this is ongoing. Soon as she says, "Stop Billy," it's like his father talking to him. I told Billy this. He says, "How do you know, Mama?" I say, "It's just because I feel that way. I put myself in your shoes," and I'm relating to him and he says, "Yes. I'm trying so hard but I can't stop myself," and I say, "Well, I'm gonna take you somewhere and maybe they can help us, help you."

Therapist: OK. I would like to have you both put yourselves in their shoes for a minute and tell me how they understand their position with you two. Do they think there is a possibility that your son could come and take them away?

Mama: But he doesn't even want them.

Therapist: But if he did. Say he and his wife broke up or something and he found somebody and he decided he wanted the kids back. What is the possibility of that happening?

Mama: I will fight it all the way. The courts know about the children. They know what was done. The children talked themselves and they had the mental hygiene over there.

Therapist: You have legal custody?

Mama: Yes.

The therapist takes a break with the team. We decide to pursue the idea that Billy's behavior may be related to his sense that nothing is certain, that all that he has at his disposal are survival skills. Mama is clearly not aware of the depths of his fears.

Therapist: I want to share with you the team's sense that the kids are very fortunate to have you and Robert. I agree very strongly.

Mama: Oh yes, very fortunate.

Therapist: I'm wondering if they know that this is permanent. Their mother kidnaps them. The court takes them away. Robert Jr. takes them from you. The court takes them back. They've been bumped around a lot in their lives.

Mama: I've been to court with them. Everytime they went to court, I went, except once. They told the court, "We want to stay with our Grandma. Our Grandma understands." I love those children.

Grandpa: She's done everything possible to make their lives good.

Therapist: I know that and I'm sure you have, too, because one person can't do that alone. But even so, when they came in here today the first thing they said was, "I want to stay with Mama," so I was just wondering.

Mama: You know!! They told me I brought them here today to take them away and I said, "NO!!"

Therapist: See, that's what I'm wondering. How safe do they feel? I'm just wondering, do they understand that they are going to be with you or do they think that people or agencies or schools can take them away from you?

Mama: That's what they are thinking, because that's what happened with their sister and the baby!

The therapist asks the grandparents to bring the children in so that they can reassure them a little about their fear.

Therapist: So one of the things that occurred to me as I was talking to Mama is that perhaps you would like to know a little bit about your future as a part of this home, because you've been bopped around a lot. You've been with many different parents and stepparents and and with your grandparents. If I were you, Billy, I would sometimes wonder and hope against hope that this was going to be a permanent situation, but I would wonder if it was. So, Mama, what I would like to ask you to do right now, and as often as you feel that it needs to be done, is to talk to the kids and tell them about what their future with you is going to be.

Mama: What your Mama tell you all the time? Where are you going? Tell the truth. Mama said you wasn't going where? Was you going anywhere or are you not going nowhere? What did I say? I says Mama's not gonna let you go nowhere because why?

Billy: Foster home or adoption?

Mama: Right. Because I'm gonna deal with you. Because if you going anywhere else with the way you are, what's gonna happen, Billy?

Billy: I'm gonna get into fights and they would send me to jail.

Mama: I told you I would never let you leave me 'cause I said I loves you. No one else know you like Mama. I says, if I let you go somewhere else, then the people will not understand you as Mama do. I says Mama loves you and Mama understands you and Mama will never leave you if you was a hundred years old.

Therapist: Mama is saying to you that she's gonna keep you forever. She'll be there for you and keep you forever because the way you are now, you would get into trouble if you didn't have Mama and Grandpa there to help you. Do you ever think about, well gee, if I was better and I behaved myself and I turned out to be the wonderful boy that I really am, then Mama would let you go or that you might be adopted?

Billy: [*Confirming Ruth's hypothesis*] I am going to stay with my grandmother 'cause the other children were good and they still got put up for adoption and foster care.

Therapist: Maybe you can appreciate that Billy sometimes thinks that, gee, as long as I'm bad, Mama will keep me because she's the only one, she says, who can understand and handle me, so I guess I'll keep being bad because it keeps Mama connected to me. But we want Billy to be able to be his natural good self. But if he does become his natural good self and lets those dukes down and starts blending in at school and playing with his friends and getting along with adults, then he wonders, would you let him go?

Mama: No, I don't want him to go. I call him "my little man." That's my baby.

Billy: I don't like to be called "little man."

Grandpa: He doesn't like that name "Billy."

Mama: What do you want me to call you?

Billy: David.

Therapist: What is David like?

Billy: A better name.

Therapist: A better name? Is he a boy who behaves?

Billy: Yeah.

Therapist: Aha! So David is your inner wonderful self.

Mama: When I call him David, he's nice.

Therapist: So you want a new identity. You don't want to be thought of as a troublesome kid. You want to be thought of as a nice kid. Billy is a nice kid. OK, so I'm going to leave it to you, Mama (because I think you know how to do this), to really sit down and talk to the kids and make them understand that this is for keeps. What is it you say to the kids when they feel a bit shaky about their permanence?

Mama speaks to the children but the grandfather does not feel heard. After all, he is a supervisor and the therapist is taking his place in the family by doing the supervision with Mama.

Grandpa: I get the feeling that he doesn't care one way or another. I try to instill in him the fact that I want him to be a decent kid, a nice kid, but I get the impression that it doesn't matter. He wants to do what he wants to do.

The grandfather has given us the clue that he has to be actively engaged in therapy and in the process of raising these kids if we are to succeed in helping this family. He rules from the sidelines. Mama is supposed to be his agent, but she is an independent spirit and does things her way, indulgently and somewhat capriciously. The children need steadiness now, as well as love. Billy needs his grandfather to be a male role model who has some love and admiration for him as well as criticism. Grandpa, faced with Mama's indulgence and indomitable optimism, as well as the history of his son's failures, becomes more disapproving and pessimistic than he would be under other circumstances. He resents Mama's control over his grandchildren, as he probably resented her role with his own children, but he will not directly confront her when he thinks that she is wrong. Instead, he tends to direct his criticism to the child, which of course brings Mama to his or her defense. Our goal is to help Grandpa take a more direct and instrumental role, within his definition as supervisor, and to balance Mama's power without directly challenging her. We also want to validate Mama's tremendous gift for nurturing.

Therapist: I think that Billy's getting himself a new name is an indication of his wanting to be a decent, respectable, good kid. Robert, when the children get scared that they will be whisked away, what do you say to them?
Grandpa: They never approach me with any questions about whether they gonna stay with us or not.
Therapist: What is your thought about whether they are going to stay? What is your intention?
Grandpa: I intend to keep them. But I also intend to have him improve his behavior.

Therapist: I want to talk to you about that, too, because I think it's important. I am talking to two men who know what it means to have to fight for themselves, for their families, and for their place in the world. There are many ways to fight. One of the ways is with their dukes up. But that often only gets us into more trouble. Robert, you know about that. I'm sure that Billy (as opposed to David) has been lectured and scolded and punished and rejected— all those things when he does something that's bad. I'm sure that he has heard those lectures a hundred times. And I'm sure that Billy sometimes has a hard time because he does do some things that people get angry at.

Grandpa: On a daily basis.

Therapist: But there must be some times, not too many times, but some times, when Billy does something good.

Mama: He does.

Therapist: And I would like to enlist your help, Robert.

Mama: Ask him. Mama says he's good. He knows it.

Therapist: What I would like is for Robert to do it, because he's a man. He's the model and he's a good model. Robert, this is what I would like you to do. Every evening, before he goes to bed, whenever it's convenient for you, sit down with Billy and talk only about the *good* things that he has done that day. Like, "You went out and picked up the garbage and took it to the incinerator. That was a very thoughtful thing to do," or, "You apologized to your sister because you said something mean to her; that was a very kind thing to do."

Grandpa: [*To Mama, sarcastically, laughing*] Does he do good things?

Mama: [*To Billy*] What does Mama say when you do something, what do I say to you?

Grandpa: "What did you do good today?" [*With sarcasm*]

Mama: [*To Billy*] What do I say to you?

Billy: You told me . . .

Mama: Well, he didn't get a chance to do anything good today because he had to write those things out for school. [*Referring to Robert*] He knows it. [*To Billy*] Sometimes, do Mama kiss you?

Billy: Sometimes when I'm good, she'll buy me ice cream or something. When we're good, she lets us watch television.

The team notices the children are caught in the subterranean warfare between the grandparents. However, this war cannot be addressed directly if we want to engage the family in treatment. The team suggests that Ruth give Robert a specific task, which by aligning him with Mama will also force him to invade her territory without her realizing that the troops have arrived.

Ruth: OK, so my partner has made a good point, which I'd like to share with you. Robert, when you see something that Billy has done that is kind or decent or good or even controlled, like not getting into a fight when he is ready to hit, holding back and . . .
Grandpa: [*Under his breath*] Oh, we hear about it!

The therapist is clear that this is an oblique reference to Mama's enthusiasm for the children, which wears on Robert. By placing the responsibility on Billy to deal directly with his grandfather, she circumvents this source of conflict.

Therapist: [*Continuing*] But it would be important also for Billy to be able to identify those things and tell you. So the conversation might go, "Billy, tell me, share with me what are the good things that you did today. What were the decent things that you did? What were the sensitive things that you did?" And then Billy will tell you about those things.
Mama: [*Eagerly, making a last play for her central place*] I do this everyday. What do I tell you when you come from school? It's really something because, Ruth, what you're telling me to do, I'm doing this already!
Therapist: Mama, this is very important and it is going to be very hard for you, because you want so much to help these kids grow straight as an oak tree. But this is something that I really want to be between *Robert* and Billy. It doesn't even necessarily have to be about a specific good thing, Robert. It can also be, "I didn't get into a fight today" or "I didn't sass the teacher even though I wanted to," because what we want you to do, Robert, is to help Billy begin to identify the good parts of himself and build on those. That really very much needs to be Robert's job. Man to man. Mama, I know how your love overflows for these kids.
Mama: [*Getting in the last word*] Starting next month he told him that they were going to go bike riding. Didn't you, Robert?

In a very simple way we have asked Robert to help Billy build a different story about himself, which we can substitute for the family's problem-saturated view. Their task is simply to talk about how Billy has succeeded rather than how he has failed.

Robert does not come to the second session, but Mama reports that he has been spending time with the children, especially with Billy. Billy is delighted. He has been telling Grandpa what he did well and his behavior has improved dramatically. He has only been in one fight. Mama thinks that it will take a while to change the school's perception of Billy, since the teachers always expect him to be in trouble.

In the third session attended by Mama and the children, Billy reported that he still had talks with Grandpa and that he received the Lollipop Award from his teacher for not fighting in school. The team had decided that the key consolidating change in this family was to make sure that Grandpa was involved with the children and with the therapy. We wrote him the following letter and gave it to the children to give to him.

Therapist: [*Reading letter*] We were very impressed by the way that you were able to help your grandson. It is clear that you helped him to develop a more positive view of himself and to handle himself strategically in a difficult world. We understand and respect the fact that you have a unique way of working with your grandchildren. We will only ask you to join us if any other issues come up at school so that we can have your ideas in addition to your wife's.

Mama: [*Applauding with the children*] Beautiful!

In the next session Mama told us how pleased Robert was with the note. He said that he intended to send us a note and that he felt that the family really needed this therapy. The children were still doing well and they were having good times playing cards and reading with their grandfather. Betty wrote on the blackboard: "Dear Grandpa, I love you a lot. I like playing cards a lot and everything you do for us."

During the team consultation we decided to ask Robert to supervise the children's progress more directly.

Therapist: We are sending Grandpa a very special kind of letter, asking him to give us some information about each of you kids from his perspective at home, OK? You don't have to share it with each other, just between each of you and Grandpa. Mama will be very curious, but when Mama comes back with you next week, we'll share it with Mama here. This one is for Billy, and there's one just like it for you, Betty, to give to your grandfather. They both say the same thing.

The letter was designed to strengthen the coalition between the grandfather and each child, and at the same time gently and respectfully to remove Mama from Grandpa's relationship with the children.

Therapist: [*Reading letter*] Dear Mr. Jefferson, [*because it's from us, right?*]
   It would be helpful to us to know how you feel the children are
   doing each week in terms of behavior from one to ten. One being
   OK and ten being terrific. [*You kids listen carefully, because this is
   going to be between you and Grandpa, not Grandma.*] Rate the week in
   terms of behavior from one to ten. [*So that on Sunday before you come
   here on Monday, you can sit down with him and say, "OK Grandpa, how
   do you rate the week?" And he might say, "Well, I rate it five for
   behavior." You might want to ask him how he came to that and what he
   thinks about a five. See if you can exchange some ideas. And maybe you
   can have some input, too.*] There are three things for you to rate. One
   is the whole week in terms of behavior. The next one is areas for
   improvement, and the third one is areas of success.

The therapist gives the children the notes for Robert (*our* supervisor)
and the next week they carefully give back sealed letters from Robert to
us. The children play an odds or evens game to determine who should go
first. They are excited and a little nervous. Billy wins. Grandpa rates
both of the children as much improved. At the end of each session we
send a rating scale to Robert and each week he returns it, with comments
about the children's successes and areas for improvement. In this section
from the next to last session, Billy can talk about the ways in which he
has internalized his conversations with Grandpa.

Therapist: OK, Billy. Areas of success. That means areas where he's very
   pleased with you. One, "taking orders and understanding."
Billy: I remember when I saw Mama and Grandpa and I said, "I don't
   think I want to be with Mama because Mama don't treat me well, I
   don't think she's gonna treat me right," but now I just take orders
   from her and started listening and say to myself, "I still gotta listen."
Therapist: Who did you tell that to?
Billy: Talking to myself. I wasn't talking out loud—just to myself, in my
   brain.
Therapist: This is something you were saying to yourself. "I have to
   listen and I have to do what I'm told to do because . . ."
Billy: No matter if I like it or not.
Therapist: 'Cause Grandpa and Grandma know what's best for you at
   this particular time. OK. And he has two areas of success for you
   where you're doing excellently. The second one is "think when in
   conversation." It means when you . . .

Billy: Think before I talk.

Therapist: Yeah, and when you're talking, you're thinking.

Billy: Or correcting.

Therapist: This is your letter, Betty. It's the same for you, right? He rated you an eight and put a "good" down. Areas for improvement—got any guesses?

Billy: I think this is a good part. She doesn't do anything bad.

Betty: What does it say?

Therapist: What do you think? Areas for improvement—there are two of them. One, "telling the truth," and the second, "playing."

Billy: I knew it.

Therapist: You knew that? Do you agree with that? What about you, Betty?

Betty: [*Silent, a little ashamed, biting her lip*]

Billy: Yes. Why not tell the truth? At first I lie, then I say OK.

Therapist: How about you, Betty? Do you think maybe there's an area for improvement there? Maybe you should talk to Grandpa. Otherwise he thinks you are doing very, very, very well. One area of success is "playing games with me and adults and children." The other area of success where you do very well is "schoolwork." So Grandpa has big eyes, huh? Grandpa knows what's going on around here.

The team asks Robert to give us another report for the next session. He does and things continue to improve.

Therapist: How are the kids doing in school? Billy, you first. How are you doing in school?

Billy: I don't know. I am good in school. I'm not having no fights or nothing.

Therapist: You're not.

Billy: No.

Therapist: You worked that out so that you're not having any more fights? How did you do that?

Billy: By talking to her and Grandpa. Anton don't bother me anymore 'cause he's scared of me.

Therapist: How come he's scared of you?

Billy: 'Cause I beat him up so many times. All those times where he be messing with me, I always be fighting. And I always win and he ends up crying.

Therapist: So now you don't play with him anymore 'cause he's not
    interested in fighting.
Billy: No.
Therapist: And the other kids? How do you manage not to get into
    fights with the other kids?
Billy: The way I act. I stop. I mean like I stop.

This time Robert has sent a note along with his report. It reads, "Dear
Mrs. Mohr: Billy's behavior has changed. I'm very delighted. I can't ask
anymore as of to date. As far as his classmates are concerned, we are
working very hard at that end. With it goes my appreciation for your
dedication and esprit de corps during a most trying period. Sincerely
yours, Mr. Robert Jefferson."

Six months later, the children were still doing well. Grandma was
enjoying a second chance with the children. She took them to Disney
World and they were doing fine. Grandpa, the supervisor, was doing
excellent work. And the brutal world of poverty and inner-city life was
kept out by the warmth and love of a new family.

PART V
AIDS and Larger Systems

CHAPTER 19

Seeding an Ecosystemic Model

A IDS HAS CREATED a health crisis that challenges the ways in which we think about illness, social deviancy, and the organization of health-care services. As we have seen in the preceding chapters, the spread of HIV infection in the urban ghettos will not be arrested unless programs also address the overarching issues of poverty, drugs, and racial discrimination. What is needed are ecosystemic approaches to care which are community based and led and which address the needs of the family within the context of everyday life (Walker & Small, 1991).

An ecosystemic/family case management model recognizes (1) that AIDS frequently infects more than one family member and always affects the psychosocial functioning of the entire family; and (2) that family members can be empowered to become problem solvers, provide adequate and loving care, counsel other families, and even become advocates for political change. Such programs would provide (1) sophisticated analysis of client needs, (2) the ability to formally conceptualize the family as the unit of care, (3) techniques for mobilizing the caregiving resources of social networks and extended kin systems to be caregivers and problem solvers, (4) techniques for negotiating the interface between the multiple agencies with which people of poverty are often involved. Because these programs would be designed to reduce the redundancy of service, they would be efficient and cost-effective and would reduce the risk of family fragmentation.

The development of ecosystemic care models will require a shift in epistemology from the categorization and segregation of social disorders to an analysis of the interaction between systems, which then leads to responses we term "disorders." The introduction of ecosystemic programs will have consequences at the political level, because they will challenge the way power is maintained by the dominant culture. The work of E. H. Auerswald at Gouverneur Hospital in New York will be used as an elegant theoretical model of an ecosytemic approach. Finally, a program design for an inner-city hospital based on Auerswald's model will be described.

CREATING SYSTEMIC SOLUTIONS IN INNER-CITY COMMUNITIES

A powerful article by Harlon Dalton, "AIDS in Blackface," poses critical issues about community attitudes toward AIDS. Dalton writes:

> The black community's impulse to distance itself from the epidemic is less a response to AIDS, the medical phenomenon, than a reaction to the myriad social issues that surround the disease and give it meaning. More fundamentally it is the predictable outgrowth of the problematic relationship between the black community and the larger society, a relationship characterized by domination and subordination, mutual fear and mutual disrespect, a sense of otherness and a pervasive neglect that rarely feels benign . . . . When we want help, white America is nowhere to be found. When, however, you decide that we need help, you are there in a flash, solution in hand. You then seek to impose that solution on us, without seeking our views, hearing our experiences, or taking account of our needs and desires. We tell you that we fear genocide and you quarrel with our use of the term. Then you try to turn our concerns back on us. "Don't you know," you ask us in an arch tone of voice, "that while you are standing on ceremony, thousands of the very people you say you care about are dying from AIDS?" Struggling to ignore the insulting implication that we are profoundly retarded or monumentally callous we respond, "Don't *you* know that they are already dying from drug overdoses, Uzis and AK-47s, joblessness, despair and societal indifference?" And white America, you sigh and say, "What's one thing got to do with the other?" Then we sigh and wonder if you truly do not understand. (pp. 218-219)

Dalton's compelling point is that the black community distances itself from AIDS as an outgrowth of its relationship to the dominant society, which threatens people of poverty and color with virtual genocide by neglecting fundamental needs for safety, employment, housing, drug programs, nutrition, education, and adequate health care. Dalton contends that white America's response to the AIDS epidemic in the inner cities is one of maintaining power and control. White America does not listen to community ideas and concerns; it does not encourage community leadership. Furthermore, it treats AIDS as a special concern, unrelated to the larger social ecology that nurtures it. These points are of critical importance when conceptualizing social service programs for AIDS patients and even when considering the definition of AIDS-related psychotherapy.

The psychiatric construction of the problems of people of color, including drug use, supports the power of the dominant white society and leads to ineffective program design that increases fragmentation and categorization. Helping professionals are trained in labeling practices that only obscure racism, sexism, and homophobia. Racism, like homophobia, is so pervasive in our culture that it contaminates the perspective of even those who want to help. Stereotypic concepts such as "the multiproblem family" or the "disintegration of the black family" that originated in proposals (Moynihan, 1965) intended to address the problems of people of color produced negative frames and expectations that limit how an individual family is perceived by the treating system.

Furthermore, therapists are trained to focus on what Michael White (White & Epston, 1990) and others have called the "problem-saturated narrative," rather than on those amazing instances of survival and health that are also present. Labeling practices lead to stigma (Imber-Black, 1988). Families in which there is a drug user are stigmatized by the label and treated as if the family as a whole were inadequate. Categories such as *drug addict, juvenile delinquent, depressive,* and *homosexual,* while they seem useful in delineating dynamics and treatment strategies, become institutionalized in programs that segregate and reify problems. Furthermore, as Michael White has noted in his application of some ideas of the French philosopher Michel Foucault, such labelings are accorded a truth status by the scientific disciplines and are subject to normalizing practices of "therapy" (White & Epston, 1990). Foucault's (1973) point is that such categorizations of deviance or "dividing practices" and their correlate, social institutions as instruments of normalization through corrective measures, are the critical method by which the dominant society maintains control.

For many years homosexuality was elaborated as a psychiatric abnormality, a "truth" which overlooked contrary evidence from other cultures as to its normalcy. Not only were many gay people subjected to normalizing procedures to change sexual orientation, but practices that grew out of life in a homophobic society – for example, "promiscuous" sexuality as opposed to settling down in a committed relationship—were described as "abnormal." Ignored in the label of abnormality was the very real fact that it was far easier for a gay man to maintain secrecy about a night life at the bars than about a committed relationship to another man. Furthermore, for many gay men, the celebration of sexuality (labeled "promiscuity") was a response to years of repression and created a sense of community and connection.

Because racism is as ubiquitous and lethal as homophobia, people who have suffered from the ravages of life in the urban ghetto are assumed to have pathologies as an inherent result of their difficult circumstances. However, reviewing the genograms of inner-city families—who live under conditions of chronic violence, ubiquitous drugs, a failing school system, and inadequate housing, health-care, and basic nutrition—what is astounding is that so many family members survive and do well. Psychotherapeutic intervention must be sensitive to context and empowering to families. The therapist must be aware of the *strengths* that are always to be found in inner-city family networks, drawing on the problem-solving ability of family members and reinforcing narratives of survival and health.

AN ECOSYSTEMIC MODEL

Critical issues dealing with the categorization of disease and the delivery of services in relation to power transactions around racial and sexual issues must be addressed if we are to develop adequate programs to deal with the AIDS crisis. A narrow focus on individuals or families leads to treatment goals that primarily involve accommodation; by contrast, an ecosystemic approach necessarily leads to the analysis of larger systems, including political systems, as an integral part of treatment. An ecosystemic approach is a radical shift in epistemology that has political consequences, because in challenging categorizations it implicitly challenges the foundations by which the dominant system retains social control.

The ecosystemic therapist is interested in the adaptive fit between individual, family, *and environment*. What was previously defined as "psychopathology" and subjected to normalizing intervention is now viewed as an attempt to fit with and to maintain integrity in a problematic environment. A psychiatric labeling intervention ignores the larger context and attempts to shape the organism to fit the dominant culture's social mores. In an ecosystemic model, intervention involves an analysis of the recursive loops between individual problem-bearer, family, environment, and culture. The goal of intervention is to disrupt critical and repetitive problem-generating premises and their resulting behaviors. This might be achieved by manipulating social conditions, by analyzing how cultural belief systems of racism, sexism, and homophobia may be problem-generating, or by introducing new "information" or narratives at the level of individual or family. Since most people (both clients and therapists) bring the prevailing epistemology of fixed pathology to counseling, a systems view would inject a powerful and mobilizing effect by providing positive, inclusive, and fluid descriptions of the situation. Furthermore, viewed within a systems context, "the problem" is no longer an "it" but a *communication* among other communications, a narrative among other narratives, which can be rewritten and changed. Because systems thinkers seek to identify those sequences of interaction that could provide different outcomes for the individual, family, or natural group, they are interested in emphasizing transactions within the various systems that do not fit with the problem-focused narrative — transactions that are nutritive, prideful, and change-promoting.

In thinking about families of people of color, for instance, a systems view would discard Moynihan's (1965) victim-blaming label of "multiproblem family," which has become the dominant cultural narrative about people of color and poverty. The systems thinker would be free to look at the history of the extraordinary resourcefulness of the African-American family, noting its strategies for surviving appalling oppression, both psychological and economic. One would see adaptive strategies that could be utilized in program development and intervention, such as the power and deep loyalty of kin ties, the embracing of related and non-related children and family members in need. One would identify coping strategies such as humor, the richness of language (Draper, 1979), the ability of the African-American church to provide meaning and experiences of positive socialization in the absence of the most basic community facilities. The community of poverty then would be seen not as a deficit-ridden, pathology-ridden group, but as a rich and varied group of people who have strong capacities for leadership, a tradition of hard work, and a long and deep history of mutual aid.

In the 1960s and early 1970s a few family therapists, influenced by the community psychiatry movement, developed some interesting ecosystemic ideas as they designed and coordinated health-care programs for inner-city populations. Instead of traditional mental health facilities, they created a model of crisis intervention therapy that utilized the resources of the client's ecosystem, and experimented with ideas such as network therapy and multisystems meetings. The programs they developed provide a useful template for the development of ecosytemic AIDS prevention and treatment programs for inner-city populations.

Perhaps the most clearly articulated community-based health program was E. H. Auerswald's crisis intervention program, which existed for five years in the late sixties at lower Manhattan's Gouverneur Hospital. Auerswald (1968, 1983) believed that the true application of systems theory could not be confined to treating family or individual dynamics in a mental health center while the larger systems that defined family life remained unaddressed. He observed that specialization had forced individuals and families with complex social, environmental, familial, and interpersonal problems to shop for pieces of help: In poor communities where once the community center provided a model of holistic care, medical, social and recreational, services had become totally fragmented. Clients journeyed large distances from agency to agency to obtain essential services, a Kafka-esque nightmare of waiting, filling out forms, waiting in clinic and welfare lines. Services were redundant and workers only knew that small piece of the puzzle which was their domain. Auerswald's crisis intervention unit was designed to provide an antidote to the fragmentation of social service. It was to be a health-care/mental-health system with a single point of entry that could respond in an integrated way to all the interrelated medical, social, and behavioral issues that created distress (Auerswald, 1983). The isolated diagnosis or single problem or request for help would not determine the location of care, but rather medical or psychiatric phenomena would be analyzed in relation to the larger context of the person's life and intervention might take place in any system which had significant impact on the problem. An important point for Auerswald was that family therapy cannot be "conceived of as an ancillary service, but the family/social system is the unit of care" (1983). One of Auerwald's metaphors is that not understanding the context is like trying to fix the fuse when, in fact, the power grid is down.

Auerswald emphasized the importance of the intake interview as changing both the client and the professional's description of the problem. "The way intake is determined determines the structure of the interventive system" (1968). Convening the family or kin-friendship network was the major tool for gathering sociocultural information about the family system. Auerswald went on to say that until network sessions were held, professionals did not see the connections between events which made up the story of which the symptom was a part, nor were they able to mobilize essential support systems.

Auerswald's belief that helping systems maintained problematic situations and that intervention to alleviate the client's problems often might take place within these very helping systems was a pivotal insight that led to critical inquiries and paradigmatic shifts in thinking and planning (Imber-Black, 1988).

Auerswald believed that a helping program should be absolutely flexible in adjusting to the needs of the client population. In order for the helping program to move into the space-time of the client who called for help, programs would be organized on an as-needed basis. Appointment times, for example, would not be fixed, teams would be interdisciplinary but not hierarchical, with the community staff having the same status as the "professionals" (Auerswald, 1968).

In the Gouverneur program interdisciplinary teams made home visits, convened networks, and facilitated the acquisition of any needed services—even if that meant inventing services that did not exist. One example of this innovative work was the creation of support groups targeted at women who had recently moved to the community from different Latin American countries and who were suffering from the depression and isolation that are a normal part of cultural transition.

While Auerswald provided valuable ideas about construction of services that located disease within a social context, his program ultimately failed. Reflecting ten years later on the collapse of the program, Auerswald wrote that it was not just that "Great Society" programs had ended, but that as his program developed within the context of the community it served, it began to take shape in accordance with the community's expression of need. In doing so, it challenged the way the dominant medical center provided pieces of service to the community. Auerswald's program joined a number of "community action" programs that were abandoned by their sponsors in the early 1970s. As Margaret Burnham wrote in *The Nation*:

> The record shows that as soon as community action projects were organized and the people started responding, many of the proponents of the new programs turned tail. They came to understand that once the poor got together, they might realize that nobody was going to solve their problems. Once they understood that—that if they were given support and encouragement in organizing—they might demand more fundamental changes.

DEVELOPING ECOSYSTEMIC
PROGRAMS FOR PEOPLE WITH AIDS

Effective prevention programs in inner-city communities should be

1. *Ecosystemic*: The program is designed to take into account the survival issues of people living in a culture of poverty where drugs are a major player.

Take, for example, a safer-sex education program: instead of merely providing information, an ecosystemic program would recognize the crucial role of childbearing in inner-city communities. It would work to strengthen a mother's bonds with existing children, by providing multi-family groups where parenting issues were discussed and mothers' networks were formed. To be effective, such programs may entail helping a mother resume care of her children by organizing meetings with child welfare and foster care agencies. A mother may need help with obtaining housing or detoxification. She may need education or help in obtaining a job so that she can leave an abusive partner who refuses to use safer sex. Or she may need counseling with her partner around reproductive issues so that gender premises linked to traditional sexual roles can be challenged.

Because the lives of people of poverty often move from crisis to crisis, appointment times should reflect client needs. Outreach teams should be able to make home visits during crises and to help clients obtain emergency concrete services.

2. *Community designed, based, and directed*: The program utilizes the talents for leadership of inner-city people for design and staffing. Programs start from focus groups which are used to engage community people from the start in development.

Most often, programs for African-American and Latino families dealing with AIDS in inner-city communities are staffed by white workers and have no community people involved. The white professionals receive no training in working with minority families, nor is consultation provided. When a family includes several drug users, frequently professionals, including professionals of color, operate on a pathology model based on a belief that these are multiproblem families, without motivation or resources. Staff attitudes create a vicious cycle that drives the client further and further from the health-care system. For example, a mother may miss her prenatal appointments out of shame about her ongoing drug use and thus fail to utilize available avenues of relief, such as acupuncture, which would help her reduce her use of drugs that are damaging her fetus.

Home visits are advantageous during an episodic disease such as AIDS because they allow treatment teams to understand family life and meet important family members who might not otherwise be available. Teams made up of professionals working in collaboration with community people can be used to provide mobile crisis intervention.

3. *Family centered*: The program must address the impact of drugs and AIDS on the complex kin networks of the ill person. Family members are trained to talk to other members, kin, and social networks about prevention and care for the ill (Landau, 1982). Families are seen as having the resources to be problem solvers and caregivers for their own system.

4. *Integrated*: All psychosocial services are coordinated by a single family case management team.

As noted in the previous chapter, redundancy of service is the norm as families scramble to enter numerous helping systems, each funded to deal with a piece of the problem. Recall the case example in the Chapter 17, in which the mother was dying of AIDS, the four-year-old child showed ARC symptoms, and the father was on crack and heroin. Over a dozen professionals were involved with the family; yet when the mother died, it was found that no provisions had been made for the child's care.

Now imagine an ecosystemic approach to this same family. The family is assigned a case manager and an outreach worker from the community. All communications from medical and social services are routed to the case manager. Perhaps the case manager is a paraprofessional versed in the problems of poverty and trained in family systems work. (The training of such a professional is neither long nor costly and has been done in various settings [Laird, 1979].) The community worker and the case manager meet frequently with the family in its apartment. An AIDS health specialist visits on occasion to monitor the medical situation. During these visits, the workers help the mother confide in other family members. The planning process begins for the little girl's care should the mother die, and the case manager initiates a relationship with family

members who indicate willingness to provide either temporary or permanent care should the father be unable to manage his drug use. The
father's family is also involved, and the community worker—himself an
ex-drug user—works with the father to get him into a drug treatment
program that will deal with his crack use. Because AIDS mothers are
isolated, the mother is invited to join a drop-in group of other family
members who have AIDS or who have a spouse with AIDS. The group
helps the mother deal with her shame and her helplessness as she
comforts other group members, and her depression lifts as the group
takes on an advocacy role on behalf of other AIDS families in need of
services.

5. *Political*: Racist policies create the environmental niche for
   AIDS in communities of poverty and of color. Ecosystemic,
   community based and directed programs would provide a location for sorely needed political advocacy. Raising community
   consciousness about AIDS and mobilizing the community to
   break the silence of shame and stigma that has paralyzed collective action would be primary goals. The founding of ecosystemic, community based and led organizations such as GMHC
   energized a gay political movement, as gay men understood the
   relationship between homophobia and the spread of AIDS.

ECOSYSTEMIC, COMMUNITY-BASED
SERVICE DELIVERY MODELS: GAY
MEN'S HEALTH CRISIS AND THE
MONTEFIORE WOMEN'S CENTER

At the beginning of the AIDS crisis in the early 1980s the gay community
developed a number of social service programs for AIDS patients. These
programs, while they lack Auerswald's conceptual clarity and emphasis
on managing the interface between larger systems, are fundamentally
holistic if not strictly ecosystemic. As such, they contain many elements
that could be applied to inner-city populations at risk. These programs
continue to demonstrate how a community whose very survival is
challenged by a disease can come together in mutual support that
ultimately catalyzes a new consciousness and a new political activism.

Not long into the AIDS epidemic it became clear that service delivery
structures pathologized gay people and were unresponsive to their needs.
The neglect of the dominant culture forced gay communities to construct

social service agencies of their own. One such agency was Gay Men's Health Crisis (GMHC), founded when the disease was so poorly understood that it was believed to attack only gay men. GMHC enlisted community volunteers to care for the sick and dying. Quite rapidly the volunteers became skilled counselors, despite a lack of official training.

Gradually it became apparent that there was a need for the coordination of all services.

GMHC's policy was that the ill person should not have to shop for "pieces of help," but that all care needs should be provided under the aegis of a single agency. People with AIDS needed legal services to help them write wills, provide instructions for medical decision-making in the event of incapacitation, plan for the future care of children, and deal with discrimination in housing and employment. Financial needs were complex, and people needed help in expediting the maze of welfare and social security bureaucracies. HIV infection meant changing sexual practices, which required sensitive sexual counseling. Ombudsmen were needed to fight for decent patient care in medical facilities, where discrimination was rampant. Clients needed access to medical information, so that they could negotiate more effectively with physicians and make choices about protocols. Crisis intervention workers were needed to convene families and other care-giving systems and negotiate with the medical and health-care provider systems. Volunteers were needed to help clients support each other in group counseling and to provide recreation as well as nutritional and spiritual counseling. Prevention was critical; educators were needed to speak to community groups, to reach out to gay men in places where they socialized, to run safer-sex workshops. Because each task was clearly defined, volunteers could be easily trained to staff the many service units.

Because these gay AIDS agencies provided a multitude of services instead of just one, they began to present an ecosystemic profile of the interaction and politics of multiple service delivery systems. Once individuals have access to more than one piece of the puzzle, once a cross-section of community people is brought together around a common task, a process of empowerment begins that leads to political activism. ACT-UP was one such off-shoot of the political activism generated by AIDS volunteerism.

In poor communities primary care facilities such as hospitals and community-based health-care clinics have the possibility of becoming the only viable centers for the dissemination of AIDS information and for changing people's attitudes toward the disease. One such project already mentioned is the Montefiore's Women's Center (Eric et al., 1989), where a group of women who were methadone patients was asked to convene to help researchers understand the needs and problems that poor, drug-using women face. This group has become the foundation for an informal AIDS prevention community outreach group in which women teach other women how to protect themselves, how to get services, how to change their lives.

This program has demonstrated the effectiveness of programs which contextualize issues such as AIDS. Clients were seen as community experts who knew what was needed. While it was acknowledged that the women were struggling with a drug problem, they were never treated as if drug use was their only narrative. The women encouraged each other to develop positive stories about themselves, as women who had knowledge to share from their experience as parents, as friends, often as caretaking daughters, as women who had aspirations for a better life for themselves and their children, as women who were struggling to raise families under extremely difficult circumstances.

The women ran peer counseling groups about HIV infection and provided mutual support both with AIDS issues and with drug use, while the professionals used their access to community resources to provide educational opportunities for women, to advocate for safe housing and child care (Eric et al., 1989). The Women's Center was based on feminist ideas that women will respond better to "care" than to "justice"; therefore, the groups were supportive, caring, and nonjudgmental. Helping women break the isolation of drug use by forming strong bonds to each other and to their families was a major building block for self-esteem.

As the program evolved, the women asked to form couples groups to deal directly with their male partners about issues of potential or actual infection. They asked for family groups to deal with issues of caretaking children when they were ill or on drugs and for future planning for their children should they die. Grandparents and siblings seemed eager to come, demonstrating the ability of networks to respond to crisis. The myth that men would not attend such programs was exploded when they saw that their women were enthusiastic and were getting concrete services, as well as support and friendship from each other. The group became enormously skillful at counseling each other and recruiting other families and couples to join.

The Montefiore Women's Center is a remarkable demonstration of what happens when the suspicion and distrust of people who have felt the burden of discrimination, lack of respect, and second-rate services are overcome. Because it was not the goal of professional staff to do therapy (to normalize), but rather to be available as respectful consultants who could learn from these women's experiences, the women felt empowered to help each other. The refusal to allow the label *drug user* to define these women and the positive frame of respect for their knowledge and power to organize and help each other and to teach the professionals had unexpected results: Women began to voluntarily enter treatment programs for polydrug abuse, to go to school, to resume caring for their children, and to seek work.

An additional grant has enabled the Women's Center and the Ackerman Institute's AIDS Team to develop a family case management program for maternal drug users located in the neonatal unit of North Central Bronx Hospital. This program, addressed to the mothers of babies who are diagnosed as "cocaine toxicology positive," would provide a full range of medical and psychosocial services to families within an ecosystemic, family case management framework, and would follow these mothers and their families over a five-year period. The network meeting developed by Auerswald is a critical element of intake, since a major goal is to coordinate service delivery at all levels of systems. These particular mothers were chosen because cocaine use puts them at risk for AIDS and because it is at the point that a baby is found to be cocaine toxicology positive that a family is threatened with the fragmentation of mandatory foster care. The goal of the family case management team, which will be composed of family therapists and Women's Center staff, will be to maintain the child in the kin system and to utilize the resources within the family to improve daily life. A major program goal is to train community people and talented family members to become the outreach workers and family case managers.

The AIDS epidemic in the gay community taught us valuable lessons about mutual aid, about the innate skills of laypeople in performing sophisticated counseling tasks and providing leadership in designing programs for their communities, about the advantages of programs that coordinate services, about the need to challenge bureaucratic procedures that prevent intelligent laypeople from having a say in policies that directly affect them. The programs discussed above are a small beginning toward creating a collaboration between health-care professionals and the people we serve in inner cities.

Bibliography

Alexander, B.K., & Dibb, O.S. (1975). Opiate addicts and their parents. *Family Process, 14,* 499–514.

Altman, D. (1982). *The homosexualization of America.* New York: Beacon.

Altman, D. (1987). *AIDS in the mind of America.* New York: Doubleday.

Altman, D. (1988). Legitimization through disaster: AIDS and the gay movement. In E. Fee & D. Fox (Eds.), *AIDS: The burdens of history* (pp. 301–315). Berkeley: University of California Press.

Altman, L. (1994, August 17). High HIV levels raise risk to newborns, 2 studies show. *New York Times,* p. C8.

Altman, L. (1995a, January 24). Long-term survivors may hold key clues to puzzle of AIDS. *New York Times,* pp. C1, C11.

Altman, L. (1995b, February 7). Protein in saliva found to block AIDS virus in test tube study. *New York Times,* p. C3.

Altman, L. (1995c, February 14). Children's AIDS study finds AZT ineffective. *New York Times,* p. C13.

Anderson, C.M., Reiss, D.J., & Hogarty, G.E. (1986). *Schizophrenia and the family.* New York: Guilford.

Angier, N. (1995). Immature immune cells may sustain brunt of HIV attack. *New York Times,* p. C3.

Annis, H. (1974). Patterns of intra-familial drug use. *British Journal of the Addictions, 69,* 361–369.

Aries, P. (1982). *The hour of our death.* New York: Vintage.

Auerswald, E.H. (1968). Interdisciplinary versus ecological approach. *Family Process, 7*(2), 202–215.

Auerswald, E.H. (1969). Cognitive development and psychopathology in the urban environment. In P. S. Graubard (Ed.), *Children against school: Education of the delinquent, disturbed, disrupted* (pp. 181–201). Chicago: Follet.

Auerswald, E.H. (1983). The Gouverneur Health Services Program: An experiment in ecosystemic community care delivery. *Family Systems Medicine, 1*(3), 5–24.

Austin, P. (1995, January 12). Medicine-Dynamics of HIV infection. *Nature News Service.*

Bartlett, J., & Finkbeiner, A. (1993). *The guide to living with HIV infection.* Baltimore, MD: Johns Hopkins Press.

Bateson, G. (1965). *Naven: A survey of the problems suggested by a composite picture of the culture of a New Guinea tribe drawn from three points of view.* Stanford: Stanford University Press.

Bateson, M.C., & Goldsby, R. (1988). *Thinking AIDS: The social response to the biological threat.* Reading, MA: Addison-Wesley.

Bayer, R. (1989). *Private acts, social consequences: AIDS and the politics of public health.* New York: Macmillan/The Free Press.

Becker, E. (1973). *The denial of death.* New York: Free Press.

Beeson, D., Zones, J., & Nye, J. (1986). *The social consequences of AIDS antibody testing: Coping with stigma.* Paper presented at the annual meeting of the Society for the Study of Social Problems, New York, NY.

Black, D. (1985). *The plague years: A chronicle of AIDS, the epidemic of our times.* New York: Simon & Schuster.

Bloch, D. (1985). The family as a psychosocial system. In S. Henao & N. Gross (Eds.), *Principles of family systems in family medicine.* New York: Brunner/Mazel.

Bloch, D. (1989). Family systems and biological processes: A coevolutionary model. In C. N. Ramsey, Jr. (Ed.), *Family systems in medicine.* New York: Guilford.

Bluebond-Langer, M. (1978). *The private worlds of dying children.* Princeton, NJ: Princeton University Press.

Blumstein, P., & Schwartz, P. (1983). *American couples: Money, work, and sex.* New York: Simon & Schuster.

Bok, S. (1978). *Lying: Moral choice in public and private life.* New York: Vintage.

Bok, S. (1983). *Secrets: On the ethics of concealment and revelation.* New York: Vintage.

Borysenko, J. (1989). Psychoneuroimmunology. In C. N. Ramsey, Jr. (Ed.), *Family systems in family medicine* (pp. 243–256). New York: Guilford.

Boscolo, L., Cecchin, C., Hoffman, L., & Penn, P. (1987). *Milan systemic family therapy. Conversations in theory and practice.* New York: Basic Books.

Boswell, J. (1980). *Christianity, social tolerance, and homosexuality: Gay people in Western Europe from the beginning of the Christian era to the fourteenth century.* Chicago: University of Chicago Press.

Bowen, M. (1978). *Family therapy in clinical practice.* New York: Aronson.

Boyd-Franklin, N. (1989). *Black families in therapy: A multisystems approach.* New York: Guilford.

Brandt, A. (1987). *No magic bullet: A social history of venereal disease in the United States since 1880.* London: Oxford University Press.

Brandt, A. (1988). AIDS from social history to social policy. In E. Fee & D. Fox (Eds.), *AIDS: The burdens of history* (pp. 147–171). Berkeley: University of California Press.

Buchanan, B., & Lapin, J. (1990). Restoring the soul of the family. *Family therapy networker, 14*(6), 46–52.

Burnham, M. (1989, July 24–31). The great society didn't fail. *The Nation*, pp. 122–126.

Camus, A. (1972). *The plague*. New York: Vintage Books.

Caplan, P. (Ed.) (1987). *The cultural construction of sexuality*. London: Tavistock.

Carl, D. (1986). Acquired immune deficiency syndrome: A preliminary examination of the effects on gay couples and coupling. *Journal of Marital and Family Therapy, 12*(3), 241–247.

Carl, D. (1990). *Counseling same-sex couples*. New York: Norton.

Carrier, J. (1976). Cultural factors of AIDS Patients. *Archives of Sexual Behavior, 5*, 103–124.

Carter, B. (1989). Societal implications of HIV infection: HIV antibody testing, health care, and AIDS education. *Marriage and Family Review, 13*(1/2), 129–185.

Carter, E., & Watney, S. (Eds.) (1989). *Taking liberties: AIDS and cultural politics*. New York: Serpents Tail.

Centers For Disease Control. (1993, 1994, 1995). HIV-AIDS surveillance report. Atlanta, GA: Author.

Clark, K. (1967). *Dark ghetto: Dilemmas of social power*. New York: Harper Torchbooks.

Clarke, L., & Potts, M. (Eds.) (1988). *The AIDS reader: Documentary history of a modern epidemic*. Boston: Branden Publishing.

Clatts, M. (1990, March). *The crack epidemic: Have we any answers?* Paper presented at the Family Therapy Networker Symposium, Washington DC.

Clumek, N. (1989, Nov. 23). A cluster of HIV infection among heterosexual people without apparent risk factors. *New England Journal of Medicine*, 1460–1462.

Cohen, J. (1995, February 17). AIDS mood upbeat—For a change. *Science, 267*, 959–960.

Coleman, S. B. (1980). Incomplete mourning and addict family transactions: A theory for understanding heroin abuse. In D. Lettieri (Ed.), *Theories of drug abuse*. Washington, DC: United States Government Printing Office, prepared by The National Institute on Drug Abuse.

Coleman, S. B., Kaplan, J. D., & Downing, R.W. (1986). Life cycle and loss: The spiritual vacuum of heroin addiction. *Family Process, 5*, 5–23.

Coleman, S. B., & Stanton, M. D. (1978). The role of death in the addict family. *Journal of Marriage and Family Counseling, 4*, 79–91.

Conner, S., & Kingman S. (1989). *The search for the virus: The scientific discovery of AIDS and the quest for a cure*. London: Penguin Books.

Crimp, D. (Ed.) (1988). *AIDS: Cultural analysis, cultural activism*. Cambridge, MA: The MIT Press.

Crimp, D. (1989, Winter). Mourning and militancy. *October, 51*, 3–18.

Cunningham, M. (1990). *At home at the end of the world*. New York: Farrar Straus Giroux.

Curran, J., Jaffe, H., Hardy, A., Morgan, W., Selik, R., & Dondero, T. (1988). Epidemiology of HIV infection and AIDS in the United States. *Science, 239*, 610–616.

Dalton, H. (1989). AIDS in Blackface. *Daedalus, 118*(2), 205–227.

DeCecco, J. P. (Ed.) (1985a). *Bashers, baiters, and bigots: Homophobia in American society.* New York: Harrington Park Press.

DeCecco, J. P. (Ed.) (1985b). *Gay Personality and sexual labeling.* New York: Harrington Park Press.

DeCecco, J. P., & Shively, M. G. (1985). *Origins of sexuality and homosexuality.* New York: Harrington Park Press.

Defoe, D. (1984). *A journal of the plague year.* New York: Meridian Classic/New American Library.

Des Jarlais, D. C., Friedman, S. R., & Hopkins, W. (1985). Risk reduction for the acquired immunodeficiency syndrome among intravenous drug users. *Annals of Internal Medicine, 1003*(5), 755–759.

Douglas, M. (1985). *Purity and danger: An analysis of concepts on pollution and taboo.* London: ARK Paperbacks.

Douglas, P., & Pinsky, L. (1989). *The essential AIDS fact book.* New York: Pocket Books.

Draper, B. (1979). Black language as an adaptive response to a hostile environment. In C. Germain (Ed.), *Social work practice: people and environments.* New York: Columbia University Press.

Drucker, E. (1986). AIDS and addiction in New York City. *American Journal of Drug and Alcohol Abuse, 12,* 165–181.

Drucker, E. (1989a, Sept/Oct). Havanna's virtue, Miami's vice, the geopolitics of cocaine. *International Journal of Drug Policy, 1*(2).

Drucker, E. (1989b). Unpublished grant proposal for Montefiore Department of Social Medicine.

Drucker, E. (1990, December). In Dickens' America. *Family Therapy Networker.* 42–45.

Dubler, N. (1987). *AIDS: Confidentiality and the duty to warn.* Unpublished manuscript.

Dunne, E., McIntosh, J., & Dunne-Maxim, K. (1987). *Suicide and its aftermath: Understanding and counseling the survivors.* New York: Norton.

Eldred, C., & Washington, M. (1976). Interpersonal relationships in heroin use by men and women and their role in treatment outcome. *International Journal of the Addictions, 11,* 117–130.

Engel, G. (1968). A life setting conducive to illness: The giving in, given up complex. *Annals of Internal Medicine, 74,* 771–772.

Eric, K., Drucker, E., Worth, D., Chabon, B., Pivnick, A., & Cochrane, K. (1989). *The Woman's Center: A model peer support program for high risk IV drug and crack using women in the Bronx.* Paper presented at the Fifth International AIDS Conference, Montreal, Canada.

Falloon, J., Eddy, J., Weiner, L., & Pizzo, P. (1989). Human immunodeficiency virus in children. *Journal of Pediatrics, 114*(1), 1–30.

Fatal triangle: Crack, syphilis and AIDS. (1989, August 20). *New York Times,* A11.

Federal study questions ability of AZT to delay AIDS symptoms. (1991, February 15). *New York Times,* A1, A22.

Fortunato, J. E. (1987). *AIDS, The spiritual dilemma.* New York: Harper & Row.

Foucault, M. (1973). *Madness and civilization: A history of insanity in the age of reason.* New York: Vintage.

Foucault, M. (1975). *The birth of the clinic: An archaeology of medical perception.* New York: Vintage.

Foucault, M. *Discipline and punish: The birth of the prison.* New York: Vintage.

Foucault, M. (1980). *The history of sexuality.* Vol. 1. New York: Vintage.

Foucault, M. (1985). *The use of pleasure: The history of sexuality.* Vol. 2. New York: Pantheon.

Foucault, M. (1988). *The care of the self: The history of sexuality.* New York: Vintage.

Fox, B. (1989). Cancer survival and the family. In C. N. Ramsey, Jr. (Ed.), *Family systems in medicine* (pp. 273–280). New York: Guilford.

Fox, R., Odaka, N., & Polk, B. (1986, June). Effect of learning HTLV-III/LAV: Antibody status on subsequent sexual activity. *Abstracts of the International Conference on AIDS.* Paris, France.

Freud, S. (1917). *Mourning and melancholia.* In J. Strachey (Ed. and Trans.), *The standard edition of the complete psychological works of Sigmund Freud,* Vol. 14 (pp. 237–258). New York: Norton.

Friedland, G. H., & Klein, R. S. (1987). Transmission of the human immunodeficiency virus. *New England Journal of Medicine, 317,* 1125–1135.

Friedman, S. R. et al. (1987). The AIDS epidemic among blacks and hispanics. *Millbank Quarterly, 65,* 477–80.

Fullilove, M. (1989). Ethnic minorities, HIV disease, and the growing underclass. In J. Dilly, C. Pies, & M. Helquist (Eds.), *Face to face: AIDS health project.* San Francisco: University of California Press.

Fullilove, M., Fullilove, R., Haynes, K., & Gross, S. (1990). Black women and AIDS prevention: A view towards understanding the gender roles. *Journal of Sex Research, 27*(1), 47–64.

Gagnon, J. (1989, Summer). Disease and desire. *Daedalus, 118*(3), 1–78.

Gallo, R. (1989, October). My life stalking AIDS. *Discover, 10*(10), 30–37.

Garcia-Preto, N. (1982). Puerto-Rican families. In M. McGoldrick, J. K. Pearce, & J. Giordano (Eds.), *Ethnicity and family therapy* (pp. 164–186). New York: Guilford.

Garret, L. (1990, June 12). AIDS: The next decade. *New York Newsday,* pp. 3–6.

Garston, L., & Curran, W. (1989, December). The limits of compulsion in controlling AIDS. *Hasting Center Report,* pp. 25–26.

Germain, C. (Ed.) (1979). *Social work practice: People and environments.* New York: Columbia University Press.

Giaquinto, C., De Rossi, A., Girotto, S., Cozzani, S., Elia, R., Chieco-Bianchi, L. (1989). *Natural history of pediatric HIV infection.* Paper presented Fifth International AIDS Conference, Montreal, Canada.

Giesecke, I. (1988). Incidence of symptoms and AIDS in 146 Swedish hemophiliacs and blood transfusion recipients infected with human immunodeficiency virus. *British Medical Journal, 297*(6641), 99–102.

Gilbert, J. (1987a, March). *Families and AIDS*. Paper presented at the Family Therapy Network Symposium, Washington, DC.

Gilbert, J. (1987b, October). *AIDS and families*. Paper presented at the American Association for Marriage and Family Therapists, Chicago, IL.

Gilbert, J. (1988, January). Coming to terms. *Family Therapy Networker, 21*(1), 42–43, 81.

Gilbert, J. (1990, March). *The therapist's use of self in work with people with AIDS*. Paper presented at the Family Therapy Networker Symposium, Washington, DC.

Gilligan, C. et al. (Eds.) (1988). *Mapping the moral domain: A contribution of women's thinking to psychological theory and education*. Cambridge, MA: Harvard University Press.

Girard, R. (1986). *The scapegoat*. Baltimore, MD: Johns Hopkins University Press.

Glazer, B., & Strauss, A. (1965). *Awareness of dying: A study of social interaction*. Chicago: Aldine.

Glazer, B. & Strauss, A. (1967). *A time for dying*. Chicago: Aldine.

Goffman, E. (1961). *Asylums: Essays on the social situation of mental patients and other inmates*. Garden City, NY: Anchor Books/Doubleday.

Goffman, E. (1972). *Relations in public*. New York: Harper & Row.

Goffman, E. (1986). *Stigma: Notes on the management of spoiled identity*. New York: Simon & Schuster.

Goldner, V., Penn, P., Sheinberg, M., & Walker, G. (1990). Love and violence: Gender paradoxes in volatile relationships. *Family Process, 29*(10), 343–364.

Goldstein, R. (1983, June 28). Fear and loving in the gay community. *Village Voice*, p. 11.

Goldstein, R. (1989). AIDS and the social contract. In E. Carter & S. Watney (Eds.), *Taking liberties* (pp. 81–94). London: Serpent Head.

Gong, V. (Ed.) (1985). *Understanding AIDS: A comprehensive guide*. New Brunswick, NJ: Rutgers University Press.

Gong, V., & Rudnick, N. (Eds.) (1987). *AIDS: Facts and issues*. New Brunswick, NJ: Rutgers University Press.

Gonsiorek, J. C. (Ed.) (1985). *A guide to psychotherapy with gay and lesbian clients*. New York: Harrington Park Press.

Gonzalez, S., Steinglass, P., & Reiss, D. (1987). *Family centered interventions for people with chronic disabilities*. Washington: George Washington University Medical Center, the Rehabilitation Research and Training Center, Department of Psychiatry and Behavioral Sciences.

Gorer, G. (1965). *Death, grief and mourning in contemporary Britain*. New York: Doubleday.

Green, R. (1987). *The "sissy boy syndrome" and the development of homosexuality*. New Haven: Yale University Press.

Greenberg, D. F. (1988). *The construction of homosexuality*. Chicago: University of Chicago Press.

Greenwich House (1988). *AIDS education for substance abusers: A comparative analysis of AIDS education in a population of methadone and non-methadone taking substance abusers*. New York: Greenwich House.

Gropman, J. E. (1985). *Clinical spectrum of HTIVIII in humans. Cancer Research*, Report No. 45, Supplement 9, 4649s & 4651s.

Gross, M. (1989). HIV antibody testing: Performance and counseling. In P. O'Malley (Ed.), *The AIDS epidemic: Private rights and the public interest* (pp. 189–212). Boston: Beacon Press.

Hamburg, M. A., & Fauci, A. S. (1989). AIDS—The challenge to biomedical research. *Daedalus, 118*(2).

Harbin, H. T., & Mazier, H. M. (1975). The families of drug abusers: A literature review. *Family Process, 14*, 411–431.

Hartman, A., & Laird, J. (1983). *Family centered social work practice*. New York: Free Press.

Hauser, M. (1983). Bereavement outcome for widows. *Journal of Psychosocial Nursing and Mental Health Services, 21*(9), 22–31.

Hauser, M. (1987). Special aspects of grief after suicide. In E. Dunne, J. McIntosh, & K. Dunne-Maxim (Eds.), *Suicide and its aftermath: Understanding and counseling the survivors*. New York: Norton.

Hay, L. (1990). *The AIDS Book*. Santa Monica, CA: Hay House Publications.

Henao, S., & Grose, N. (Eds.) (1985). *Principles of family systems in family medicine*. New York: Brunner/Mazel.

Hendin, D. (1973). *Death as a fact of life*. New York: Norton.

Hepworth, S., & Shernoff, M. (1989). Strategies for AIDS education and prevention. In E. Machlin (Ed.), *AIDS and families*. New York: Haworth Press.

Hessol, N. et al. (1988). *The natural history of HIV infection in a cohort of homosexual and bisexual men: A decade of followup*. Paper presented at the Fourth International Conference on AIDS, Abstract 4096, Stockholm, Sweden.

Hilts, P. (1990, June 22). Evidence is said to increase in microbes' role in AIDS. *New York Times*, A1.

Hines, P. M., & Boyd-Franklin, N. (1982). Black families. In M. McGoldrick, J. K. Pearce, & J. Giordano (Eds.), *Ethnicity and family therapy* (pp. 84–107). New York: Guilford.

Ho, D., Neuman, A., Perelson, A., WenChen, Leonard, J., & Markowirtz, M. (1995, January 12). Rapid turnover of plasma virons and CD4 lymphocytes in HIV 1 infection. *Nature, 373*, 123–125.

Illich, I. (1976). *Medical nemesis: The exploration of health*. New York: Pantheon.

Imber-Black, E. (1988). *Families and larger systems: A family therapist's guide through the labyrinth*. New York: Guilford.

Imber-Black, E. (1990). Multiple embedded systems. In M. P. Mirkin (Ed.), *The social and political contexts of family therapy* (pp. 193–214). Boston: Allyn & Bacon.

Inclan, J., & Ferran, E. (1990). Poverty, politics and family therapy: A role for systems theory. In M. P. Mirkin (Ed.), *The social and political contexts of family therapy* (pp. 193–214). Boston: Allyn & Bacon.

Institute of Medicine, National Academy of Sciences (1986). *Confronting AIDS: Directions for public health, health care, and research*. Washington, DC: National Academy Press.

Isay, R. A. (1989). *Being homosexual: Gay men and their development*. New York: Farrar Straus Giroux.

Kaplan, L. (1988, January). AIDS and guilt. *Family Therapy Networker, 12*(12), 40–41, 80.

Kaplan, L., & Patten, J. (1989, October). *AIDS and the gay man*. Paper presented at the American Association of Marriage and Family Therapists conference, San Francisco.

Kaufman, E., & Kaufmann, P. (1979a). From a psychodynamic orientation to a structural family therapy approach in the treatment of drug dependency. In E. Kaufman & P. Kaufmann (Eds.), *Family therapy of drug and alcohol abuse*. New York: Gardner.

Kaufman, E., & Kaufmann, P. (Eds.) (1979b). *Family therapy of drug and alcohol abuse*. New York: Gardner.

Kaufmann, P. (1979). Family therapy with adolescent substance abusers. In E. Kaufman & P. Kaufmann (Eds.), *Family therapy of drug and alcohol abuse*. New York: Gardner.

Kerr, B. (1974). *Strong at the broken places: Women who have survived drugs*. Chicago: Follet.

Kessler, H. et al. (1987). Diagnosis of human immunodeficiency virus in seropositive homosexuals presenting with an acute viral symptom. *Journal of the American Medical Association, 258*, 1196–1199.

Khantzian, T. E. J. (1985). The self medication hypothesis of addictive disorders: Focus on heroin and cocaine dependence. *American Journal of Psychiatry, 142*, 1259–1264.

Kinsey, A. C., Pomeroy, W. B., & Martin, C. E. (1948). *Human sexuality in the human male*. Philadelphia: Saunders.

Klagsburn, M., & Davis, D. I. (1977). Substance abuse and family interaction. *Family Process, 16*, 149–173.

Kleinman, A. (1988). *The illness narratives: Suffering, healing and the human condition*. New York: Basic Books.

Kolata, G. (1995a, January 12). New AIDS findings on why drugs fail. *New York Times*, pp. A1, B9.

Kolata, G. (1995b, January 29). Researchers find early battlers with HIV. *New York Times*, A1, B9.

Kramer, L. (1985). *The normal heart*. New York: New American Library.

Kübler-Ross, E. (1970). *On death and dying: What the dying have to teach doctors, nurses, clergy, and their own families*. New York: Macmillan.

Kübler-Ross, E. (1982). *Living with death and dying*. New York: Macmillan.

Kuklin, S. (1989). *Fighting back: What some people are doing about AIDS*. New York: G.P. Putnam.

Laird, J. (1979). An ecological approach to child welfare issues of family identity and community. In C. Germain (Ed.), *Social work practice: People and environments* (pp. 174–213). New York: Columbia University Press.

Lambert, B. (1988, January 13). Study finds antibodies for AIDS in 1 in 61 babies in New York City. *New York Times*, A1.

Lambert, B. (1990, June 22). Relapse into risky sex found in AIDS studies. *New York Times*, A27.

Landau, J. (1982). Therapy with families in cultural transition. In M. McGoldrick, J. Pearce, & J. Giordaino (Eds.), *Ethnicity and family therapy.* New York: Guilford.

Landau-Stanton, J., Clements, C., et al. (1993). *AIDS health and mental health: A primary sourcebook.* New York: Brunner/Mazel.

Leeper, M. A. (1990). Preliminary evaluation of Reality, a condom for women. *AIDS Care, 2*(3), 287–301.

Lemann, N. (1986, June). The origins of the underclass. Part I. *Atlantic Monthly,* 31–53.

Lemann, N. (1986, July). The origins of the underclass. Part II. *Atlantic Monthly,* 54–68.

Levine, M. P. (Ed.) (1971). *Gay men: The sociology of male homosexuality.* New York: Harper & Row.

Lewes, K. (1988). *The psychoanalytical theory of male homosexuality.* New York: Simon & Schuster.

Liebow, E. (1968). *Tally's Corners: A study of Negro streetcorner men.* Boston: Little, Brown.

Lifson, A., Ancelle-Park, R., Brunet, J. P., & Curran, J. (1986). The epidemiology of AIDS worldwide. In A. J. Pinching (Ed.), *Clinics in immunology and allergy: AIDS and HIV infection* (pp. 442–446) London: W. B. Saunders.

Lifson, A., Rutherford, G., & Jaffe, H. (1988). The natural history of human immunodeficiency virus infection. *Journal of Infectious Diseases, 158,* 1362.

Lifton, R. (1983). *The broken connection: On death and the continuity of life.* New York: Basic Books.

Lindemann, E. (1944). Symptomatology and management of acute grief. *American Journal of Psychiatry, 101,* 141–148.

Lyter, D., Valdessari, R., Kingsley, L., Amoroso, W., & Rimaldo, C. (1987). The antibody test: Why gay and bisexual men want or do not want to know their results. *Public Health Representative, 102,* 168–474.

Macklin, E. D. (Ed.) (1989). AIDS and families: Report on the AIDS task force, Groves Conference on Marriage and the Family. *Marriage and Family Review, 13*(1 & 2). New York: Haworth.

Madanes, C., Dukes, J., & Harbin, H. (1980). Family ties of heroin addicts. *Archives of General Psychiatry, 37,* 889–894.

Mallory, M., & Allan, L. (1993). The HIV infected child. In T. Eidson (Ed.), *The AIDS caregivers handbook.* New York: St. Martins Press.

Mayer, K. (1989). The clinical spectrum of HIV infections. In P. O'Malley (Ed.), *The AIDS epidemic: Private rights and the public interest* (pp. 37–58). Boston: Beacon Press.

McClusker, J., Stoddard, A., Mayer, R., Zapka, G., Morrison, C., & Saltzman, S. (1988). Effects of HIV antibody test on sexual behaviors on a cohort of homosexually active men. *American Journal of Public Health, 78*:462–467.

McEwen, B., & Schmeck, H. (1994). *The hostage brain.* New York: Rockefeller University Press.

McGoldrick, M., Pearce, J. K., Giordano, J. (Eds.) (1982). *Ethnicity and family therapy.* New York: Guilford.

McKusick, L. (1986). *What to do about AIDS: Physicians and mental health professionals discuss the issues.* Berkeley, CA: University of California Press.

McKusick, L., Horstman, W., & Coates, T. J. (1985). AIDS and sexual behavior reported by gay men in San Francisco. *American Journal of Public Health, 75,* 493–496.

McKusick, L., Horstman, W., & Coates, T. J. (1987, June). *Prevention of HIV infection among gay and bisexual males: Two longitudinal studies.* Paper presented at the Third International Conference on AIDS, Washington, DC.

McKusick, L., Horstman, W., Coates, T. J., Wiley, J., Stall, R., Saika, G., Morin, S., Charles, K., & Conant, M. A. (1985, November/December). Reported changes in the sexual behavior of men at risk for AIDS, San Francisco, 1982–1984: The AIDS research project. *Public Health Reports, 100,* 622–629.

McNeill, W. H. (1976). *Plagues and peoples.* Garden City, NY: Anchor Books/ Doubleday.

McWhirter, D., & Mattison, A. (1984). *The male couple.* New York: Prentice-Hall.

Michaels, D., & Levine, C. (1993). The youngest survivors: Estimate of the number of motherless youth orphaned by AIDS in New York city. In C. Levine (Ed.), *A death in the family: Orphans of the HIV epidemic.* New York: United Hospital Fund.

Millar, D. (1986). The management of AIDS patients. In S. Cochran & V. Mays (Eds.), *Women and AIDS-related concerns: Roles for psychologists in helping the worried well* (pp. 131–149). London: Macmillan.

Mirkin, M. P. (Ed.) (1990). *The social and political contexts of family therapy.* Boston: Allyn & Bacon.

Mofenson, L. M., Hoff, R., & Grady, G. F. (1989). *Trends in newborn HIV rates reveal the true proportions seen clinically.* Paper presented at Fifth Annual AIDS Conference, Montreal, Canada.

Mohr, R. (1988, January). Deciding what's do-able. *Family Therapy Networker, 12*(1), 34–36.

Mohr, R. (1987). *Lovers, spouses, families and AIDS.* Paper presented at the Ackerman Institute for Family Therapy, New York, NY.

Monette, P. (1990). *Borrowed time: An AIDS memoir.* New York: Avon.

Money, J. (1988). *Gay, straight and in-between: The sexology of erotic orientation.* New York: Oxford University Press.

Monte, T. (1990). *The way of hope.* New York: Wagner Books.

Morawetz, A. (1988). Speaking personally. *Family Systems Medicine, 6*(3), 349–360.

Morley, J. (1989, October 2). The contradictions of cocaine capitalism. *The Nation, 24*(10), 341–347.

Moynihan, D. P. (1965). *The Negro family: The case for national action.* Washington DC: Department of Labor.

Murphy, J. M. (1988). *Santeria: An African religion in America.* Boston: Beacon Press.

Needle, R., Leach, S., & Graham-Tomasi, R. (1989). HIV Epidemic: Epidemiological implications for family professionals. In E. Macklin (Ed.), AIDS and families: Report of the AIDS task force, Groves Conference on Marriage and the Family. *Marriage and Family Review, 13*(1 & 2).

Nichols, E. (1986). *Mobilizing against AIDS: The unfinished story of a virus.* Cambridge, MA: Harvard University Press.

Noone, R. J. (1979). *Drug abuse behavior in relation to change in the family structure.* Paper presented at the Third Pittsburgh Family Systems Symposium, Western Psychiatric Institute and Clinic, University of Pittsburgh.

Noone, R. J., & Redding, R. L. (1976). Case studies in the family treatment of drug abuse. *Family Process, 15*, 325–332.

Novick, L., Berns, D., Stroud, R., Stevens, R., Pass, K., & Wethers, J. (1989). HIV seroprevalence in newborns in New York State. *Journal of the American Medical Association, 261*(12), 1745.

Nunes, E. V., & Klein, D. (1987). Research issues in cocaine abuse. In H. Spitz & J. Rosecan (Eds.), *Cocaine abuse: New directions in treatment and research.* New York: Brunner/Mazel.

Nunes, E. V., & Rosecan, J. (1987). Human neurobiology of cocaine. In H. Spitz & J. Rosecan (Eds.), *Cocaine abuse: New directions in treatment and research.* New York: Brunner/Mazel.

O'Connor, C. (1987a, October). *AIDS and family therapy: An overview.* Paper presented at the American Association for Marriage and Family Therapy Conference, Chicago, IL.

O'Connor, C. (1987b). *Families, couples, lovers, and AIDS: A gay couple copes with AIDS.* Paper presented at the Gay Men's Health Crisis in-staff training seminar, New York, NY.

O'Connor, C. (1990, March). *AIDS and families: Three Women.* Paper presented at the Family Therapy: Networker Symposium, Washington, DC.

O'Malley, P. (Ed.) (1989). *The AIDS epidemic: Private rights and the public interest.* Boston: Beacon Press.

Orwell, G. (1983). *1984.* New York: NAL.

Osborn, J. (1989). Public health and the politics of AIDS prevention. *Daedalus, 118*(3), 123–145.

Padian, N., Marquis, L., Francis, D., Anderson, R., Rutherford, G., O'Malley, P., & Winkelstein, W. (1987). Male-to-female transmission of HIV. *Journal of the American Medical Association, 258*, 788–790.

Palacios-Jimenez, L., & Shernoff, M. (1986). *Eroticizing safer sex.* Facilitator's guide to eroticizing safer sex: A psychoeducational workshop to safer sex education. New York: Gay Men's Health Crisis.

Paracelsus. (1969). *Selected writings: Bollingen series XXVIII.* (N. Gutterman, Trans.). Princeton, NJ: Princeton University Press.

Parkes, C. (1982). *Bereavement: Studies of grief in adult life.* New York: International University Press.

Parkes, C., & Weiss, R. (1983). *Recovery from bereavement.* New York: Basic Books.

Patten, J. (1987a, March). *Families and AIDS: Family of choice, family of origin.*

Paper presented at the Family Therapy Networker Symposium, Washington, DC.

Patten, J. (1987b, October). *AIDS and families*. Paper presented at the Association for Marriage and Family Therapists, Chicago, IL.

Patten, J. (1988, January). AIDS and the gay couple. *Family Therapy Networker, 12*(1), 37–39.

Patten, J., & Walker, G. (1989). *Gay couples: Family of origin, family of choice*. Presentation at the Fifth International Conference on AIDS, Montreal, Canada.

Patton, C. (1985). *Sex and germs: The politics of AIDS*. Boston: South End Press.

Patton, C. & Kelley, J. (1987). *Making it: A woman's guide to sex in the age of AIDS*. Ithaca, NY: Firebrand Books.

Paver, L. (1988). *Medicine and culture: Varieties of treatment in the United States, England, West Germany, and France*. New York: Hoet.

Penn, P. (1982). Circular questioning. *Family Process, 21*(3), 267–280.

Penn, P. (1983). Coalitions and binding interactions in families with chronic illness. *Family Systems Medicine, 1*(1), 16–25.

Penn, P. (1985). Feed-forward, future questions, future maps. *Family Process, 24*(3), 299–310.

Pharr, S. (1988). *Homophobia: A weapon of sexism*. Inverness: Chardon Press.

Pinderhughes, E. (1982). Afro-American families and victim system. In M. McGoldrick, J. K. Pearce, & J. Giordano (Eds.), *Ethnicity and family therapy* (pp. 108–122) New York: Guilford.

Pinderhughes, E. (1989). *Understanding race, ethnicity, and power*. New York: Free Press.

Pivnick, A., Jacobsen, A., Eric, K., Hsu, M., & Drucker, E. (1990). *Reproductive decision making among HIV positive women*. Paper presented at the New York Public Health Association's 118th Annual Meeting, New York, NY.

Plummer, K. (1981). *The making of the modern homosexual*. Totowa, NJ: Barnes & Noble Books.

Porter, V. (1989). Minorities and HIV infection. In P. O'Malley (Ed.), *The AIDS epidemic: Private rights and the public interest*. Boston: Beacon Press.

Powell, L. (1983). Black macho and black feminism. In B. Smith (Ed.), *Home girls: A black feminist anthology*. Kitchen Table Press.

Price, M.E. (1989). *Shattered mirrors: Our search for identity and community in the AIDS era*. Cambridge, MA: Harvard University Press.

Rabinow, P. (Ed.) (1984). *Foucault reader*. New York: Pantheon.

Rampton, D. (1989). Quoted in L. Segal, Lessons from the past: Feminism, sexual politics and the challenge of AIDS. In S. Watney (Ed.), *Taking liberties* (pp. 133–146). London: Serpents Tail.

Ramsey, C. N., Jr. (1989). *Family systems in medicine*. New York: Guilford.

Ranki, K. (1987). Long latency precedes overt sero-conversion in sexually transmitted human immunodeficiency virus infection. *Lancet, 2*, 589–583.

Ransom, D. (1985). Evolution from an individual to a family approach. In S. Henao & N. Grose (Eds.), *Principles of family systems in family medicine* (pp. 5–23). New York: Brunner/Mazel.

Reed, P. (1989). *Serenity: Challenging the fear of AIDS—From despair to hope.* Berkeley, CA: Celestial Arts.

Reider, I., & Ruppelt, P. (1988). *AIDS: The women.* San Francisco: Cleiss Press.

Reilly, D. M. (1976). Family factors in the etiology and treatment of youthful drug abuse. *Family Therapy, 2,* 149–171.

Reiss, D. (1981). *The family's construction of reality.* Cambridge, MA: Harvard University Press.

Reiss, D. (1989). Families and their paradigms: An ecological approach to understanding the family in its social world. In C. N. Ramsey, Jr. (Ed.), *Family systems in medicine* (pp. 127–132). New York: Guilford.

Reiss, D., Gonzalez, S., & Kramer, N. (1986). Family process, chronic illness and death: On the weakness of strong bonds. *Archives of General Psychiatry, 43,* 795–804.

Reiss, D., & Kaplan-DeNour, A. (1989). The family and medical team in chronic illness: A transactional and developmental perspective in C. N. Ramsey, Jr. (Ed.), *Family systems in medicine* (pp. 435–444). New York: Guilford.

Remier, R., & Wagner, G. (1995). Counseling long-term survivors of HIV/AIDS. In W. Odets & M. Shernoff (Eds.), *The second decade of AIDS.* New York: Hatherleigh Press.

Richardson, D. (1988). *Women and AIDS.* New York: Methuen.

Rogers, M., Thomas, P., Starcher, E., Noa, M., Bush, T., & Jaffe, H. (1987). Aquired immunodeficiency syndrome in children. Report of the Centers for Disease Control: National surveillance 1982–1985. *Pediatrics, 79,* 1, 8–14.

Rolland, J. S. (1984). Toward a psychosocial typology of chronic and life-threatening illness. *Family Systems Medicine, 2*(3), 245–263.

Rolland, J. S. (1987a). Family systems and chronic illness: A typological model. *Journal of Psychotherapy and the Family, 3,* 143–168.

Rolland, J. S. (1987b). Family illness paradigms: Evolution and significance. *Family Systems Medicine, 5*(4), 482–503.

Rolland, J. S. (1987c). Chronic illness and the life cycle: A conceptual framework. *Family Process, 26*(2), 203–221.

Rosecan, J., Spitz, H., & Gross, B. (1987). Contemporary issues in the treatment of cocaine abuse. In H. Spitz & J. Rosecan (Eds.), *Cocaine abuse: New directions in treatment and research.* New York: Brunner/Mazel.

Rosenberg, C. (1988). Disease and social order in America: Perceptions and expectations. In E. Fee & D. Fox (Eds.), *AIDS: The burdens of history* (pp. 12–32). Berkeley: University of California Press.

Rosman, B. (1988, June). Paper presented on the Philadelphia Child Guidance Clinic hemophilia program at the American family therapy association, Montreal.

Ross, M. W. (Eds.) (1985). *Homosexuality, masculinity and femininity.* New York: Harrington Park Press.

Ruitenbeek, H. M. (Ed). *The problem of homosexuality in modern society.* New York: Dutton.

Ruse, M. (1988). *Homosexuality: A philosophical inquiry.* Oxford: Basil Black-well.

Saint-Exupery, A. de (1943). *The little prince.* New York: Harcourt Brace Jo-vanovich.

Saint Phalle, N. (1987). *AIDS: You can't catch it holding hands.* San Francisco: Lapis Press.

Scagliotti, J. (1985). *Before stonewall.* A film.

Schletter, S., Keller, S., & Stein, M. (1989). Bereavement and immune func-tions. In C. N. Ramsey, Jr. (Ed.), *Family systems in medicine* (pp. 257–262). New York: Guilford.

Schmidt, D., & Schmidt, P. (1989). Family systems, stress and infectious dis-ease. In C. N. Ramsey, Jr. (Ed.), *Family systems in medicine* (pp. 263–272). New York: Guilford.

Schwartzman, J. (1975). The addict, abstinence and the family. *American Jour-nal of Psychiatry, 132,* 154–157.

Schwartzman, J. (Ed.) (1985). *Families and other systems.* New York: Guilford.

Scopetta, M. A., King, O. E., & Szapocznik, J. (1977). Relationship of accul-turation, incidence of drug abuse and effective treatment of Cuban-Ameri-cans: Final report. National Institute on Drug Abuse, Contract No. 271-75-4136.

Sedgewick, E. K. (1985). *Between men: English literature and male homosexual desire.* New York: Columbia University Press.

Sedgewick, E. K. (1990). *Epistemology of the closet.* Berkeley: University of Cali-fornia Press.

Selvini Palazzoli, M., Boscolo, L., Cecchin, G. F., & Prata, G. (1980). Hy-pothesizing, circularity, neutrality: Three guidelines for the conduct of the session. *Family Process, 19*(1), 7–19.

Shaw, G., et al. (1995, January 12). Viral dynamics in human immunodefi-ciency virus type 1 infection. *Nature, 373,* 117–122.

Sheinberg, M. (1983a). The family and chronic illness: A treatment diary. *Family Systems Medicine, 1*(2), 26–36.

Sheinberg, M. (1983b). Creating a context of observation and the separation of patterns in chronic illness families. *Journal of Strategic and Systematic Thera-pies, 5*(4), 409–425.

Shilts, R. (1988). *And the band played on: Politics, people, and the AIDS epi-demic.* New York: Penguin.

Siegel, L. (Ed.) (1988). *AIDS and substance abuse.* New York: Harrington Park Press.

Simonton, O., Simonton, S., & Creighton, J. (1978). *Getting well again.* Los Angeles: Tarcher.

Sontag, S. (1979). *Illness as metaphor.* New York: Vintage.

Sontag, S. (1989). *AIDS and its metaphors.* New York: Farrar Straus Giroux.

Speck, R., & Attneave, C. (1973). *Family networks.* New York: Vintage.

Stanton, M. D. (1985). The family and drug abuse, concepts and rationale. In T. E. Bratter, & G. G. Forrest (Eds.), *Alcoholism and substance abuse in New York.* New York: Free Press.

Stanton, M.D., & Todd, T.C. (1979). Structural family therapy with drug addicts. In E. Kaufman & P. Kaufmann (Eds.), *Family therapy of drug and alcohol abuse*. New York: Gardner.

Stanton, M.D., & Todd, T. (1982). *The family therapy of drug abuse and addiction*. New York: Guilford.

Stoller, R. J. (1986). *Sexual excitement: Dynamics of erotic life*. Washington, DC: American Psychiatric Press, Inc.

Stone, A. (1976). The Tarasoff decisions: Suing psychotherapy to safeguard society. *Harvard Law Review, 90*, 358–378.

Stuntzner-Gibson, D. (1991). Women and HIV disease: An emergency social crisis. *Social Work, 36*(1), 22–27.

Szasz, T. S. (1971). *Law, liberty and psychiatry: An inquiry into the social uses of mental health practices*. New York: Collier Books.

Szasz, T. S. (1977). *The manufacture of madness: A comparative study of the institution and the mental heath movement*. New York: Harper Colophon Books/Harper & Row.

Tanner, W., & Pollack, R. (1987). *The effect of condom use and sensuous instruction on attitudes towards condoms*. Paper presented at the Annual Meeting of the Society for the Scientific Study of Sex, Atlanta, Georgia.

Tasker, M. (1988). *Jimmy and the eggs virus*. Newark, NJ: Children's Hospital AIDS Program.

Thomas, M., Mundy, L., Lieb, J., Ward, B., Allen, M., Oxtoly, J., & Fanes, M. (1989). *Seven year followup of HIV infection in neonatal transfusion*. Paper presented at the Fifth International Conference on AIDS, Montreal, Canada.

Tiblier, K., Walker, G., & Rolland, J. (1989). Therapeutic issues when working with families of persons with AIDS. In E. D. Macklin, (Ed.), AIDS and families: Report on the AIDS task force, Groves Conference on Marriage and the Family. *Marriage & Family Review, 13*(1 & 2), 81–128.

Tolstoy, L. (1963). *The death of Ivan Illich*. In M. Wettlen (Trans.), *Six Short Masterpieces by Tolstoy*. New York: Dell.

Treichler, P. (1989). AIDS: Gender and biomedical discourse: Current contexts for meaning. In E. Fee & D. Fox (Eds.), *AIDS: The burdens of history* (pp. 190–261). Berkeley: University of California Press.

Tsiantis, T., Anastasopolos, D., Meyer, M., Pantiz, D., Lanes, V., Platakouk, N., Aroni, S., & Kattamis, C. (1990). A multi-level intervention approach for care of HIV positive hemophiliacs and thalassaemic patients and their families. *AIDS Care, 2*(3), 253–266.

Turner, C., Millar, H., & Moses, L. (Eds.) (1989). *AIDS: Sexual behavior and intravenous drug use. Report to the National Research Council*. Washington, DC: National Academy Press.

Ulene, A. (1987). *Safe sex in a dangerous world: Understanding and coping with the threat of AIDS*. New York: Vintage Books.

Vaillant, G. E. (1966). A 12-year follow-up of New York narcotic addicts: Some social and psychiatric characteristics. *Archives of General Psychiatry, 15*, 599–609.

Walker, G. (1987, April/June). AIDS and family therapy. *Family Therapy Today*, 2(2), 6.

Walker, G. (1988). An AIDS journal. *Family Therapy Networker*, 12(1), 20–33.

Walker, G. (1983). The pact: The caretaker parent/ill child coalition in families with chronic illness. *Family Systems Medicine*, 1(3), 6–29.

Walker, G., & Small, S. (1991). AIDS, crack, poverty and race in the African American community: The need for an ecosystemic approach. In K. Lewis (Ed.), *Family system approach to social work: Teaching and clinical practice*. New York: Haworth.

Wallace, J. (1988, June). HIV exposure among the clients of prostitutes. Paper presented at the Fourth International Conference on AIDS, Abstract 4055, Stockholm, Sweden.

Watney, S. (1987). *Policing desire: Pornography, AIDS, and the media*. Minneapolis: University of Minnesota Press.

Weeks, J. (1983). *Coming out: Homosexual politics in Britain, from the nineteenth century to present*. London: Quartet Books.

Weeks, J. (1985). *Sexuality and its discontents: Meanings, myths and modern sexualities*. London: Routledge, Chapman, & Hall.

White, E. (1983). *States of desire: Travels in gay America*. New York: Dutton.

White, E., & Mars-Jones, A. (1988). *The darker proof. Stories from a crisis*. New York: NAL.

White, M. (1988). The process of questioning: A therapy of literary merit? *Dulwich Centre Newsletter*, Winter, 8–14.

White, M. (1989). *Saying hello again: The incorporation of the lost relationship in the resolution of grief*. In M. White, *Selected papers*. Adelaide, South Australia: Dulwich Centre.

White, M., & Epston, D. (1990). *Narrative means to therapeutic ends*. New York: Norton.

Williams, T. (1989). *The cocaine kids*. Reading, MA: Addison-Wesley.

Winkler, J. J. (1990). *Constraints of desire: The anthropology of sex and gender in ancient Greece*. New York: Routledge.

Woffard, C. (1991, February). The bisexual revolution: Deluded closet cases or the vanguard of the movement outward. *Outweek*, 33–80.

Worth, D. (1989). *The relationship between crack using mothers and the men they live with*. Women's Center of Montefiore Hospital Methadone Maintenance Program. Unpublished study.

Worth, D., Drucker, E., Eric, K., & Pivnick, A. (1990). *Sexual and physical abuse factors in continuous risk behavior of women HIV drug users in a South Bronx methadone clinic*. Sixth International Conference on AIDS, San Francisco, California, June 20–24.

Worth, D., & Rodriguez, R. (1987, January/February). Latino women and AIDS. *SIECUS Report*, 5–7.

Wyatt, G.E. (1988). Ethnic and cultural differences in women's sexual behavior. In S. J. Blumenthal & A. Eichler, Chairpersons, *NIMH/NIDA National Institute of Mental Health/National Institute of Drug Abuse Workshop on Women and AIDS: Promoting Healthy Behaviors* (pp. 9–11). Rockville, MD: National Institute of Mental Health.

Zahn, M., & Ball, J. (1972). Factors related to the cure of opiate addiction among Puerto Rican addicts. *International Journal of the Addictions, 7,* 237–245.

Zeig, J. K. (1980). *A teaching seminar with Milton H. Erickson.* New York: Brunner/Mazel.

Zinberg, N.E. (1989). Social policy: AIDS and intravenous drug use. *Daedalus, 118*(3), 23–46.

Index